2005
YEAR BOOK OF
DERMATOLOGY
AND
DERMATOLOGIC
SURGERY™

The 2005 Year Book Series

Year Book of Allergy, Asthma, and Clinical Immunology™: Drs Rosenwasser, Boguniewicz, Milgrom, Routes, and Weber

Year Book of Anesthesiology and Pain Management™: Drs Chestnut, Abram, Black, Gravlee, Mathru, Lee, and Roizen

Year Book of Cardiology®: Drs Gersh, Cheitlin, Graham, Kaplan, Sundt, and Waldo

Year Book of Critical Care Medicine®: Drs Dellinger, Parrillo, Balk, Bekes, Dorman, and Dries

Year Book of Dentistry®: Drs Zakariasen, Horswell, McIntyre, Scott, and Zakariasen Victoroff

Year Book of Dermatology and Dermatologic Surgery™: Drs Thiers and Lang

Year Book of Diagnostic Radiology®: Drs Osborn, Birdwell, Dalinka, Gardiner, Levy, Maynard, Oestreich, and Rosado de Christenson

Year Book of Emergency Medicine®: Drs Burdick, Cydulka, Hamilton, Handly, Quintana, and Werner

Year Book of Endocrinology®: Drs Mazzaferri, Bessesen, Howard, Kannan, Kennedy, Leahy, Miekle, Molitch, Rogol, and Rubin

Year Book of Family Practice®: Drs Bowman, Apgar, Bouchard, Dexter, Miser, Neill, and Scherger

Year Book of Gastroenterology™: Drs Lichtenstein, Burke, Dempsey, Drebin, Ginsberg, Katzka, Kochman, Morris, Nunes, Shah, and Stein

Year Book of Hand and Upper Limb Surgery®: Drs Berger and Ladd

Year Book of Medicine®: Drs Barkin, Frishman, Klahr, Loehrer, Mazzaferri, Phillips, Pillinger, and Snydman

Year Book of Neonatal and Perinatal Medicine®: Drs Fanaroff, Maisels, and Stevenson

Year Book of Neurology and Neurosurgery®: Drs Gibbs and Verma

Year Book of Nuclear Medicine®: Drs Coleman, Blaufox, Royal, Strauss, and Zubal

Year Book of Obstetrics, Gynecology, and Women's Health®: Dr Shulman

Year Book of Oncology®: Drs Loehrer, Arceci, Glatstein, Gordon, Hanna, Morrow, and Thigpen

Year Book of Ophthalmology®: Drs Rapuano, Cohen, Eagle, Grossman, Hammersmith, Myers, Nelson, Penne, Sergott, Shields, Tipperman, and Vander

Year Book of Orthopedics®: Drs Morrey, Beauchamp, Peterson, Swiontkowski, Trigg, and Yaszemski

Year Book of Otolaryngology-Head and Neck Surgery®: Drs Paparella, Otto, and Keefe

2005

The Year Book of DERMATOLOGY AND DERMATOLOGIC SURGERY™

Editor-in-Chief
Bruce H. Thiers, MD
Professor and Chair, Department of Dermatology, Medical University of South Carolina, Charleston, South Carolina

Associate Editor
Pearon G. Lang, Jr, MD
Professor of Dermatology, Pathology, Otolaryngology, and Communicative Sciences, Medical University of South Carolina, Charleston, South Carolina

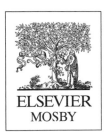

ELSEVIER
MOSBY

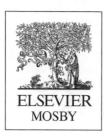

ELSEVIER
MOSBY

Vice President, Continuity Publishing: Timothy M. Griswold
Publishing Director, Continuity: J. Heather Cullen
Senior Manager, Continuity Production: Idelle L. Winer
Developmental Editor: Ali Gavenda
Senior Issue Manager: Pat Costigan
Senior Illustrations and Permissions Coordinator: Kimberly E. Denando

Printed in the United States of America
Composition by Thomas Technology Solutions, Inc.
Printing/binding by Sheridan Books, Inc.

Editorial Office:
Elsevier, Inc.
Suite 1800
1600 John F. Kennedy Boulevard
Philadelphia, PA 19103-2899

International Standard Serial Number: 0093-3619
International Standard Book Number: 0-323-02105-0

Contributors

Margaret M. Boyle, BS
Research Associate, Dermatoepidemiology Unit, Brown University, Providence, Rhode Island

Antonio A. T. Chuh, MD, MRCP, FRCP, MRCPCH
Honorary Clinical Assistant Professor, Department of Medicine, University of Hong Kong and Queen Mary Hospital, Pokfulam; and Part-time Clinical Assistant Professor, Department of Community and Family Medicine, Chinese University of Hong Kong and Prince of Wales Hospital, Shatin, Hong Kong SAR, China

Joel Cook, MD
Associate Professor, Department of Dermatology, Medical University of South Carolina, Charleston, South Carolina

Gillian M. P. Galbraith, MD
Professor and Chair of Biomedical Sciences, University of Las Vegas School of Dental Medicine, Las Vegas, Nevada

Ronald L. Moy, MD
Clinical Professor, David Geffen School of Medicine at UCLA, Los Angeles, California

Sharon Raimer, MD
Professor of Dermatology and Pediatrics; Chair, Department of Dermatology, University of Texas Medical Branch, Galveston, Texas

Jean-Francois Tremblay, MD, CM, FRCPC
Clinical Faculty, Division of Dermatology, University of Montreal Hospital Centre, Montreal, Quebec, Canada

Martin A. Weinstock, MD, PhD
Professor of Dermatology and Community Health, Brown University; Chief of Dermatology, VA Medical Center; Director, Dermatoepidemiology, Pigmented Lesion, and Photomedicine Units, Rhode Island Hospital, Providence, Rhode Island

Table of Contents

Journals Represented

Journals represented in this YEAR BOOK are listed below.

American Journal of Clinical Pathology
American Journal of Emergency Medicine
American Journal of Epidemiology
American Journal of Human Genetics
American Journal of Medicine
American Journal of Obstetrics and Gynecology
American Journal of Public Health
American Journal of Surgery
American Surgeon
Annals of Internal Medicine
Annals of Surgical Oncology
Archives of Dermatology
Archives of Disease in Childhood
Archives of Facial Plastic Surgery
Archives of Pediatrics and Adolescent Medicine
Archives of Surgery
Arthritis and Rheumatism
British Journal of Cancer
British Journal of Dermatology
British Journal of Plastic Surgery
British Journal of Surgery
British Medical Journal
Cancer
Cancer Research
Clinical Cancer Research
Clinical Infectious Diseases
Clinical Pharmacology and Therapeutics
Critical Care Medicine
Dermatologic Surgery
Dermatology
European Journal of Nuclear Medicine and Molecular Imaging
European Journal of Surgical Oncology (London)
Headache
International Journal of Cancer
International Journal of Gynaecology and Obstetrics
Journal of Allergy and Clinical Immunology
Journal of Clinical Endocrinology and Metabolism
Journal of Clinical Investigation
Journal of Clinical Oncology
Journal of Immunology
Journal of Infectious Diseases
Journal of Investigative Dermatology
Journal of Nuclear Medicine
Journal of Pathology
Journal of Pediatric Gastroenterology and Nutrition
Journal of Pediatrics
Journal of the American Academy of Dermatology
Journal of the American Board of Family Practice
Journal of the American Geriatrics Society

Journal of the American Medical Association
Journal of the National Cancer Institute
Lancet
Mayo Clinic Proceedings
Medical Care
Medical Journal of Australia
Modern Pathology
Nephrology, Dialysis, Transplantation
Neurology
Neuroradiology
New England Journal of Medicine
Pediatric Dermatology
Pediatric Infectious Disease Journal
Pediatrics
Plastic and Reconstructive Surgery
Science
The Journal of Investigative Dermatology. Symposium Proceedings
Transplantation

STANDARD ABBREVIATIONS

The following terms are abbreviated in this edition: acquired immunodeficiency syndrome (AIDS), cardiopulmonary resuscitation (CPR), central nervous system (CNS), cerebrospinal fluid (CSF), computed tomography (CT), deoxyribonucleic acid (DNA), electrocardiography (ECG), health maintenance organization (HMO), human immunodeficiency virus (HIV), intensive care unit (ICU), intramuscular (IM), intravenous (IV), magnetic resonance (MR) imaging (MRI), ribonucleic acid (RNA), ultrasound (US), and ultraviolet (UV).

NOTE

The YEAR BOOK OF DERMATOLOGY AND DERMATOLOGIC SURGERY™ is a literature survey service providing abstracts of articles published in the professional literature. Every effort is made to assure the accuracy of the information presented in these pages. Neither the editors nor the publisher of the YEAR BOOK OF DERMATOLOGY AND DERMATOLOGIC SURGERY™ can be responsible for errors in the original materials. The editors' comments are their own opinions. Mention of specific products within this publication does not constitute endorsement.

To facilitate the use of the YEAR BOOK OF DERMATOLOGY AND DERMATOLOGIC SURGERY™ as a reference tool, all illustrations and tables included in this publication are now identified as they appear in the original article. This change is meant to help the reader recognize that any illustration or table appearing in the YEAR BOOK OF DERMATOLOGY AND DERMATOLOGIC SURGERY™ may be only one of many in the original article. For this reason, figure and table numbers will often appear to be out of sequence within the YEAR BOOK OF DERMATOLOGY AND DERMATOLOGIC SURGERY™.

COLOR PLATE I

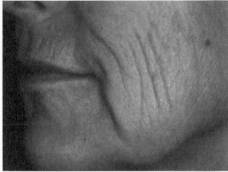

Tremblay Fig 1A

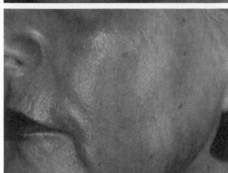

Tremblay Fig 1B

Tremblay Fig 2A

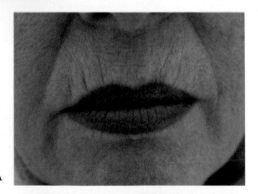

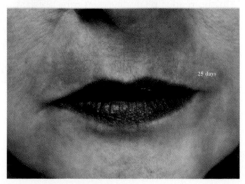

Tremblay Fig 2B

COLOR PLATE II

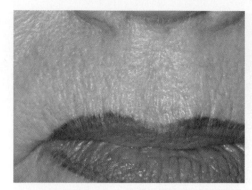

Tremblay Fig 3A

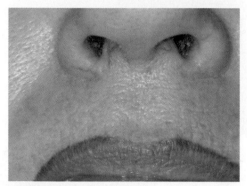

Tremblay Fig 3B

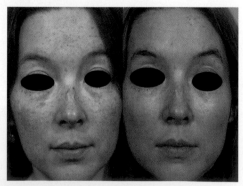

Tremblay Fig 4

COLOR PLATE III

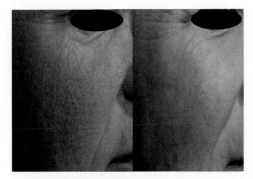

Tremblay Fig 5

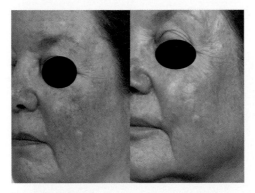

Tremblay Fig 6

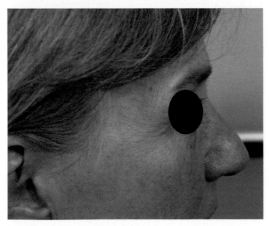

Tremblay Fig 7A

COLOR PLATE IV

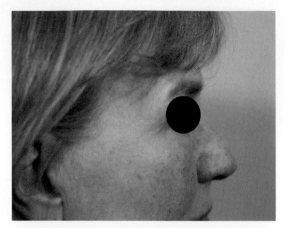

Tremblay Fig 7B

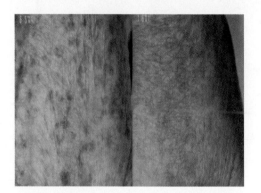

Tremblay Fig 8

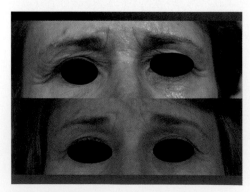

Tremblay Fig 9

COLOR PLATE V

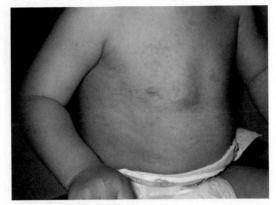

Chuh Fig 1B

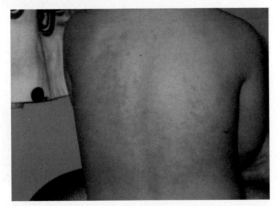

Chuh Fig 1B

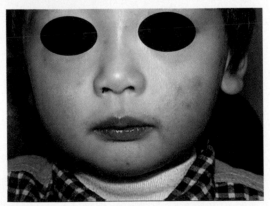

Chuh Fig 2A

COLOR PLATE VI

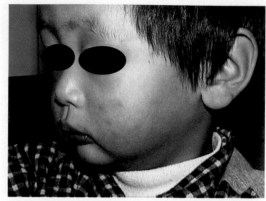

Chuh Fig 2B

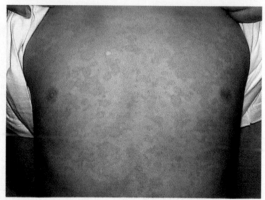

Chuh Fig 3

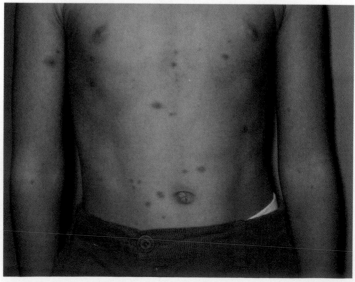

Chuh Fig 4A

COLOR PLATE VII

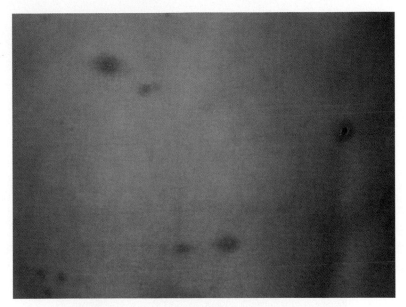

Chuh Fig 4B

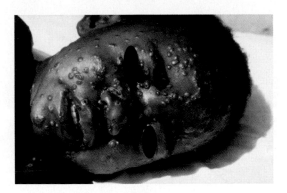

Chuh Fig 5

COLOR PLATE VIII

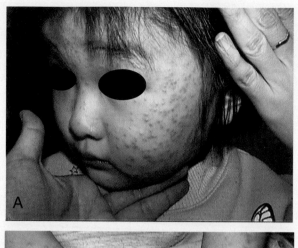

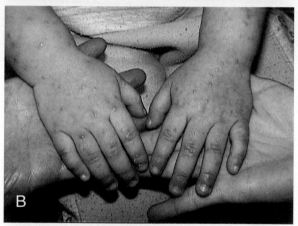

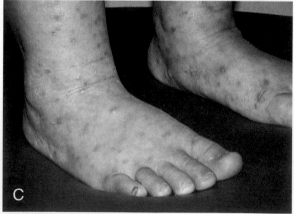

Chuh Fig 6A,B, C

COLOR PLATE IX

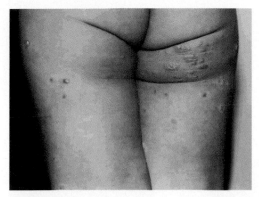

Chuh Fig 7A

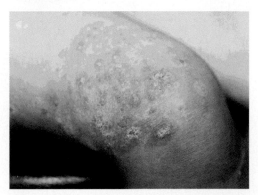

Chuh Fig 7B

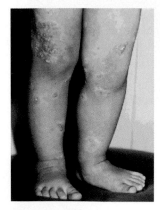

Chuh Fig 7C

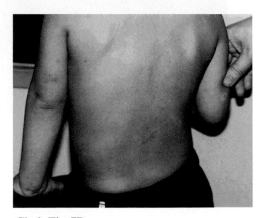

Chuh Fig 7D

COLOR PLATE X

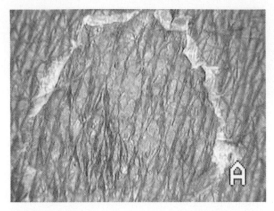

Chuh Fig 8

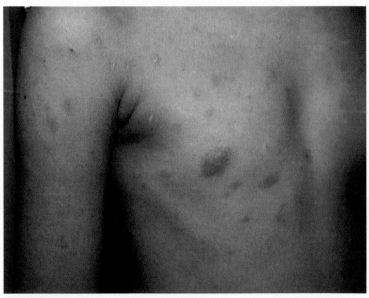

Chuh Fig 9A

COLOR PLATE XI

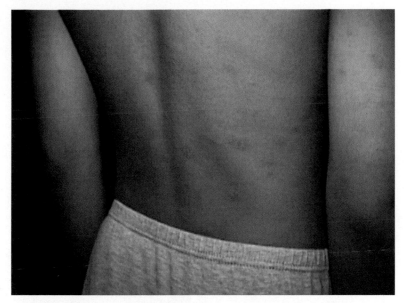

Chuh Fig 9B

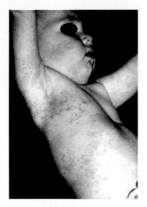

Chuh Fig 10A

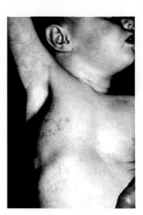

Chuh Fig 10B

COLOR PLATE XII

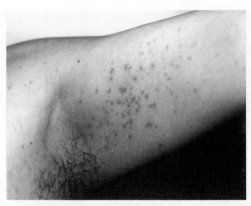

Chuh Fig 11A

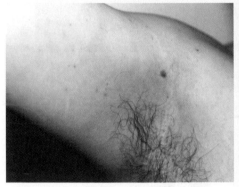

Chuh Fig 11B

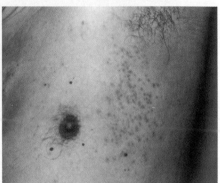

Chuh Fig 11C

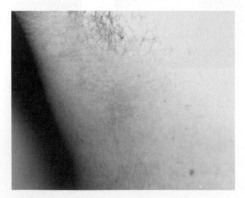

Chuh Fig 11D

COLOR PLATE XIII

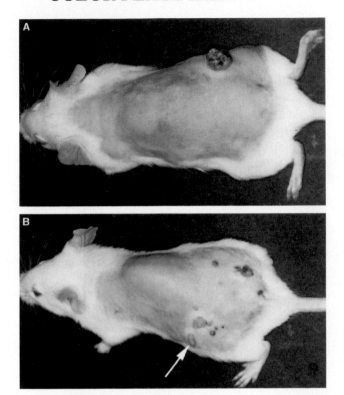

Abstract 1-16   Fig 2, A, B

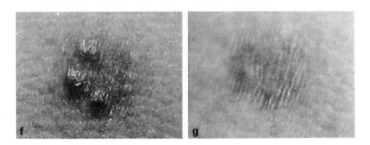

Abstract 2-3   Fig 1, f, g

COLOR PLATE XIV

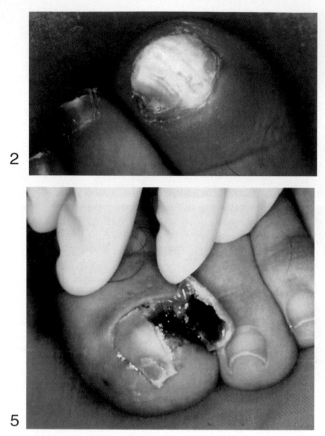

Abstract 3-18 Fig 2, Fig 5

COLOR PLATE XV

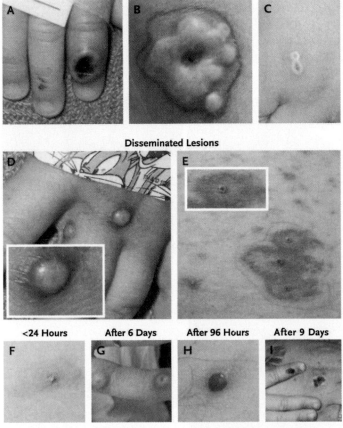

Disseminated Lesions

<24 Hours   After 6 Days   After 96 Hours   After 9 Days

Abstract 4-13 Fig 2, A-I

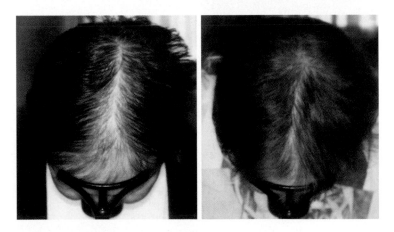

Abstract 7-13 Fig 1

COLOR PLATE XVI

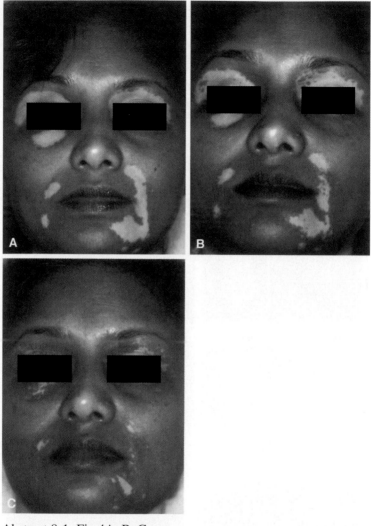

Abstract 8-1 Fig 4A, B, C

COLOR PLATE XVII

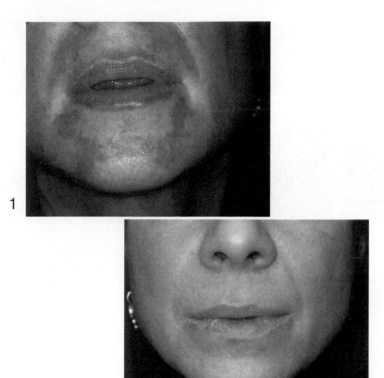

1

2

Astract 8-4 Fig 1, Fig 2

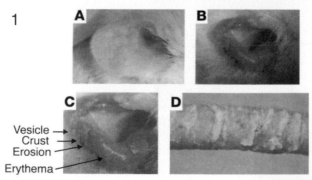

1

A

B

C

Vesicle →
Crust →
Erosion →
Erythema →

D

Abstract 10-1 Fig 1,A-D Fig 2B

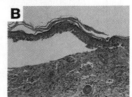

B

2

COLOR PLATE XVIII

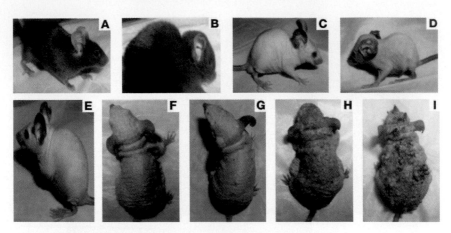

Abstract 16-7 Fig 1, A-I

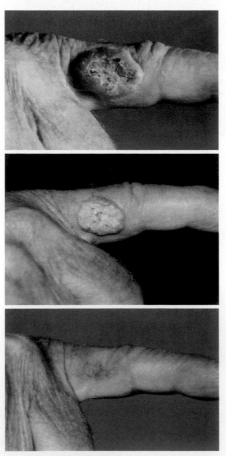

Abstracts 16-21 Fig 17

COLOR PLATE XIX

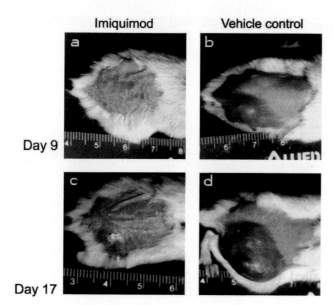

Abstracts 20-11 Fig 2a, b, c, d

COLOR PLATE XX

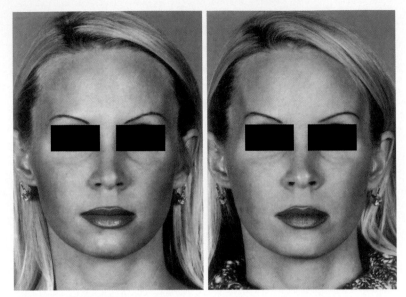

Abstracts 20-16 Figure

Nonablative Photorejuvenation: A Review

JEAN-FRANCOIS TREMBLAY, MD, CM, FRCPC
Clinical Faculty, Division of Dermatology, University of Montreal Hospital Centre, Montreal, Quebec, Canada

RONALD L. MOY, MD
Clinical Professor, David Geffen School of Medicine at UCLA, Los Angeles, California

Introduction

Nonablative photorejuvenation was initially defined as laser treatments of the skin for wrinkle and scar reduction as well as skin tightening involving stimulation of dermal collagen production without epidermal destruction. Over time, this definition has been broadened to include technologies that address other aspects of skin photoaging, including dyspigmentation, dilated capillaries, and actinic keratosis (AK) with minimal discomfort, downtime, and lack of significant epidermal wounding. The goal of this article is to provide an updated review on the mechanism of action and indications of currently available and emerging laser, intense pulsed light, radiofrequency, plasma, fractional photothermolysis, and light-emitting diode technologies in the treatment of photoaged skin (see Table 1 for summary of technologies discussed).

Background

Until recently, ablative laser technologies including carbon dioxide (CO_2) and Er:YAG had been the mainstay of skin photorejuvenation. They largely started to replace dermabrasion and chemical peels some 15 years ago because of their increased efficacy, reproducibility, and control in depth of tissue damage. CO_2 (10,600 nm) and Er:YAG (2940 nm) lasers produce infrared radiation that is highly absorbed by water. A rapid increase in skin temperature results in rapid tissue vapor pressure buildup and tissue vaporization. The superficial layer of the skin where the greatest amount of energy is deposited is instantly vaporized, resulting in measurably reproducible tissue ablation with each pass. Er:YAG laser has significantly greater water absorption compared with CO_2 laser, resulting in less collateral thermal damage (10-30 μm for Er:YAG versus 80-150 μm for CO_2). The 3 main mechanism of action in ablative photorejuvenation are (1) epidermal ablation, (2) immediate dermal collagen contraction, and (3) delayed dermal collagen remodeling.[1-3] Epidermal ablation using CO_2 and Er:YAG lasers is very effective at eliminating solar pigmentation, actinic dyskeratosis, and superficial textural irregularities (Figs 1 and 2; see color plate I).

The best biological effects of ablative laser photorejuvenation occur in the dermis. Acute tissue contraction is observed with 1 to 2 passes using CO_2 laser or when using long-pulsed Er:YAG lasers. This immediate tissue effect results from thermal denaturation of collagen that has been correlated with the amount of the collagen formation in the superficial dermis. The exact role of immediate tissue contraction on long-term skin tightening and

1

TABLE 1

Technologies	Energy Sources	Clinical Indications	Mechanism of Action
Intense pulsed-light technologies	500-1200 nm	Dyspigmentation Ectatic capillaries Minor collagen remodelling	Targets chromophores (Melanin and oxyhemoglobin) Some dermal collagen heat injury Heat shock protein activation Fibroblast growth factor release
Yellow lasers Potassium titanyl phosphate (KTP) Pulsed dye laser (PDL) N-Lite laser	532 nm 585-600 nm 585 nm (short pulse)	Ectatic capillaries Minor textural improvement	Targets oxyhemoglobin, some melanin Fibroblast growth factor release Heat shock protein activation
Infrared lasers Cooltouch TM Gentle YAG/Coolglide Vantage Smoothbeam (diode) Aramis (erbium-glass)	1320 nm 1064 nm 1450 nm 1540 μm	Fine wrinkles Acne scars Acne Dilated skin pores	Targets water to induce tissue thermal damage Stimulates collagen remodelling Induces shrinking of sebaceous glands
Radiofrequency devices Thermage TM	Monopolar radiofrequency and cryogen cooling	Facial and extrafacial skin tightening and tissue elevation; Acne and acne scars	Volumetric dermal heating Dermal collagen tightening Deep fibrous septae tightening Sebaceous gland shrinking
Plasma skin resurfacing Portrait TM	Non-contact plasma beam	Dyspigmentation Textural improvement Collagen remodelling	Photothermal damage to epidermis and dermo-epidermal junction (increase epidermal turnover and elimination of pigment and actinically damaged cells) Stimulates collagen formation in papillary dermis Stimulate elimination of elastotic material in dermis
Light emitting diode (LED) Omnilux TM Blue-Red-Infrared Lumpiphase TM Gentlewave TM	410-633 nm	Collagen remodelling	Photomodulation of inflammation and wound healing Upregulation of pro-collagen I synthesis Downregulation of metalloproteinases activity
Broad-band infrared (Titan)	1100-1800 nm	Facial and extrafacial tissue tightening and elevation	Deep thermal heating targetting water Fibroblast activation
Fractional resurfacing	1550 nm infrared laser	Dyspigmentation Wrinkles Skin tightening? Collagen remodelling	Microthermal zone of collagen denaturation Increased epidermal turnover and pigment elimination Wound healing cascade activation Superficial and deep dermal collagen remodelling
Photodynamic therapy ALA-PDT (aminolevulinic acid) IPL PDL LED		Solar pigmentation Dilated capillaries Actinic keratoses Sebaceous hyperplasia Skin pore dilatation Collagen remodelling	Selective uptake by actinically damaged epithelium and sebaceous glands–destruction of atypical keratinocytes; amplifies effect of IPL and LED

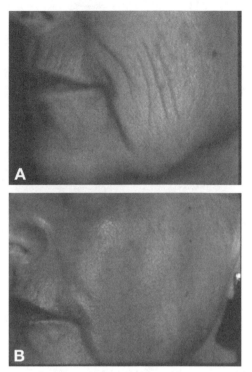

FIGURE 1A and 1B.—Significant improvement in facial wrinkles, texture, and skin tightening after full-face CO_2 laser resurfacing.

wrinkle improvement, however, is unclear. On the other hand, delayed collagen remodeling and synthesis of new collagen and extracellular matrix resulting from the wound healing reaction, activation of fibroblasts, and resorption of elastotic collagen fibers seem most important.

However, ablative laser technologies are far from ideal. Epidermal wounding is associated with postoperative discomfort and necessary downtime from work and social life that may last 7 to 14 days. Extrafacial applications are extremely limited because of the high incidence of scarring. The use of ablative laser therapies for skin phototypes IV to VI is also impractical because of the high incidence of postinflammatory hyperpigmenation. In addition, potential complications that include infection, scarring, pigmentation irregularities, delayed healing, and prolonged erythema may occur.

Therefore, an ideal photorejuvenation treatment would feature the following characteristics: (1) non-painful, (2) no downtime, (3) high safety profile in all skin types, (4) high efficacy and reproducibility, and (5) comprehensive improvement of all aspects of skin aging.

The nonablative photorejuvenation devices aim at improving epidermal and dermal skin characteristics without significant alteration of skin integrity and function, which translates clinically in minimal downtime and patient discomfort. Epidermal features that can be targeted and improved in-

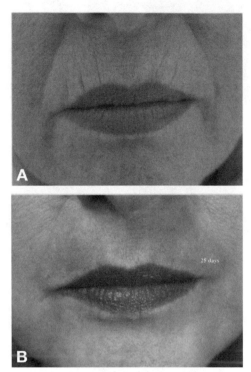

FIGURE 2A and 2B.—Improvement of perioral wrinkles after long-pulse Er:YAG resurfacing of the upper lip.

clude skin pigmentation, ectatic vessels, fine superficial textural irregularity and actinic roughness. Dermal and subcutaneous age-related changes that can be addressed include solar elastosis, wrinkling, skin laxity, and scars.

Nonablative photorejuvenation devices have been classified into 3 different categories. We are adding a fourth one to include newer modalities (Table 2).

Type I photorejuvenation involves the rejuvenation of vascular damage (telangiectases, grade 1 rosacea, angiomas) and solar pigmentation (solar lentigines, dyschromia, melasma). Type II photorejuvenation involves

TABLE 2

Type I	Type II	Type III	Type IV
IPL	LED photomodulation	ALA-PDT	Monopolar
PDL	IPL	with Blue light	radiofrequency
ALA-PDT	Infrared lasers	LED	skin tightening
Plasma resurfacing	PDL	IPL	
Fractional	ALA-PDT	PDL	Deep infrared skin
photothermolysis	Plasma resurfacing		tightening
	Fractional photothermolysis		

wrinkle reduction, improvement of skin textures, and collagen remodeling without epidermal damage. Type III photorejuvenation involves wrinkle reduction and skin texture and pigment improvement using photodynamic therapy. Type IV photorejuvenation involves deep tissue skin tightening and elevation without epidermal damage or skin surgery.

Infrared Lasers

One of the first lasers developed for nonablative photorejuvenation was the 1320-nm Nd:YAG laser (Cooltouch). Several studies have shown measurable but subtle improvement in wrinkles and skin texture with repeated treatments.[4-6] Histologic evidence of fibroblast stimulation and neocollagenogenesis has also been demonstrated. The 1450-nm diode laser (Smoothbeam) was also developed and introduced for nonablative photorejuvenation and later on applied as well for the treatment of acne. Modest improvement in fine wrinkling was reported after repeated treatment as well as decreased skin pore size and sebaceous glands.[7] However, discomfort during the procedure is an issue for most patients. The Er:glass 1540-nm laser with contact cooling (Aramis) has also shown some efficacy in treating periorbital and perioral wrinkles. Mild improvement may be observed after 3 to 4 treatments with some histologic evidence of new collagen formation.[8] More recently, long-pulsed Nd:YAG technologies have been introduced

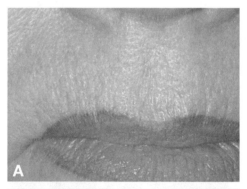
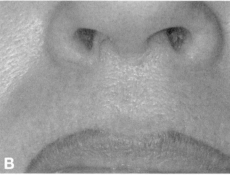

FIGURE 3A and 3B.—Moderate improvement in wrinkles and texture after a series of 4 treatments using long-pulse Nd:YAG laser.

that provide similar results (Fig 3; see color plate II). The infrared remodeling may be useful in clinical practice as adjuncts to other treatments. Although results are modest compared with CO_2 and Er:YAG lasers, they improve overall texture, elasticity, and skin tone in a subjective and objective manner. All infrared laser technologies appear to be somewhat similar in efficacy.[9]

Yellow Lasers

A number of small studies have shown the modest clinical effect of pulsed-dye laser (PDL) 585-nm and short pulse 585-nm as well as long pulsed 595-nm laser in improving skin texture and fine wrinkles after repeated subpurpuric treatments.[10,11] Recently, results of PDL photorejuvenation was also further improved when combined with aminolevulinic acid. (see below).

Intense Pulsed-Light (IPL)

Intense pulsed-light (IPL) devices produce broadband light within the 500- to 1200-nm range. Different filter sets cut off shorter or longer wavelength to allow more specific targeting of different chromophores including melanin, hemoglobin, and water. Studies on various different commercial devices have demontrated IPL efficacy at improving solar pigmentation and ectatic blood vessels[12-14] (Fig 4; see color plate II). Temporary darkening with mild erythema and subsequent peeling is expected especially after the initial treatments. Response with ectatic blood vessels is progressive and rarely purpuric. The longer wavelength within the infrared spectrum targets tissue water and allows for some deeper dermal heating affecting collagen production and remodeling.[15] Heat-shock protein and fibroblastic growth factors may also be released as a result of vascular endothelial injury and secondarily boost collagen remodeling. Repeated IPL treatments have been shown to have beneficial effects on skin texture, pore size, and skin elasticity.[12,13] IPL in combination with aminolevulinic acid has recently been shown to augment this effect (see discussion below).

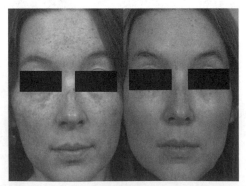

FIGURE 4.—Significant improvement of solar pigmentation after a series of 4 IPL treatments.

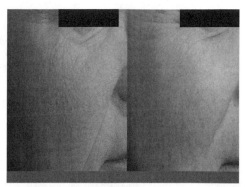

FIGURE 5.—Improvement of skin texture, pore size, fine wrinkles, and elasticity after a series of 12 treatments using 633-nm LED light (Omnilux Revive).

Light-Emitting Diode (LED) Photomodulation

A number of light-emitting diode (LED) devices have emerged on the market that capitalize on the nonthermal properties of light energy on fibroblast and inflammatory cell activity in photorejuvenation. In vitro studies have shown the effect of LED light on skin, including the increased production of pro-collagen I and the downregulation of metalloproteinase I (MMP-I). Blue and red light have been extensively tested for the treatment of acne. Modest but measurable improvement in skin texture, elasticity, and fine wrinkles have also been reported in a number of oral and written communications[16,17] (Fig 5; see color plate III). The effect of LED may also be augmented with levulinic acid.

Aminolevulinic Acid Photodynamic Therapy (ALA-PDT)

Photodynamic therapy using topical aminolevulinic acid (ALA) activated by blue visible light IPL, PDL, and LED light has been found to be effective in treating actinic keratoses, acne, hyperseborrhea, dilated skin pores, sebaceous hyperplasia as well as to enhance the effects of IPL on pigmentation and dilated capillaries[18-26] (Fig 6; see color plate III). It appears that ALA ac-

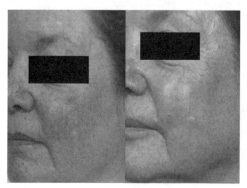

FIGURE 6.—Significant improvement in ectatic capillaries, skin texture, and color after 2 treatments using IPL with ALA-PDT.

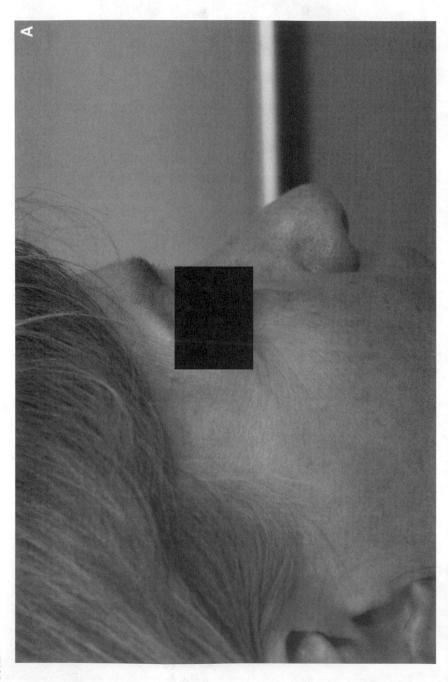

FIGURE 7

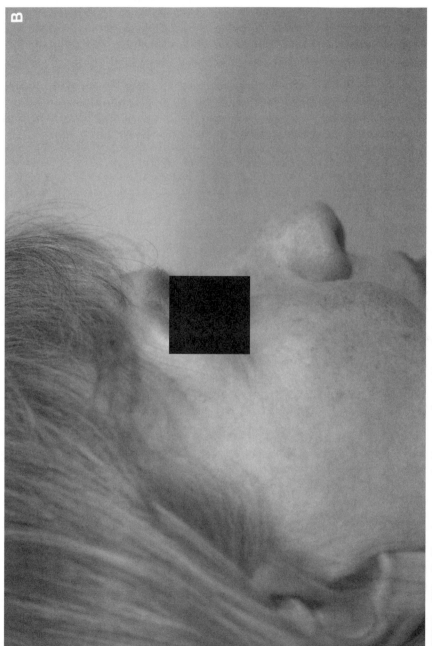

FIGURE 7A and 7B.—Significant improvement in skin texture, fine wrinkles, and solar pigmentation after 2 nonablative treatments with plasma skin resurfacing.

cumulates in dysplastic epidermal cells secondary to low iron stores, resulting in some degree of selectivity in targeting and killing of those cells. The diminished epidermal barrier effect of actinically damaged epidermis may also contribute to the selective uptake of ALA. ALA is also selectively uptaken by pilosebaceous glands and helps shrink sebaceous glands and diminish *Propionibacterium acnes* in pilosebaceous units. Different treatment protocols using ALA for photorejuvenation have been described. Limitations of this procedure include patient discomfort that may vary from mild to severe, depending on patient individual sensitivity, degree of actinic damage, duration of incubation of the medication, and type of light source being used. The traditional protocol that uses Levulan ALA-PDT involves a 12-hour incubation period followed by blue light exposure for the treatment of AK. Patients with AK experience significant discomfort, erythema, swelling, and crusting. Repeated gentler treatments either decreasing the incubation period (from 30 minutes to 3 hours) have been described as effective in treating AK and other aspects of photoaging.

Plasma Skin Resurfacing (PSR)

The plasmakinetic skin resurfacing (PSR) has recently been introduced under the name of Portrait™ and is a unique surgical tool that uses pulsed nitrogen plasma to deliver energy to target tissue. The hand-piece is used with a noncontact technique. The PSR device can be used ablatively and nonablatively. Nonablative tissue response characterized by mild erythema and desquamation is obtained when using less than 2-J settings. Deeper erythema with delayed epidermal sloughing 48 hours posttreatment is obtained when using greater than 2-J/cm settings. Low energy setting results in thermal damage limited to the epidermis and dermoepidermal junction. Depth of immediate dermal collagen denaturation remains superficial even with high energy settings averaging 8-12 μm with 3-4-J energy settings. Repeated low energy nonablative full-face treatments (4 treatments spaced 3 weeks apart) have shown significant improvement in skin pigmentation, texture, and fine lines but no significant measurable skin tightening in one multicentre open-label trial (Fig 7; see color plates III and IV). The procedure is well tolerated with topical anesthesia alone. Evidence of new collagene formation is observed on skin biopsy 4 weeks after a single treatment. At day 90, epidermal thickening, collagen remodeling in the mid-dermis, and decreased elastotic material is observed (personal communication). Greater improvement is obtained with high-energy ablative PSR treatments however. One periorbital study showed improvement in pigmentation and wrinkle lines similar to CO_2 laser with significantly shorter recovery time and no prolonged postoperative erythema (personal communication). Another study looking at perioral wrinkles also showed significant improvement in number and depth albeit more modest than expected with CO_2 laser (oral communication Fitzpatrick, Kilmer et al). Anecdotal reports suggested good results in treating facial acne scars. Further studies are necessary to better quantify the long-term efficacy of nonablative plasma photorejuvenation and other therapeutic applications.

Fractional Photothermolysis

Fractional photothermolysis is another new concept in photorejuvenation. The fractional photothermolysis device commercially known as Fraxel relies on a 1550-nm infrared laser technology to induce microscopic thermal denaturation zones in the epidermis and dermis in order to induce controlled collagen matrix denaturation and collagen remodeling.[27] The diameter of the columns of thermal denaturation varies between 50-120 μm in diameter and 400-1000 μm in depth depending on the energy settings chosen. The microscopic wound size allows for rapid and complete reepithelialization of microperforations with no significant visible superficial wounding.

The procedure alone can be painful and require topical or systemic analgesia. The recovery period is associated with some mild erythema and desquamation that may last up to 1 week. Treatments can be spaced 7-14 days apart with no significant downtime. The procedure consists initially in cleansing the skin with a mild abrasive solution followed by the application of the Optiguide Blue substance on the area to be treated. The exact optimal treatment parameters have not yet been firmly established, and clinical trials are still ongoing. Excellent results have been reported in the treatment of solar pigmentation and poikiloderma of Civatte in facial and extrafacial locations, including neck, chest, hands, and forearms (Fig 8; see color plate IV). Reported results on facial wrinkles are also interesting, although they appear to be inferior to CO_2 and Er:YAG laser using today's energy parameters. Comparative studies and long-term follow-up data are lacking right now to substantiate the precise comparative value of this new technology with currently available devices and treatments.

Monopolar Radiofrequency Photorejuvenation

The Thermacool II or Thermage device uses radiofrequency via a capacitative coupling tip in order to induce uniform deep volumetric tissue heating and thermal injury to superficial and deep collagen structures. No epidermal injury occurs as a result of concurrent cooling of the epidermis by direct contact with a cryogen-cooled handpiece. The 1-cm handpiece can deliver heat

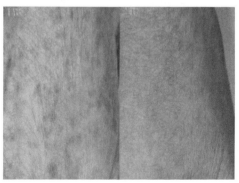

FIGURE 8.—Marked improvement in skin texture and pigmentation after 4 fractional photothermolysis treatment on the back of hands.

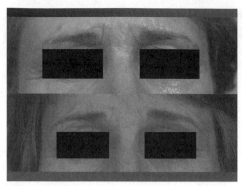

FIGURE 9.—Noticeable improvement in brow elevation and upper eyelid laxity after monopolar radio-frequency skin tightening of the upper face.

as far as 2500 μm deep. Animal studies have shown evidence of initial tissue contraction, activation of fibroblasts, and collagen remodeling as well as some degree of fat lysis.

Monopolar radiofrequency skin tightening results clinically in tissue tightening and elevation in areas that could only be approached by cutting surgery in the past. Several published and unpublished studies have shown measurably significant tissue tightening and elevation in the brow area, crow's feet, cheek, and neck areas of the face[28-30] (Fig 9; see color plate IV). More anecdotal reports have suggested the beneficial use of this device for extrafacial locations such as abdomen, arms, and chest. Successful results have also been reported in combination with liposuction for neck rejuvenation. Most patients also report improvement in skin texture and pore size, which may be related to shrinkage of sebaceous glands also having a beneficial impact on acne and hyperseborrhea.

The treatment itself is uncomfortable for most patients. Different oral analgesic protocols have been reported as well as topical analgesia, although the latter is not recommended by the manufacturer. Lack of predictability and reproducibility of results is also an issue with this technology. Newer algorithms suggest the use of multiple lower energy treatment passes with a treatment grid for better and more reproducible results. This method also makes the procedure more tolerable for patients as pain is energy-level dependent. The characteristics of the ideal candidate for radiofrequency skin tightening still remains to be established.

Broadband Deep Infrared

The Titan™ phototightening device broadband infrared light energy is used to induce sustained deep thermal injury to superficial and deep dermis. The energy output window produced ranges from 1100 nm to 1800 nm, which is mostly absorbed by water and reaches 1-2 mm in depth. Multi-second pulsing results in sustained heating of the treated area resulting in collagen denaturation and immediate tissue contraction. The procedure consists of precooling, treatment and postcooling phases to protect the epidermis from excessive heating and is associated with no epidermal wound or downtime. The treatments algorithms consist of 2 to 4 passes per treatment with 1 to 3 treatments performed at monthly intervals. Most patients require no analgesia or mild oral sedation and analgesia. Reports have suggested impressive results in skin tightening and tissue elevation in facial and extrafacial locations. However, optimal patient selection criteria and treatment protocols are areas that still require further study.

Conclusion

To this day, ablative CO_2 laser and long-pulsed Er:YAG laser technologies still remain the most effective treatment for severe facial photoaging. However, with the increasing demand for less-invasive procedures with minimal, more effective technologies have emerged and treatment protocols have improved. For better patient satisfaction, the best approach is one involving combination therapies and repeated treatment sessions as no single treatment can offer comprehensive full-facial or extrafacial rejuvenation. IPL and ALA-PDT using IPL or pulsed-dye laser may offer the best currently available treatment for photorejuvenation of pigmentation and ectatic blood vessels. Newer technologies such as plasmakinetic skin resurfacing and fractional photothermolysis appear to approach better the effect of ablative lasers in terms of dermal collagen remodeling and tissue tightening at the cost of little to no downtime. In addition, their use on extrafacial locations may represent promising new applications, although further studies will be required to better define their efficacy. Monopolar radiofrequency skin tightening and deep infrared skin tightening devices offer new alternatives for skin tightening and tissue elevation, delaying the need for cutting surgery by a few years in patient with facial and extrafacial skin laxity. Improvement of these technologies and of treatment parameters is likely to improve the efficacy and reproducibility of those techniques that are often operator-dependent.

Patient education of the therapeutic effect and realistic expected outcome of each procedure is also imperative to maximize patient satisfaction. Adequate daily at-home skin care, sun protection, botulinum toxin therapy, and soft tissue fillers are also excellent adjuncts that help improve the overall beneficial effects of nonablative photorejuvenation therapies.

References

1. Fitzpatrick RE, Rostan EF, Marchell N: Collagen tightening induced by carbon dioxide laser versus erbium:YAG laser. *Lasers Surg Med* 27:232-241, 2000.
2. Cotton J, Hood AF, Gonin R, et al: Histologic evaluation of preauricular and postauricular human skin after high energy, short-pulse carbon dioxide laser. *Arch Dermatol* 132:425-428, 1996.
3. Kuo T, Speyer MT, Ries WR, et al: Collagen thermal damage and collagen synthesis after cutaneous laser resurfacing. *Laser Surg Med* 23:66-71, 1998.
4. Kelly KM, Nelson JS, Lask GP: Cryogen spray cooling in combination with nonablative laser treatment of facial rhytides. *Arch Dermatol* 135:691-694, 1999.
5. Goldberg DJ: Full-face non-ablative dermal remodeling with 1320 nm Nd:YAG laser. *Dermatol Surg* 26:915-918, 2000.

6. Menaker GM, Wrone DA, Williams RM, et al: Treatment of facial rhytides with non-ablative laser: a clinical and histologic study. *Dertmatol Surg* 25:440-444, 1999.
7. Hardaway CA, Ross EV, Paithankar DY: Non-ablative cutaneous remodeling with 1.45 µm mid-infrared diode laser phase II. *J Cosmet Laser Ther* 4:9-14, 2002.
8. Fournier N, Dahan S, Barneaon G, et al: Nonablative remodeling: Clinical, histologic, ultrasound imaging, and profilometric evaluation of a 1540 nm Er:glass laser. *Dermatol Surg* 27:799-806, 2001.
9. Alster TS, Lupton JR: Are all infrared lasers equally effective in skin rejuvenation. *Sem Cut Med Surg* 21(4):274-279, 2002.
10. Bjerring P, Clement M, Heickedorff L, et al: Selective non-ablative wrinkle reduction by laser. *J Cut Laser Ther* 2:9-15, 2000.
11. Rostan E, Bowes LE, Iyer S, et al: A double-blind, side-by-side comparison study of low fluence long pulse dye laser to coolant treatment for wrinkling of the cheeks. *J Cosmet Laser Ther* 3:129-136, 2001.
12. Bitter PH: Noninvasive rejuvenation of photodamaged skin using serial, full-face intense pulsed light treatments. *Dermatol Surg* 26:835-842, 2000.
13. Goldberg DJ, Cutler KB: Nonablative treatment of rhytids with intense pulsed light. *Lasers Med Surg* 26:196-200, 2000.
14. Goldman MP: Non-ablative laser treatment of wrinkles. *Cosmet Dermatol* 15:17-20, 2000.
15. Goldberg DJ: New collagen formation after dermal remodeling with an intense pulsed light source. *J Cutan Laser Ther* 2:59-61, 2000.
16. Weiss RA, McDaniel DH, Geronemus RG, et al: Clinical trial of a novel non-thermal LED array for reversal of photoaging: clinical, histologic, and surface profilometric results. *Lasers Surg Med* 36(2):85-91, 2005.
17. Weiss RA, Weiss MA, Geronemus RG, et al: A novel non-thermal non-ablative full panel LED photomodulation device for reversal of photoaging: Digital microscopic and clinical results in various skin types. *J Drugs Dermatol* 3(6):605-610, 2004.
18. Gold MH, Bradshaw VL, Boring MM, et al: Treatment of sebaceous gland hyperplasia by photodynamic therapy with 5-aminolevulinic acid and a blue light source or intense pulsed light source. *J Drugs Dermatol* 3(6 Suppl):S6-S9, 2004.
19. Alster TS, Tanzi EL, Welsh EC: Photorejuvenation of facial skin with topical 20% 5-aminolevulinic acid and intense pulsed light treatment: A split-face comparison study. *J Drugs Dermatol* 4(1):35-38, 2005.
20. Taub AF: Photodynamic therapy for the treatment of acne: a pilot study. *J Drugs Dermatol* 3(6 Suppl):S10-S14, 2004.
21. Gold MH, Bradshaw VL, Boring MM, et al: The use of a novel intense pulsed light and heat source and ALA-PDT in the treatment of moderate to severe inflammatory acne vulgaris. *J Drugs Dermatol* 3(6 Suppl):S15-S19, 2004.
22. Alam M, Dover JS: Treatment of photoaging with topical aminolevulinic acid and light. *Skin Therapy Lett* 9(10):7-9, 2005.
23. Lang K, Schulte KW, Ruzicka T, et al: Aminolevulinic acid (Levulan) in photodynamic therapy of actinic keratoses. *Skin Therapy Lett* 6(10):1-2, 5, 2001.
24. Goldman MP, Boyce SM. A single-center study of aminolevulinic acid and 417 NM photodynamic therapy in the treatment of moderate to severe acne vulgaris. *J Drugs Dermatol* 2(4):393-396, 2003.
25. Touma DJ, Gilchrest BA: Topical photodynamic therapy: a new tool in cosmetic dermatology. *Semin Cutan Med Surg* 22(2):124-130, 2003.
26. Avram DK, Goldman MP: Effectiveness and safety of ALA-IPL in treating actinic keratoses and photodamage. *J Drugs Dermatol* 3(1 Suppl):S36-S39, 2004.
27. Manstein D, Herron GS, Sink RK, et al: Fractional photothermolysis: A new concept for cutaneous remodeling using microscopic patterns of thermal injury. *Lasers Surg Med* 34(5):426-438, 2004.

28. Nahm WK, Su TT, Rotunda AM, et al: Objective changes in brow position, superior palpebral crease, peak angle of the eyebrow, and jowl surface area after volumetric radiofrequency treatments to half of the face. *Dermatol Surg* 30(6):922-928; discussion, 928, 2004.
29. Alster TS, Tanzi E: Improvement of neck and cheek laxity with a nonablative radiofrequency device: a lifting experience. *Dermatol Surg* 30(4 Pt 1):503-507; discussion, 507, 2004.
30. Ruiz-Esparza J, Gomez JB: The medical face lift: a noninvasive, nonsurgical approach to tissue tightening in facial skin using nonablative radiofrequency. *Dermatol Surg* 29(4):325-332; discussion, 332, 2003.

Pediatric Viral Exanthems

ANTONIO A. T. CHUH, MD, MRCP, FRCP, MRCPCH
Honorary Clinical Assistant Professor, Department of Medicine, University of Hong Kong and Queen Mary Hospital, Pokfulam, Hong Kong SAR, China; Part-time Clinical Assistant Professor, Department of Community and Family Medicine, Chinese University of Hong Kong and Prince of Wales Hospital, Shatin, Hong Kong SAR, China

Introduction

Exanthem denotes a skin eruption occurring as a symptom of an acute viral or coccal disease, as in scarlet fever or measles.[1] This term comes from the Greek word *exanthema*, meaning a breaking out. Anthos describes a flower blossom in Greek. As flower blossoming comprises a spontaneous chain of events, early physicians were obviously impressed by the apparently pre-programmed course of events in exanthematous diseases.

In this article, we concentrate on dermatologic aspects of common or important exanthems in childhood of viral (or probably viral) origin.

Roseola Infantum

Human herpesvirus 6 (HHV-6) was isolated from 4 infants with roseola infantum, also known as *exanthem subitum*, by Yamanishi et al[2] in 1988. The clinical course and complications of primary HHV-6 infection were further reported by Hall et al[3] in 1994. Primary HHV-6 infection commonly occurs in infants and children younger than 3 years. HHV-6 then replicates in the salivary glands and is secreted in saliva. It remains latent in peripheral blood mononuclear cells and various body tissues and is reactivated in immunocompromised states. Primary human herpesvirus 7 (HHV-7) infection was subsequently shown to be another cause of roseola.[4] Both HHV-6 and HHV-7 belong to the *Roseolovirus* genus of the *Betaherpesvirinae* subfamily.[5] HHV-6 is further classified into HHV-6A and HHV-6B. Most cases of roseola in infants and children are related to HHV-6B infection. The age of primary infection of HHV-7 is likely to be older than that for HHV-6B.[6]

Infants and children with roseola infantum typically have sudden onset of high fever but remain clinically well, playful and active. Some may have vomiting, runny nose, and cough. Uvulopalatoglossal junctional ulcers may be observed.[7] On the fifth day of fever, erythematous macules appear on the trunk and neck (Fig 1A and 1B; see color plate V), which may spread to the face and extremities. The fever subsides within a few hours of rash eruption. The rash then becomes confluent, and fades in 2 to 5 days without scarring or hyperpigmentation.

Complications of roseola are uncommon, and include febrile convulsion,[8] otitis media,[8] encephalitis and encephalopathy,[9] thrombocytopenia,[10] Guillain-Barré syndrome,[11] and myocarditis.[12] Febrile convulsion may be more likely for HHV-7 infection.[6]

The diagnosis of roseola is clinical. The detection of HHV-6 DNA by polymerase chain reaction (PCR) in the plasma, HHV-6 DNA in whole blood in the absence of IgG, or high HHV-6 viral DNA load in the acute whole blood specimen are indicative of active HHV-6 infection.[13] Seroconversion

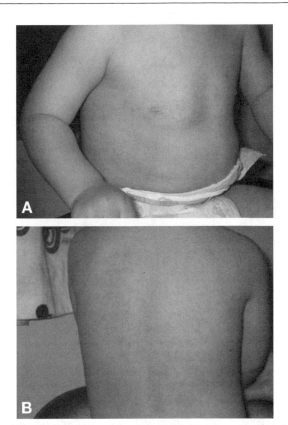

FIGURE 1A and 1B.—Erythematous macules on the trunk of an infant with roseola infantum.

on parallel testing of acute and convalescent sera indicates primary infection.[13] The management of roseola is symptomatic and supportive.

Erythema Infectiosum

Erythema infectiosum (EI), also known as the *fifth disease*, was discovered to be due to parvovirus B19 infection by Anderson et al in 1983.[14,15] B19 belongs to the family *Parvoviridae*, the subfamily *Parvovirinae*, and the genus *Erythrovirus*.[5] The virus is spread from person to person by direct contact with secretions such as saliva, sputum, or nasal discharge. In response to a common question by residents, we list the historical against modern nomenclature for the first to sixth diseases in Table 1.

EI is probably the commonest viral rash in school children in the United States.[16] The child may have low-grade fever, malaise, and sore throat. The characteristic facial erythema traditionally termed *slapped cheek* consists of erythematous papules that coalesce to form plaques (Fig 2A and 2B; see color plates V and VI). A lacy, reticular, or maculopapular rash on the trunk and extremities usually follows 2 days later (Fig 3; see color plate VI). The rash on face, trunk, and extremities may fade and re-erupt over the next 2 to 3 weeks.

TABLE 1.—Historical and Modern Nomenclature of Exanthematous Diseases

Historical Name	Modern Name	Causative Agent(s)
First disease	Measles	Measles virus
Second disease	Scarlet fever	*Streptococcus pyogenes*
Third disease	Rubella	Rubella virus
Fourth disease	Viral rash	Coxsackievirus or Echovirus
Fifth disease	Erythema infectiosum	Parvovirus B19
Sixth disease	Roseola infantum	Human herpesvirus 6 or human herpesvirus 7

Complications are rare. Arthralgia and arthritis are more common in adults than in children, and can become chronic in some adults.[17] Children with sickle cell anemia, thalassemia major, and hereditary spherocytosis may have severe aplastic crisis after parvovirus B19 infection, but the characteristic rash may not be present.[18] It is likely that parvovirus B19 infection is an important contributing factor to aplastic anaemia and chronic aplastic

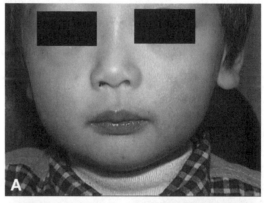

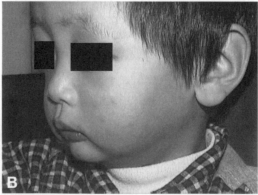

FIGURE 2A and 2B.—The *slapped cheek* appearance. The facial erythema in a child with erythema infectiosum consists of erythematous papules which coalesce to form plaques.

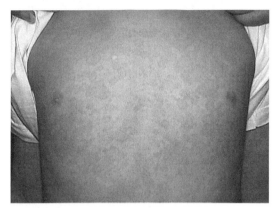

FIGURE 3.—Lacy and reticular rash on the trunk of a child with erythema infectiosum.

anaemia in children and adults alike.[19] Because of facial rash, fever, arthralgia, arthritis, and effects on the hemopoietic system, EI may cause diagnostic confusions with systemic lupus erythematosus.[20] Whether parvovirus B19 infection can trigger systemic lupus erythematous, however, still remains controversial.

The diagnosis of EI is mainly clinical, supplemented by demonstration of the specific IgM or detection of parvovirus B19 DNA by PCR, if necessary. Treatment for children with EI is entirely symptomatic, for the febrile symptoms and for pruritus. As the child is contagious only before the rash erupts, excluding the child from child care centers or schools is not likely to prevent the spread of the virus.[21] Pregnant women who have been in contact with the child before the eruption appears should be advised to consult their obstetricians, as infection during pregnancy may lead to spontaneous abortion, hydrops fetalis, congenital anomalies, and intrauterine fetal death.[22] About one third of pregnant women with parvovirus B19 are asymptomatic and the absence of symptoms should not deter referral.[23]

Chickenpox

Chickenpox is caused by the varicella zoster virus. This virus (human herpesvirus 3) belongs to the *Varicellovirus* genus of the *Alphaherpesvirnae* subfamily.[5] It spreads by direct contact with the vesicles or vesicular fluid or through the air when the infected person coughs or sneezes. The vesicles usually first erupt on the trunk and face (Fig 4A and 4B; see color plates VI and VII) and then spread centrifugally to the extremities. The scalp, genitalia, and mucous membranes including oral cavity and vagina can be affected. The vesicles, which can number 250 to 500 in some children, are 5 to 10 mm in diameter with an erythematous base. They erupt in crops and can be intensely pruritic. Secondary impetiginization is common. Affected children may have fever and malaise. Systemic symptoms usually last for 3 to 5 days. Younger children seem to have fewer vesicles and less severe systemic symptoms.

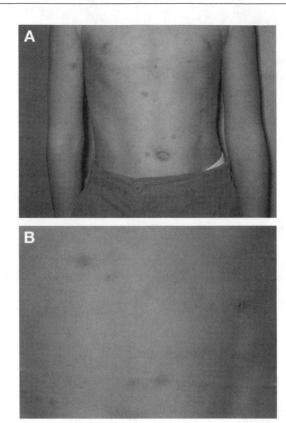

FIGURE 4A and 4B.—Vesicles on the trunk of a child with chickenpox. Vesicles can be seen to be in different stages of development in Fig 4B.

Common complications of chickenpox include impetiginization of skin lesions, respiratory tract infections, vomiting, and diarrhea. Rare and serious complications including viral pneumonitis, encephalitis, and disseminated varicella are usually related to immunodeficiency states. Chickenpox is the commonest cause of post-infectious acute cerebellar ataxia in children.[24] Chickenpox during pregnancy might lead to congenital varicella syndrome. The risk is estimated to be 0.78% for disease onset in the first trimester, 1.52% in the second trimester, and negligibly small (0.00%) in the third trimester.[25]

The incubation period is 10 to 21 days. The infectious period is 1 to 2 days before the rash appears to until all vesicles have become scabs. Immunity is usually lifelong after primary infection, with reactivation causing varicella zoster later in life.

Chickenpox can be prevented by vaccinating children above the age of 12 months. The protection seems to be long-term. The estimated vaccine efficacy in a 10-year follow-up study was 94.4% for 1 injection and 98.3% for

2 injections.[26] Breakthrough disease is possible, but most cases are mild. If the vaccine is administered at younger than 15 months, the effectiveness may be lower in the first year after vaccination.[27]

Symptomatic treatment is adequate for most children with chickenpox. Oral paracetamol might be prescribed for fever. Parents should be explicitly warned not to give the child aspirin in view of the risk of Reye's syndrome. Topical emollients and bath oils may soothe the itch. Some pediatricians recommended that nails should be trimmed. While the child should be discouraged from excessive scratching if at all possible, we have seen parents trimming the nails of children so enthusiastically that ingrown fingernails developed. Complications such as chest infection and dehydration from nausea and vomiting require specific treatment.

Systemic acyclovir can be prescribed for adolescents, children with preexisting chronic chest problems such as cystic fibrosis, children with extensive atopic dermatitis, children on systemic corticosteroids, and children with immunodeficiencies.[28] For immunocompetent children, acyclovir may reduce the duration of fever. Impacts on the number of days of new lesions erupting, the severity of pruritus, and the maximum number of lesions are controversial.[29] There is also no evidence that the spread of virus by the airborne route can be reduced by administering oral acyclovir to children with chickenpox.[30]

Smallpox

In view of the threat of bioterrorism,[31] we briefly discuss here the clinical manifestations of smallpox. Case definitions, investigations, vaccination policies, and community protective issues will not be covered.

Smallpox is caused by the variola virus, a member of the *Orthopoxvirus* genus, *Chordopoxvirinae* subfamily of the *Poxviridae* family.[5] Fever, myalgia, vomiting, rigor, and sometimes delirium were the major symptoms during the prodromal phase of a child with smallpox.[32] An enanthem as erythematous spots on the tongue and in the buccal cavity might be the first sign. These soon became ulcerated. The exanthem began as small macules on the face (Fig 5; see color plate VII), then spreading to trunk and extremities.

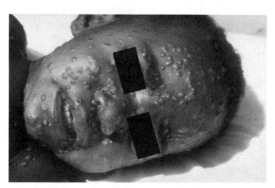

FIGURE 5.—Vesicles on the face of a child with smallpox. The lesions usually first erupt on the face and have a characteristic umbilicated appearance. The lesions are synchronous.

These became papules and then pustules and finally scabs. The scabs then fell off and formed depressed scars.

The umbilicated appearance of the pustules was characteristic of small-pox.[32] The cutaneous lesions were synchronous, unless in those in chickenpox erupting in crops.[33,34] Smallpox lesions evolved centripetally and lesions appeared on the palms and soles, unlike chickenpox with truncal lesions being more prominent.[33,34] Chickenpox lesions are also more superficial than smallpox lesions. The overall mortality rate for smallpox was about 30%.[35] Variants of classical smallpox included hemorrhagic smallpox with a high mortality, flat smallpox with almost 100% mortality, and variola minor with less lesions. The clinical severity was dependent on the virus load and the immunological responses.[36]

The incubation period was 7 to 17 days. The infectious period commenced from the prodromal phase until all scabs had fallen off, a fact again distinct from chickenpox. The peak was when the enanthem became ulcerated.

Rashes Due to the Enteroviruses

Viral rashes are commonly due to enteroviruses, including echoviruses, Coxsackie viruses, and other enteroviruses. They were known as the *fourth disease, Duke's disease*, or *epidemic pseudoscarlantina*. Enteroviruses are spread by direct contact with saliva, sputum, or nasal mucous from an infected person, or by contact with contaminated objects. The incubation period is 3 to 6 days.

The child may have fever, vomiting, diarrhea, sore throat, and cervical lymphadenopathy. The time of rash onset and the rash morphology are variable. It is mostly erythematous and maculopapular but may sometimes be urticarial, vesicular, petechial,[37] or hemorrhagic.[38] The face, trunk, and extremities including palmoplantar surfaces can be involved.

Complications include myocarditis, viral encephalitis, and paralysis. Neonates may develop severe infection with sepsis, meningoencephalitis, myocarditis, pneumonia, hepatitis, and coagulopathy.[39] The mortality rate can be substantial. For hand, foot, and mouth disease, the risk factors for a fatal course include vomiting, absence of mouth ulcers, atypical presentation, and leukocytosis.[40] An association between early enterovirus infection and type 1 diabetes mellitus has been suspected[41] but still remains controversial.[42]

Hand, foot, and mouth disease is usually caused by Coxsackie virus A16 and enterovirus 71, but Coxsackie viruses A4-A7, A9, A10, B1-B3, and B5 are also implicated. The exanthem affects the hands, feet, and buttocks. Individual lesions are erythematous macules developing into round or oval vesicles. The oval lesions may orient along lines of skin cleavage. The oral lesions are also erythematous macules developing into painful vesicles on the tongue, palate, buccal mucosa and gingiva. By the time the child is seen by the physician, vesicles are usually ruptured. The exanthem lasts for 7 to 10 days. The virus may be detectable in the stool for up to 1 month.

The diagnosis of viral rashes due to enteroviruses is mainly clinical. Investigations might be performed to exclude other infections. Serum viral culture or paired serum samples for serology might be performed. PCR might be used if available.[39]

There is no active vaccination for these enteroviruses. Commonsense hygiene practices are the most pertinent preventive strategies. Enterovirus 71 is particularly highly contagious. Intrafamilial and kindergarten transmissions are prominent.[43] The transmission rate to household contacts was estimated to be 52%, that to siblings being as high as 83%.[44] Some physicians would recommend exclusion from school for 2 to 3 days after onset of the exanthem and enanthem. Exclusion for longer periods are generally not required. If at all possible, the child should be discouraged from rupturing the blisters to reduce viral shedding.

No specific antiviral therapy is yet available for enterovirus infections. Clinical trials on the use of pleconaril, which inhibits viral attachment to host cell receptors and uncoating of viral nucleic acid, in neonates with severe enterovirus infections are being conducted.[39] Acyclovir has been reported to be useful for immunocompromised host with hand, foot, and mouth disease.[45] Low level laser therapy may shorten the painful period in stomatitis in hand, foot, and mouth disease.[46]

Infectious Mononucleosis

Infectious mononucleosis (IM) is caused by active primary infection of Epstein-Barr virus (EBV). EBV (human herpesvirus 4) belongs to the *Lymphocryptovirus* genus of the *Gammaherpesvirinae* subfamily.[5] The child or adolescent may have fever, sore throat, cervical or generalized lymphadenopathy, headache, anorexia, abdominal discomfort, and cough. Palatal petechiae and periorbital edema may be seen. About 5% to10% of patients have jaundice of varying degrees. Splenomegaly or hepatomegaly is sometime noted.

Complications including meningitis, encephalitis, and hepatitis are rare in children. Fatality is rare in IM, with virus-associated hemophagocytic syndrome being a major cause.[47] Like other herpesviruses, EBV infection is lifelong, with latent infection and reactivations. Chronic infection is associated with Burkitt's lymphoma, Hodgkin's disease, non-Hodgkin's lymphoma, and nasopharyngeal carcinoma.[48] The association of chronic EBV infection and chronic fatigue syndrome remains controversial.[49]

Two types of exanthem may be seen in IM. The first is the viral rash itself. This presents as a nonpruritic faint generalized maculopapular rash. It usually occurs early in the disease course, and lasts for only 24 to 48 hours. This rash can closely mimic that in secondary syphilis,[50] and VDRL (Venereal Disease Research Laboratory test) should be considered for adolescents if clinically indicated.

The second form erupts after administration of antibiotics. Such are usually ampicillin or amoxycillin, but cephalexin,[51] erythromycin,[52] azithromycin,[53] and levofloxacin[54] have also been implicated. This exanthem is usually a pruritic maculopapular rash and is often prolonged. The trunk and upper extremities are mostly affected.[55] The children and their parents should be reassured that in the absence of further evidence, the child should not be assumed to be allergic to beta-lactams. The mechanism of such rash is unknown. It is likely that real sensitization to beta-lactams may occur, as reported by investigations using prick, intradermal, and patch tests in vivo and using lymphocyte transformation tests in vitro.[56]

The diagnosis of IM is usually clinical, supported by leukocytosis, lymphocytosis, atypical lymphocytes of more than 10%, and a positive monospot test. Clinical diagnosis alone is unlikely to be reliable,[57] and primary infection of HIV can cause very similar symptoms.[58]

The interpretation of EBV serological results is complex. In short, the profiles compatible with primary infection are (1) positive IgM against viral capsid antigen in the absence of antibodies against EBV nuclear antigen, or (2) a very high or rising titer of IgG against viral capsid antigen in the absence of antibodies against EBV nuclear antigen after at least 4 weeks of onset of symptoms. IgG in the early disease phase is not likely to be detectable.[59] The detection of antibodies against EBV early antigen alone is unreliable as such can persist for years after primary infection.

EBV is spread by intimate contact with saliva, thus the nickname *kissing disease*. Airborne transmission does not normally occur. The incubation period is 4 to 6 weeks. Children with IM are potentially infectious. However, as viral shedding is also present in saliva of normal people, isolation is not generally recommended. The child is fit to attend childcare or school once he is physically well enough.

Measles

Measles is caused by the measles virus, a paramyxovirus, genus *Morbillivirus*.[5] Children with measles have prodromal symptoms including cough and coryza, conjunctivitis, and fever. Koplik's spots may be seen on day 2 or 3 of fever and is pathognomonic of measles. These are whitish spots with a red halo on the buccal mucous membrane opposite to the premolar teeth. The exanthem appears on day 4 or 5 of fever. First appearance on the face and behind the ears is typical. It then spreads to the trunk and extremities. The rash consists of maculopapular lesions around 0.1 to 1.0 cm. They are frequently confluent on the face and trunk. Lesions are blanchable initially, but not after 4 to 5 days of rash onset.

Even in developed countries, measles can run a severe course with significant mortality.[60] The commonest complications are diarrhea, otitis media, and pneumonia. Pneumonia, frequently due to bacterial superinfection,[61] accounts for 60% of deaths from measles. There exists no definite evidence that giving antibiotics to all children with measles decreases the risk of pneumonia.[62] Other complications include febrile convulsion, encephalitis, and myelitis. Residual neurological damage occurs in as many as 25% after encephalitis, while most patients with myelitis suffer no residual disability.[63] Subacute sclerosing panencephalitis is believed to be related to persistent measles virus infection of the brain. Progressive deterioration of intellect is followed by ataxia, myoclonic seizures, and death. Children below 2 years have a higher risk of serious complications from measles.

Measles is spread by droplets and contact with nasal and throat secretions. The incubation period from exposure to onset of fever is about 10 to 14 days. The infectious period is from 4 days before rash onset to 4 days after rash onset. It is highly infectious. Airborne transmission has been documented in examination room for up to 2 hours after a person with measles occupied the room. Local measles transmission is now rare in the United States, and most measles outbreaks were caused by imported cases.[64]

Passive immunity offers some protection in the first 6 to 8 months of life. Such immunity lasts longer in infants born to mothers who have had measles than those born to vaccinated mothers.[65] Vaccination as a 2-dose regimen confers active immunity for older children. It seems that measles and measles-mumps-rubella vaccinations are unlikely to be associated with autism[66,67] or asthma.[68] A recent report[69] on the association of measles-mumps-rubella vaccination and atopic dermatitis might, however, commence yet another controversy over long-term effects of the such vaccinations.

The diagnosis is usually clinical, supplemented by IgM serology, viral culture, or reverse-transcriptase PCR if necessary.[70] Paired serum samples for rising IgG must be performed in parallel, limiting the usefulness of the test.

Rubella

Rubella is caused by the rubella virus, a togavirus, genus *Rubivirus*.[5] The rash usually erupts on the first day of fever and constitutional symptoms. It is a macular rash first appearing on face, and then spreading to neck, trunk and the extremities. It is fainter than that in measles. Coalescence is infrequently seen. Forschheimer's spots which are small macules or petechiae over the soft palate and uvula may be seen but are nonspecific for rubella. Generalized lymphadenopathy involving especially the suboccipital and postauricular nodes is characteristic. Conjunctivitis and testalgia are occasionally present.

Arthralgia and arthritis commonly seen in adult females with rubella are less common in children with rubella.[71] Encephalitis is also less frequently seen in children. Other complications include thromobocytopenia, orchitis, neuritis, and late progressive panencephalitis.[72]

Of particular concern is congenital rubella syndrome. Despite global efforts, it is estimated that there are still more than 100,000 infants born with such syndrome worldwide each year.[73] Fetal infection can occur throughout pregnancy, but the first trimester incurs the highest risk. Sensorineural hearing impairment, cataracts, glaucoma, retinopathy, congenital cardiac defects, and mental retardation are the traditionally described manifestations. Neonatal thrombocytopenic purpura, hepatitis, bone lesions, meningoencephalitis, diabetes mellitus, and progressive rubella panencephalitis being the more recently known effects of congenital rubella infection.[74]

The incubation period of rubella is 14 to 21 days. It is spread by airborne transmission or droplets from nasal and throat secretions, and is less contagious than measles. Rubella is prevented by active immunization, as 2 doses of measles-mumps-rubella vaccine. Vaccination is contraindicated in pregnancy, but inadvertent administration of such should not be considered an indication for termination of pregnancy.[75]

The diagnosis of rubella is clinical, supplemented by specific IgM. Viral culture and reverse-transcriptase PCR can also be performed if available. Clinical diagnosis alone is unreliable, and laboratory confirmation is necessary should there be any complications or risk of transmission to a pregnant woman. Immunity status should be ascertained by serology and not by history of clinical diagnosis of rubella.[76] However, a case of congenital rubella syndrome was reported to be born by a mother vaccinated for rubella with documented seropositivity against rubella.[77] A test of for detecting rubella IgG in oral fluid reported a sensitivity of 94.4% and a specificity of 90.0%.[78]

Gianotti-Crosti Syndrome

Gianotti-Crosti syndrome (GCS) was first described by Gianotti in 1965.[79] Also known as *papular acrodermatitis of childhood*, it is an acrally distributed papular eruption occurring mainly in infants and children.

The 3 cardinal characteristics originally described include an erythematous papular eruption on the face and limbs, paracortical hyperplasia of lymph nodes, and acute, usually anicteric, hepatitis.[80] Earlier reports established an association between GCS and hepatitis B virus infection.[81-83] Recent reports suggest that in developed countries, papular acrodermatitis in childhood might more closely be associated with EBV infection.[84-86] Lymphadenopathy and hepatitis are no longer mandatory for diagnosis. Spontaneous remission within 2 to12 weeks is the rule for these children, but the range of rash duration can be wide.[87] Truncal lesions do not exclude the diagnosis.[88] Complications are rarely seen.

Other viruses including coxsackievirus,[89] cytomegalovirus,[90] hepatitis A virus,[91] HIV,[92] parvovirus B19,[93] rotavirus,[94] and HHV-6B[95] have also been implicated in the etiology of GCS. It is thus likely that GCS represents a final common pathway for a number of viral infections. The underlying immunopathogenesis is unknown. GCS has been reported to be more prevalent in children with atopic tendency.[96] Thus, IgE and immediate hypersensitivity might have a role.

The diagnosis of GCS is based on clinical grounds (Figs 6A-6C, 7A-7D; see color plates VIII and IX). Lesional histopathological changes are nonspecific and rarely indicated for young children. A set of diagnostic criteria (Table 2) has been proposed and validated and might be helpful for a more objective diagnosis to be made.[97]

The management of GCS is symptomatic. Topical emollients are adequate for most children. For children with severe pruritus, topical corticosteroids might have a role in symptomatic relief, although there is no evidence that the disease course is modified by such therapy. Parents should be reassured that the rash is self-limiting, is highly unlikely to be contagious, has very low risk of complications, and does not cause permanent scarring.

Pityriasis Rosea

Pityriasis rosea (PR), also known as *pityriasis rosea of Gibert* (not *Gilbert*), was first termed as such by Gibert in 1860.[98] A characteristic herald

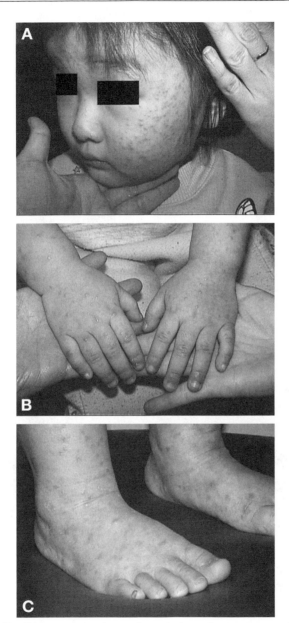

FIGURE 6A-6C.—Erythematous papular eruption on the face and extensor aspects of 4 extremities in a child with Gianotti-Crosti syndrome.

patch reported to be present in 40% to 60% of all patients is followed 7 to 14 days later by a generalized secondary eruption. Lesions exhibit a collarette scaling pattern (Fig 8; see color plate X), affect mostly the trunk and proximal aspects of 4 extremities, and generally orientate themselves along skin

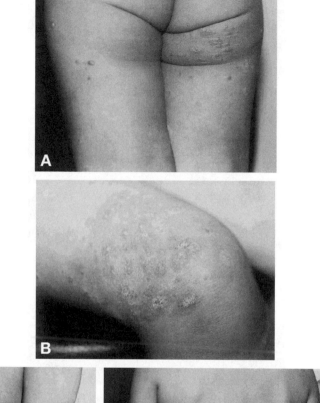

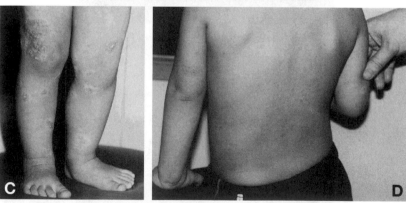

FIGURE 7A-7D.—Erythematous papulovesicular lesions on the buttocks and lower limbs of a child with Gianotti-Crosti syndrome. Calamine lotion was applied. The presence of minimal truncal lesions in Fig 7D does not exclude the diagnosis.

cleavage lines.[99] In a series of 247 patients, 50 (18%) had severe pruritus, 99 (36%) had moderate pruritus, 64 (23%) had mild pruritus, and 61 (22%) had no pruritus.[100] Spontaneous remission in 2 to 12 weeks is the rule. Relapse is rare. *Pityriasis circinata et marginata of Vidal* is likely to be a variant

TABLE 2.—Diagnostic Criteria of Gianotti-Crosti
Syndrome[97]

Essential clinical features:
Monomorphous, flat-topped, pink-brown papules or papulovesicles
  1-10 mm in diameter.
At least 3 of the following 4 sites involved: (1) cheeks, (2) buttocks, (3)
  extensor surfaces of forearms, and (4) extensor surfaces of legs.
Being symmetrical.
Lasting for at least 10 days.

Exclusional clinical features:
Extensive truncal lesions.
Scaly lesions.

of PR, with fewer and larger lesions often localized at the axillae and groins.[101]

PR is fairly common in children. A cross sectional study based on 1-day surveys in secondary schools in Burkina-Faso reported the prevalence of PR to be 0.6% for children and young adults aged between 10 and 29 years.[102] The youngest reported patient was 3 months old.[103] Of the numerous atypical forms of PR that have been described, the vesicular variant is said to be commoner in children and young adults.[104]

The cause of PR is unknown. The *programmed* clinical course with a herald patch followed by a secondary eruption, the spontaneous resolution, the lack of recurrence for most patients, and the presence of temporal case clustering[105,106] all substantiate an infectious, possible viral, etiology. Further evidence for an infectious cause comes from seasonal variation and the associations with respiratory tract infections,[107] unfavorable social and economic background of patients,[102] and a history of contact for some patients with PR.[108]

Recent focus has been on the association of PR and human herpesvirus 7 infection. Despite early encouraging results by several investigators,[109-113]

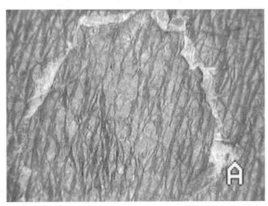

FIGURE 8.—Peripheral collarette (collar-like) scaling with *hanging curtains* in a lesion of a patients with pityriasis rosea.

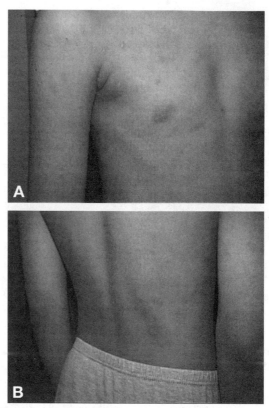

FIGURE 9A and 9B.—Generalized discrete scaly patches on the trunk and proximal aspects of upper limbs of a child with pityriasis rosea.

other investigators[114-121] were not able to confirm the positive findings. Such association is best considered controversial at present. It is also highly unlikely that PR is associated with infections of cytomegalovirus,[122] EBV,[122] parvovirus B19,[122] picornaviruses,[123] influenza and parainfluenza viruses,[124] *Legionella spp*,[125] *Mycoplasma spp*,[125] and *Chlamydia spp*.[125]

PR remains a clinical diagnosis (Figs 9A and 9B; see color plates X and XI). Lesional histopathological changes are nonspecific and can only support but not confirm a diagnosis of PR. A set of diagnostic criteria (Table 3) has been proposed for PR.[126]

As the eruption is self limiting, symptomatic relief for pruritus by emollients and topical corticosteroids is adequate for most patients. Oral sedating antihistamines as a single nocturnal dose might be considered for patients with severe pruritus at night. Studies on the efficacy of ultraviolet radiation[127,128] have reported conflicting results. Beneficial effect has been reported for systemic corticosteroids for patients with particularly recalcitrant eruption.[129] However, systemic corticosteroids have been reported to exacerbate PR as well.[130] Their routine use thus cannot be recommended.

TABLE 3.—Diagnostic Criteria of Pityriasis Rosea[126]

Essential clinical features:
Discrete circular or oval lesions.
Scaling on most lesions.
Peripheral collarette scaling with central clearance on at least 2 lesions

Optional clinical features (at least one has to be present):
Truncal and proximal limb distribution, with less than 10% of lesions
  distal to mid-upper-arm and mid-thigh.
Orientation of most lesions along direction of the ribs.
A herald patch (not necessarily the largest) appearing at least 2 days
  before the generalized eruption.

Exclusional clinical features:
Multiple small vesicles at the center of 2 or more lesions.
Most lesions on palmar or plantar skin surfaces.
Clinical or serological evidence of secondary syphilis.

A double-blind, placebo-controlled clinical trial was reported on the efficacy of oral erythromycin in PR.[131] The study adopted a pseudorandomized method of alternatively allocating patients to treatment and placebo groups, instead of the conventional true randomization procedures. Adverse gastrointestinal reactions were reported to be very low (4%) in the study, much lower than that expected in routine administration of the macrolide. Further clinical trials are necessary to confirm the results of this study.

Individual investigators have reported the use of acyclovir in PR.[132] Whether the effect was genuinely due to treatment or related to spontaneous rash resolution is unknown. Acyclovir has little in vitro action against HHV-7.[133] As the association between PR and HHV-7 infection is still controversial, further studies are necessary before adopting antiviral treatment in PR.

Papular Purpuric Gloves and Socks Syndrome

Harms et al[134] first described first young adults with swollen and pruritic hands and feet in 1990. Involved areas were erythematous and subsequently became purpuric. Sharp demarcations at the wrists and ankles were characteristic. The rash was therefore termed *papular purpuric gloves and socks syndrome* (PPGSS).

Involvements of the mouth and lips in form of aphtoid ulcers, and the perioral areas are sometimes described.[135] A prodromal syndrome with fever and fatigue is frequently reported. Spontaneous resolution in 1 to 2 weeks was the rule. Skin exfoliation was reported to accompany rash resolution in some cases. In one reported case,[136] the rash was accompanied by dysuria, vulval erythema and unilateral petechiae on the breast. In one case, resolution of the purpuric lesions on feet was accompanied by superficial skin necrotic changes.[137] In another case, the rash was accompanied by multiple hemorrhagic bullae on the toes.[138] One patient with PPGSS had palatal petechiae.[139] However, as the patient had von Willebrand disease, whether the oral manifestation is genuinely related to PPGSS is unknown.

The diagnosis of PPGSS is clinical. Lesional histopathological changes are nonspecific and can only support, but not confirm, the diagnosis.[140] An interface dermatitis, vacuolar degeneration at the dermoepidermal junction, and a superficial perivascular lymphocytic infiltrate sometimes with exocytosis, are reported.[136,141]

The apparently "programmed" sequence of events led investigators to suspect a role of viruses. Other supporting evidence are that children and young adults are mostly affected, and that most cases occur in spring and summer. The association of PPGSS with parvovirus B19 infection was documented by seroconversion in many reports,[135,142-144] involving a mother and daughter both with PPGSS in one such report.[145] Antibodies against parvovirus B19 were found by intracytoplasmic staining in dermal endothelial cells, keratinocytes, and sweat glands.[141] Parvovirus B19 DNA was also detectable in lesional biopsy specimens by PCR.[136,141] In one reported case, PPGSS was seen concomitantly with EI in a patient with parvovirus B19 infection.[146]

PPGSS was also reported to be associated with infections by cytomegalovirus,[147] measles,[148] hepatitis B,[149,150] rubella,[151] Coxsackie virus B6,[140] HHV-6,[152] HHV-7,[153] and HIV.[154] Some cases of PPGSS are believed to be drug-induced, such as by sulphonamides.[155]

As PPGSS is a self-limiting eruption, the management is largely symptomatic. For patients diagnosed to have parvovirus B19 infection, contact tracing should be conducted for especially vulnerable groups, such as patients with hematological disorders, under immunosuppressive therapy, or pregnant women.

Asymmetric Periflexural Exanthem (Unlitaral Laterothoracic Exanthem)

Bodemer and de Prost[156] reported in 1992 a series of 18 children with a rash which they termed *unilateral laterothoracic exanthema*. In 1993, Taieb et al[157] reported 21 children with similar eruption, which they termed *asymmetric periflexural exanthem of childhood* (APE). It is believed that these conditions are variations of the same disease.[158,159]

The eruption often commences as small papular lesions, sometimes surrounded by a pale halo, on unilateral axilla or groin regions (Fig 10A and 10B; see color plate XI). The lesions gradually become patchy scaly. The patches may appear in circular or reticular patterns. The rash might then spread centrifugally during the first 8 days. In approximately 50% of all cases, the rash become generalized to involve the face, genitalia, hands, or feet on days 10-15, while still remaining mostly unilateral. However, minor lesions on the contralateral side are commonly seen.[160,161] Vesicles and hemorrhagic bullae are sometimes present. Pruritus of moderate to severe intensity is usually reported.

As with other paraviral rashes, prodromal symptoms such as fever, sore throat, chills, and gastrointestinal disturbances are frequently reported. Axillary and inguinal lymphadenitis is sometimes present. The mean rash duration is 5 weeks.[162] Spontaneous remission within 3 months is the rule.

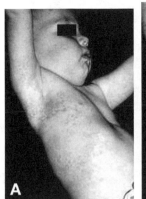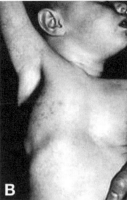

FIGURE 10A and 10B.—Small papular lesions on axilla and lateral trunk of a child with asymmetric periflexural exanthem.

APE mainly occurs in winter and spring. The male to female ratio is approximately 1:2.[141] Most affected children are between 1 and 5 years old, but adults can also be affected (Fig 11A-11D; see color plate XII).[159,163-165]

The lesional histopathology of APE is nonspecific, although a perisudoral interface CD8+ infiltrate has been reported as a relatively specific change.[162,166]

The cause of APE is unknown. Epidemiological study has reported no triggering factor, no interhuman transmission, and no demonstrable association with PR.[166] Microbiological evidence for a viral etiology is slim. In a series of 187 patients with APE,[161] virological investigations were performed on 34 cases. Two children were found to have evidence of parainfluenzavirus 2 infection, 2 children had parainfluenzavirus 3, and 2 children had adenovirus infections. In another series of 37 children with APE and 37 age-matched controls,[167] no significant difference was noted for the viruses and bacteria investigated. In another study involving 48 children with APE,[162] no infectious agent and no significant epidemiological factor were identified. Evidence of parvovirus B19 infection was found in an adult patient with APE.[168]

The management of APE is largely symptomatic. The pruritus may be relieved by topic emollients and oral sedative antihistamines. The rash resolution may be hastened by topical corticosteroids for some patients.[162]

Eruptive pseudoangiomatosis

Eruptive pseudoangiomatosis (EP) was first described by Cherry et al[169] in 1969. The eruption consists of small erythematous papules on the face, trunk, and extremities. The lesions resemble cherry angiomas and are surrounded by white halos. A characteristic clinical sign is the fading of the lesions on digital pressure and re-engorgement from the center on release. There are usually less then 10 lesions, and spontaneous rash remission within 10 days is the rule. Accompanying constitutional symptoms includ-

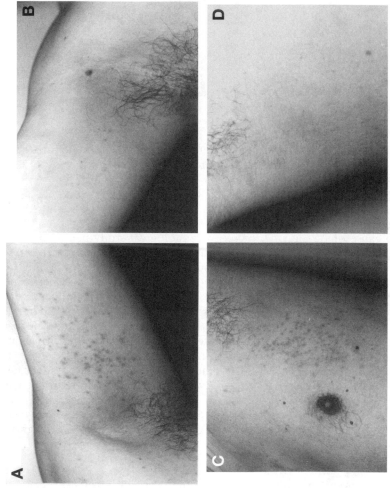

FIGURE 11A–11D.—Small papular lesions on left axilla and left lateral trunk of an adult with asymmetric periflexural exanthem. The right side of the body is relatively spared of lesions.

ing fever, sore throat, and gastrointestinal disturbances are frequently reported.[170]

Most cases of EP affect children,[171,172] but adult cases have also been reported,[170,173] including 1 post-renal transplantation adult.[174] Adult cases were reported to run a longer course.[170] It is exceptional to find clustering of cases, but familial occurrence has been reported.[175]

Lesional histopathological examination revealed mainly dermal changes. The epidermis is relatively unaffected. Dilated blood vessels with plump hobnail-shaped endothelial cells are most characteristic.[172,176] There is no evidence of vasculitis. Owing to the absence of proliferation of blood vessels, Prose et al[176] termed the disease *EP*. The changes are nonspecific otherwise and include perivascular infiltrates with lymphocytes and polymorphs in the superficial dermis.

The initial 4 cases of EP reported by Cherry et al[169] were believed to be associated with echovirus infection. Similar virological findings have not been reported otherwise.[170,176,177] A multifactorial viral etiology has been proposed for EP.[178] No active intervention has been reported to affect the course of EP.

Acknowledgments

We thank the CDC for authorizing us to reproduce Fig 5. We also thank Dr Ellen Szalinski, Children's Memorial Hospital, Chicago, for allowing us to reproduce Figs 9A and 9B. All other photographs were taken by the author on his own patients.

Figs 6B and 6C have been published by us in *International Pediatrics* (2002; 17:45-48), and are reproduced in this article with the kind permission of Mr Rolando Irizarry, Managing Editor. Figs 7A-7D have been published by us in the *Australasian Journal of Dermatology* (2003; 44:215-216), and Fig 11A has been published by us in *Clinical and Experimental Dermatology* (2004; 29:320-321). We thank Ms Zoë Ellams, Permissions Coordinator, Blackwell Publishing, for granting us permission to reproduce them in this article.

Table 2 has been published by us in *Cutis* (2001; 68:201-213) and is reproduced here with the kind permission of Ms Sharon Finch, Group Publisher. Table 3 was published by us in the *Journal of European Academy of Dermatology and Venereology* (2003; 17:101-103), and is reproduced with the authorization of Ms Laura Wilson, Permissions Coordinator, Blackwell Publishing.

References

1. Stedman's medical dictionary. Available at www.stedmans.com/section.cfm/45.
2. Yamanishi K, Okuno T, Shiraki K, et al: Identification of human herpesvirus-6 as a causal agent for exanthem subitum. *Lancet* 1:1065-1067, 1988.
3. Hall CB, Long CE, Schnabel KC, et al: Human herpesvirus-6 infection in children. A prospective study of complications and reactivation. *N Engl J Med* 331:432-438, 1994.
4. Tanaka K, Kondo T, Torigoe S, et al: Human herpesvirus 7: another causal agent for roseola. *J Pediatr* 125:1-5, 1994.

5. The universal virus database of the International Committee on Taxonomy of Viruses. Available at www.ictvdb.iacr.ac.uk/index.htm.
6. Caserta MT, Hall CB, Schnabel K, et al: Primary human herpesvirus 7 infection: a comparison of human herpesvirus 7 and human herpesvirus 6 infections in children. *J Pediatr* 133:386-389, 1998.
7. Chua KB: The association of uvulo-palatoglossal junctional ulcers with exanthem subitum: A 10-year paediatric outpatient study. *Med J Malaysia* 54:58-64, 1999.
8. Barone SR, Kaplan MH, Krilov LR: Human herpesvirus-6 infection in children with first febrile seizures. *J Pediatr* 127:95-97, 1995.
9. Suga S, Yoshikawa T, Asano Y, et al: Clinical and virological analyses of 21 infants with exanthem subitum (roseola infantum) and central nervous system complications. *Ann Neurol* 33:597-603, 1993.
10. Hashimoto H, Maruyama H, Fujimoto K, et al: Hematologic findings associated with thrombocytopenia during the acute phase of exanthem subitum confirmed by primary human herpesvirus-6 infection. *J Pediatr Hematol Oncol* 24:211-214, 2002.
11. Miyake F, Yoshikawa T, Suzuki K, et al: Guillain-Barré syndrome after exanthem subitum. *Pediatr Infect Dis J* 21:569-570, 2002.
12. Yoshikawa T, Ihira M, Suzuki K, et al: Fatal acute myocarditis in an infant with human herpesvirus 6 infection. *J Clin Pathol* 54:792-795, 2001.
13. Chiu SS, Cheung CY, Tse CYC, et al: Early diagnosis of primary human herpesvirus 6 infection in childhood: serology, polymerase chain reaction, and virus load. *J Infect Dis* 178:1250-1256, 1998.
14. Anderson MJ, Jones SE, Fisher-Hoch SP, et al: Human parvovirus, the cause of erythema infectiosum (fifth disease)? *Lancet* 1:1378, 1983.
15. Anderson MJ, Lewis E, Kidd IM, et al: An outbreak of erythema infectiosum associated with human parvovirus infection. *J Hyg (Lond)* 93:85-93, 1984.
16. CDC: Rashes among schoolchildren – 14 states, October 4, 2001-February 27, 2002. *MMWR Morb Mortal Wkly Rep* 51:161-164, 2002.
17. Lennerz C, Madry H, Ehlhardt S, et al: Parvovirus B19-related chronic monoarthritis: immunohistochemical detection of virus-positive lymphocytes within the synovial tissue compartment: Two reported cases. *Clin Rheumatol* 23:59-62, 2004.
18. Kellermayer R, Faden H, Grossi M: Clinical presentation of parvovirus B19 infection in children with aplastic crisis. *Pediatr Infect Dis J* 22:1100-1101, 2003.
19. Qian X, Zheng Y, Zhang G, et al: Relationship between human parvovirus B19 infection and aplastic anemia. *Chin Med Sci J* 16:172-174, 2001.
20. Severin MC, Levy Y, Shoenfeld Y: Systemic lupus erythematosus and parvovirus B-19: Casual coincidence or causative culprit? *Clin Rev Allergy Immunol* 25:41-48, 2003.
21. CDC: Parvovirus B19 (fifth disease). Available at www.cdc.gov/ncidod/dvrd/revb/respiratory/parvo_b19.htm.
22. Crane J, for the Society of Obstetricians and Gynaecologists of Canada. Parvovirus B19 infection in pregnancy. *J Obstet Gynaecol Can* 24:727-743, 2002.
23. Wong SF, Chan FY, Cincotta RB, et al: Human parvovirus B19 infection in pregnancy: Should screening be offered to the low-risk population? *Aust N Z J Obstet Gynaecol* 42:347-351, 2002.
24. Nussinovitch M, Prais D, Volovitz B, et al: Post-infectious acute cerebellar ataxia in children. *Clin Pediatr (Phila)* 42:581-584, 2003.
25. Koren G: Risk of varicella infection during late pregnancy. *Can Fam Physician* 49:1445-1446, 2003.
26. Kuter B, for the Study Group for Varivax: Ten year follow-up of healthy children who received one or two injections of varicella vaccine. *Pediatr Infect Dis J* 23:132-137, 2004.
27. Vazquez M, LaRussa PS, Gershon AA, et al: Effectiveness over time of varicella vaccine. *JAMA* 2004; 291:851-855, 2004.
28. American Academy of Pediatrics: Chickenpox. [serial online] 1999. Available at: www.medem.com.

29. Klassen TP, Belseck EM, Wiebe N, et al: Acyclovir for treating varicella in otherwise healthy children and adolescents. *Cochrane Database Syst Rev* 4:CD002980, 2002.
30. Suzuki K, Yoshikawa T, Ihira M, et al: Spread of varicella-zoster virus DNA to the environment from varicella patients who were treated with oral acyclovir. *Pediatr Int* 45:458-460, 2003.
31. Pennington H: Smallpox and bioterrorism. *Bull World Health Organ* 81:762-767, 2003.
32. Lofquist JM, Weimert NA, Hayney MS: Smallpox: A review of clinical disease and vaccination. *Am J Health Syst Pharm* 60: 749-756, 2003.
33. Noeller TP: Biological and chemical terrorism: recognition and management. *Cleve Clin J Med* 68:1001-1009, 1013, 2001.
34. Varkey P, Poland GA, Cockerill FR III, et al: Confronting bioterrorism: Physicians on the front line. *Mayo Clin Proc* 77:661-672, 2002.
35. Guharoy R, Panzik R, Noviasky JA, et al: Smallpox: Clinical features, prevention, and management. *Ann Pharmacother* 38:440-447, 2004.
36. Bray M, Buller M: Looking back at smallpox. *Clin Infect Dis* 38:882-889, 2004.
37. Sukhai RN, Munneke R: Enteroviral meningitis with a petechial rash in three children. *Eur J Pediatr* 161:226-227, 2002.
38. Nielsen HE, Andersen EA, Andersen J, et al: Diagnostic assessment of haemorrhagic rash and fever. *Arch Dis Child* 85:160-165, 2001.
39. Abzug MJ: Presentation, diagnosis, and management of enterovirus infections in neonates. *Paediatr Drugs* 6:1-10, 2004.
40. Chong CY, Chan KP, Shah VA, et al: Hand, foot and mouth disease in Singapore: A comparison of fatal and non-fatal cases. *Acta Paediatr* 92:1163-1169, 2003.
41. Ylipaasto P, Klingel K, Lindberg AM, et al: Enterovirus infection in human pancreatic islet cells, islet tropism in vivo and receptor involvement in cultured islet beta cells. *Diabetologia* 47:225-239, 2004.
42. Viskari H, Ludvigsson J, Uibo R, et al: Relationship between the incidence of type 1 diabetes and enterovirus infections in different European populations: Results from the EPIVIR project. *J Med Virol* 72:610-617, 2004.
43. Chang LY, King CC, Hsu KH, et al: Risk factors of enterovirus 71 infection and associated hand, foot, and mouth disease/herpangina in children during an epidemic in Taiwan. *Pediatrics* 109:e88, 2002.
44. Chang LY, Tsao KC, Hsia SH, et al: Transmission and clinical features of enterovirus 71 infections in household contacts in Taiwan. *JAMA* 291:222-227, 2004.
45. Faulkner CF, Godbolt AM, DeAmbrosis B, et al: Hand, foot and mouth disease in an immunocompromised adult treated with aciclovir. *Australas J Dermatol* 44:203-206, 2003.
46. Toida M, Watanabe F, Goto K, et al: Usefulness of low-level laser for control of painful stomatitis in patients with hand-foot-and-mouth disease. *J Clin Laser Med Surg* 21:363-367, 2003.
47. Mroczek EC, Weisenburger DD, Grierson HL, et al: Fatal infectious mononucleosis and virus-associated hemophagocytic syndrome. *Arch Pathol Lab Med* 111:530-535, 1987.
48. Thompson MP, Kurzrock R: Epstein-Barr virus and cancer. *Clin Cancer Res* 10:803-821, 2004.
49. Soto NE, Straus SE: Chronic fatigue syndrome and herpesviruses: The fading evidence. *Herpes* 7:46-50, 2000.
50. Kato H, Kitajima Y, Yaoita H, et al: Atypical exanthema in a patient with infectious mononucleosis. *J Dermatol* 20:365-368, 1993.
51. McCloskey GL, Massa MC: Cephalexin rash in infectious mononucleosis. *Cutis* 59:251-254, 1997.
52. Pendleton N, Mallik LJ, Williams JG: Erythromycin rash in glandular fever. *Br J Clin Pract* 43:464-465, 1989.
53. Dakdouki GK, Obeid KH, Kanj SS: Azithromycin-induced rash in infectious mononucleosis. *Scand J Infect Dis* 34:939-941, 2002.

54. Paily R: Quinolone drug rash in a patient with infectious mononucleosis. J Dermatol 27:405-406, 2000.
55. Ikediobi NI, Tyring SK: Cutaneous manifestations of Epstein-Barr virus infection. *Dermatol Clin* 20:283-289, 2002.
56. Renn CN, Straff W, Dorfmuller A, et al: Amoxicillin-induced exanthema in young adults with infectious mononucleosis: Demonstration of drug-specific lymphocyte reactivity. *Br J Dermatol* 147:1166-1170, 2002.
57. Crespin FH Jr, Gordon RC: Infectious mononucleosis in the community hospital. *J Fam Pract* 16:703-708, 1983.
58. Gaines H, von Sydow M, Pehrson PO, et al: Clinical picture of primary HIV infection presenting as a glandular-fever-like illness. *BMJ* 297:1363-1368, 1988.
59. Krabbe S, Hesse J, Uldall P: Primary Epstein-Barr virus infection in early childhood. *Arch Dis Child* 56:49-52, 1981.
60. Van Den Hof S, Smit C, Van Steenbergen JE, et al: Hospitalizations during a measles epidemic in the Netherlands, 1999 to 2000. *Pediatr Infect Dis J* 21:1146-1150, 2002.
61. Duke T, Mgone CS: Measles: not just another viral exanthem. *Lancet* 361:763-773, 2003.
62. Shann F, D'Souza RM, D'Souza R: Antibiotics for preventing pneumonia in children with measles. *Cochrane Database Syst Rev* 4:CD001477, 2000.
63. Gunaratne PS, Rajendran T, Tilakaratne S: Neurological complications of measles. *Ceylon Med J* 46:48-50, 2001.
64. CDC: Measles outbreak associated with an imported case in an infant—Alabama, 2002. *MMWR Morb Mortal Wkly Rep* 53:30-33, 2004.
65. Szenborn L, Tischer A, Pejcz J, et al: Passive acquired immunity against measles in infants born to naturally infected and vaccinated mothers. *Med Sci Monit* 9:CR541-CR546, 2003.
66. DeStefano F, Thompson WW: MMR vaccine and autism: An update of the scientific evidence. *Expert Rev Vaccines* 3:19-22, 2004.
67. Jacobson RM: Association of autistic spectrum disorder and the measles, mumps, and rubella vaccine—A systematic review of current epidemiological evidence. *Child Care Health Dev* 30:91-92, 2004.
68. Maher JE, Mullooly JP, Drew L, et al: Infant vaccinations and childhood asthma among full-term infants. *Pharmacoepidemiol Drug Saf* 13:1-9, 2004.
69. Olesen AB, Juul S, Thestrup-Pedersen K: Atopic dermatitis is increased following vaccination for measles, mumps and rubella or measles infection. *Acta Derm Venereol* 83:445-450, 2003.
70. van Binnendijk RS, van den Hof S, van den Kerkhof H, et al: Evaluation of serological and virological tests in the diagnosis of clinical and subclinical measles virus infections during an outbreak of measles in The Netherlands. *J Infect Dis* 188:898-903, 2003.
71. Masuko-Hongo K, Kato T, Nishioka K: Virus-associated arthritis. *Best Pract Res Clin Rheumatol* 17:309-318, 2003.
72. Frey TK: Neurological aspects of rubella virus infection. *Intervirology* 40:167-175, 1997.
73. Robertson SE, Featherstone DA, Gacic-Dobo M, et al: Rubella and congenital rubella syndrome: Global update. *Rev Panam Salud Publica* 14:306-315, 2003.
74. Cooper LZ: The history and medical consequences of rubella. *Rev Infect Dis* 7 Suppl 1:S2-S10, 1985.
75. Sur DK, Wallis DH, O'Connell TX: Vaccinations in pregnancy. *Am Fam Physician* 68:299-304, 2003.
76. Palihawadana P, Wickremasinghe AR, Perera J: Seroprevalence of rubella antibodies among pregnant females in Sri Lanka. *Southeast Asian J Trop Med Public Health* 34:398-404, 2003.
77. Ushida M, Katow S, Furukawa S: Congenital rubella syndrome due to infection after maternal antibody conversion with vaccine. *Jpn J Infect Dis* 56:68-69, 2003.

78. Ben Salah A, Zaatour A, Pomery L, et al: Validation of a modified commercial assay for the detection of rubella-specific IgG in oral fluid for use in population studies. *J Virol Methods* 114:151-158, 2003.

79. Gianotti F: [Viral anicteric hepatitis in infantile papular acrodermatitis]. *Epatologia* 12:171-191, 1966.

80. Gianotti F: Papular acrodermatitis of childhood and other papulo-vesicular acro-located syndromes. *Br J Dermatol* 100:49-59, 1979.

81. Claudy AL, Ortonne JP, Trepo C, et al: Papular acrodermatitis associated with hepatitis B virus infection. *Arch Dermatol* 115:931, 1979.

82. Colombo M, Rumi MG, Sagnelli E, et al: Acute hepatitis B in children with papular acrodermatitis. *Pediatr Pathol* 6:249-257, 1986.

83. Kanzaki S, Kanda S, Terada K, et al: Detection of hepatitis B surface antigen subtype adr in an epidemic of papular acrodermatitis of childhood (Gianotti's disease). *Acta Med Okayama* 35:407-410, 1981.

84. Hofmann B, Schuppe HC, Adams O, et al: Gianotti-Crosti syndrome associated with Epstein-Barr virus infection. *Pediatr Dermatol* 14:273-277, 1997.

85. Drago F, Crovato F, Rebora A: Gianotti-Crosti syndrome as a presenting sign of EBV-induced acute infectious mononucleosis. *Clin Exp Dermatol* 22:301-302, 1997.

86. Smith KJ, Skelton H: Histopathologic features seen in Gianotti-Crosti syndrome secondary to Epstein-Barr virus. *J Am Acad Dermatol* 43:1076-1079, 2000.

87. Chuh AAT: Gianotti-Crosti syndrome—The extremes in rash duration. *Int Pediatr* 17:45-48, 2002.

88. Chuh AAT: Truncal lesions do not exclude a diagnosis of Gianotti-Crosti syndrome. *Australas J Dermatol* 44:215-216, 2003.

89. James WD, Odom RB, Hatch MH: Gianotti-Crosti-like eruption associated with coxsackievirus A-16 infection. *J Am Acad Dermatol* 6:862-866, 1982.

90. Berant M, Naveh Y, Weissman I: Papular acrodermatitis with cytomegalovirus hepatitis. *Arch Dis Child* 58:1024-1025, 1983.

91. Sagi EF, Linder N, Shouval D: Papular acrodermatitis of childhood associated with hepatitis A virus infection. *Pediatr Dermatol* 3:31-33, 1985.

92. Blauvelt A, Turner ML: Gianotti-Crosti syndrome and human immunodeficiency virus infection. *Arch Dermatol* 130:481-483, 1994.

93. Carrascosa JM, Just M, Ribera M, et al: Papular acrodermatitis of childhood related to poxvirus and parvovirus B19 infection. *Cutis* 61:265-267, 1998.

94. Di Lernia V: Gianotti-Crosti syndrome related to rotavirus infection. *Pediatr Dermatol* 15:485-486, 1998.

95. Chuh AAT, Chan HHL, Chiu SSS, et al: A prospective case control study on the association of Gianotti-Crosti syndrome with human herpesvirus 6 and human herpesvirus 7 infections. *Pediatr Dermatol* 19:492-497, 2002.

96. Ricci G, Patrizi A, Neri I, et al: Gianotti-Crosti syndrome and allergic background. *Acta Derm Venereol* 83:202-205, 2003.

97. Chuh AAT: Diagnostic criteria for Gianotti-Crosti syndrome—A prospective case control study for validity assessment. *Cutis* 68:207-213, 2001.

98. Percival GH: Pityriasis rosea. *Br J Dermatol* 44:241-253, 1932.

99. Chuh AAT: Rash orientation in pityriasis rosea—A qualitative study. *Eur J Dermatol* 12:253-256, 2002.

100. Björnberg A, Hellgren L: Pityriasis rosea. A statistical, clinical and laboratory investigation of 826 patients and matched healthy controls. *Acta Derm Venereol* 42:50, 1962.

101. Klauder JV: Pityriasis rosea with particular reference to its unusual manifestations. *JAMA* 82:178-183, 1924.

102. Traore A, Korsaga-Some N, Niamba P, et al: Pityriasis rosea in secondary schools in Ouagadougou, Burkina Faso. *Ann Dermatol Venereol* 128:605-609, 2001.

103. Hyatt H: Pityriasis rosea in a three month old. *Arch Pediatr* 77:364, 1960.

104. Bari M, Cohen BA: Purpuric vesicular eruption in a 7-year-old girl. Vesicular pityriasis rosea. *Arch Dermatol* 126:1497, 1500-1501, 1990.

105. Messenger AG, Knox EG, Summerly R, et al: Case clustering in pityriasis rosea: support for role of an infective agent. *Br Med J (Clin Res Ed)* 284:371-373, 1982.
106. Chuh A, Lee A, Molinari N: Case clustering in pityriasis rosea—A multi-center epidemiological study in primary care settings in Hong Kong. *Arch Dermatol* 139:489-493, 2003.
107. Chuang TY, Perry HO, Ilstrup DM, et al: Recent upper respiratory tract infection and pityriasis rosea: A case-control study of 249 matched pairs. *Br J Dermatol* 108:587-591, 1983.
108. McPherson A, McPherson K, Ryan T: Is pityriasis rosea an infectious disease? *Lancet* 2:1077, 1980.
109. Drago F, Ranieri E, Malaguti F, et al: Human herpesvirus 7 in pityriasis rosea. *Lancet* 349:1367-1368, 1997.
110. Drago F, Ranieri E, Malaguti F, et al: Human herpesvirus 7 in patients with pityriasis rosea. Electron microscopy investigations and polymerase chain reaction in mononuclear cells, plasma and skin. *Dermatology* 195:374-378, 1997.
111. Watanabe T, Sugaya M, Nakamura K, et al: Human herpesvirus 7 and pityriasis rosea. *J Invest Dermatol* 113:288-289, 1999.
112. Drago F, Malaguti F, Ranieri E, et al: Human herpes virus-like particles in pityriasis rosea lesions: an electron microscopy study. *J Cutan Pathol* 29:359-361, 2002.
113. Watanabe T, Kawamura T, Jacob SE, et al: Pityriasis rosea is associated with systemic active infection with both human herpesvirus-7 and human herpesvirus-6. *J Invest Dermatol* 119:793-797, 2002.
114. Kempf W, Adams V, Kleinhans M, et al: Pityriasis rosea is not associated with human herpesvirus 7. *Arch Dermatol* 135:1070-1072, 1999.
115. Yoshida M: Detection of human herpesvirus 7 in patients with pityriasis rosea and healthy individuals. *Dermatology* 199:197, 1999.
116. Yasukawa M, Sada E, Machino H, et al: Reactivation of human herpesvirus 6 in pityriasis rosea. *Br J Dermatol* 140:169-170, 1999.
117. Kosuge H, Tanaka-Taya K, Miyoshi H, et al: Epidemiological study of human herpesvirus-6 and human herpesvirus-7 in pityriasis rosea. *Br J Dermatol* 143:795-798, 2000.
118. Offidani A, Pritelli E, Simonetti O, et al: Pityriasis rosea associated with herpesvirus 7 DNA. (correspondence) *J Eur Acad Dermatol Venereol* 14:313-314, 2000.
119. Wong WR, Tsai CY, Shih SR, et al: Association of pityriasis rosea with human herpesvirus-6 and human herpesvirus-7 in Taipei. *J Formos Med Assoc* 100:478-483, 2001.
120. Chuh AAT, Chiu SSS, Peiris JSM: Human herpesvirus 6 and 7 DNA in peripheral blood leukocytes and plasma in patients with pityriasis rosea by polymerase chain reaction—A prospective case control study. *Acta Derm Venereol* 81:289-290, 2001.
121. Karabulut AA, Kocak M, Yilmaz N, et al: Detection of human herpesvirus 7 in pityriasis rosea by nested PCR. *Int J Dermatol* 41:563-567, 2002.
122. Chuh AAT: The association of pityriasis rosea with cytomegalovirus, Epstein-Barr virus and parvovirus B19 infections—A prospective case control study by polymerase chain reaction and serology. *Eur J Dermatol* 13:25-28, 2003.
123. Aractingi S, Morinet F, Mokni M, et al: Absence of picornavirus genome in pityriasis rosea. *Arch Dermatol Res* 289:60-61, 1996.
124. Hudson LD, Adelman S, Lewis CW: Pityriasis rosea. Viral complement fixation studies. *J Am Acad Dermatol* 4:544-546, 1981.
125. Chuh AAT, Chan HHL: Prospective case-control study of chlamydia, legionella and mycoplasma infections in patients with pityriasis rosea. *Eur J Dermatol* 12:170-173, 2002.
126. Chuh AAT: Diagnostic criteria for pityriasis rosea—A prospective case control study for assessment of validity. *J Eur Acad Dermatol Venereol* 17:101-103, 2003.
127. Arndt KA, Paul BS, Stern RS, et al: Treatment of pityriasis rosea with UV radiation. *Arch Dermatol* 119:381-382, 1983.

128. Leenutaphong V, Jiamton S: UVB phototherapy for pityriasis rosea: a bilateral comparison study. *J Am Acad Dermatol* 33:996-999, 1995.

129. Tay YK, Goh CL: One-year review of pityriasis rosea at the National Skin Centre, Singapore. *Ann Acad Med Singapore* 28:829-831, 1999.

130. Leonforte JF: Pityriasis rosea: Exacerbation with corticosteroid treatment. *Dermatologica* 163:480-481, 1981.

131. Sharma PK, Yadav TP, Gautam RK, et al: Erythromycin in pityriasis rosea: A double-blind, placebo-controlled clinical trial. *J Am Acad Dermatol* 42:241-244, 2000.

132. Castanedo-Cazares JP, Lepe V, Moncada B: Should we still use phototherapy for Pityriasis rosea? *Photodermatol Photoimmunol Photomed* 19:160-161, 2003.

133. Zhang Y, Schols D, De Clercq E: Selective activity of various antiviral compounds against HHV-7 infection. *Antiviral Res* 43:23-35, 1999.

134. Harms M, Feldmann R, Saurat JH: Papular-purpuric "gloves and socks" syndrome. *J Am Acad Dermatol* 23:850-854, 1990.

135. Harel L, Straussberg I, Zeharia A, et al: Papular purpuric rash due to parvovirus B19 with distribution on the distal extremities and the face. *Clin Infect Dis* 35:1558-1561, 2002.

136. Grilli R, Izquierdo MJ, Farina MC, et al: Papular-purpuric "gloves and socks" syndrome: polymerase chain reaction demonstration of parvovirus B19 DNA in cutaneous lesions and sera. *J Am Acad Dermatol* 41:793-796, 1999.

137. Passoni LF, Ribeiro SR, Giordani ML, et al: Papular-purpuric "gloves and socks" syndrome due to parvovirus B19: report of a case with unusual features. *Rev Inst Med Trop Sao Paulo* 43:167-170, 2001.

138. Higashi N, Fukai K, Tsuruta D, et al: Papular-purpuric gloves-and-socks syndrome with bloody bullae. *J Dermatol* 29:371-375, 2002.

139. Sklavounou-Andrikopoulou A, Iakovou M, Paikos S, et al: Oral manifestations of papular-purpuric 'gloves and socks' syndrome due to parvovirus B19 infection: the first case presented in Greece and review of the literature. *Oral Dis* 10:118-122, 2004.

140. Vargas-Diez E, Buezo GF, Aragues M, et al: Papular-purpuric gloves-and-socks syndrome. *Int J Dermatol* 35:626-632.

141. Aractingi S, Bakhos D, Flageul B, et al: Immunohistochemical and virological study of skin in the papular-purpuric gloves and socks syndrome. *Br J Dermatol* 135:599-602, 1996.

142. Labbe L, Mortureux P, Leaute-Labreze C, et al: Cutaneous parvovirus infections: "gloves and socks" syndrome. *Ann Dermatol Venereol* 121:553-556, 1994.

143. Feldmann R, Harms M, Saurat JH: Papular-purpuric "gloves and socks" syndrome: not only parvovirus B19. *Dermatology* 188:85-87, 1994.

144. Smith PT, Landry ML, Carey H, et al: Papular-purpuric gloves and socks syndrome associated with acute parvovirus B19 infection: Case report and review. *Clin Infect Dis* 27:164-168, 1998.

145. Alfadley A, Aljubran A, Hainau B, et al: Papular-purpuric "gloves and socks" syndrome in a mother and daughter. *J Am Acad Dermatol* 48:941-944, 2003.

146. Sato A, Umezawa R, Kurosawa R, Kajigaya Y: [Human parvovirus B19 infection which first presented with petechial hemorrhage, followed by papular-purpuric gloves and socks syndrome and erythema infectiosum.] *Kansenshogaku Zasshi* 76:963-966, 2002.

147. Carrascosa JM, Bielsa I, Ribera M, et al: Papular-purpuric gloves-and-socks syndrome related to cytomegalovirus infection. *Dermatology* 191:269-270, 1995.

148. Perez-Ferriols A, Martinez-Aparicio A, Aliaga-Boniche A: Papular-purpuric "gloves and socks" syndrome caused by measles virus. *J Am Acad Dermatol* 30:291-292, 1994.

149. Guibal F, Buffet P, Mouly F, et al: Papular-purpuric gloves and socks syndrome with hepatitis B infection. *Lancet* 347:473, 1996.

150. Velez A, Fernandez-de-la-Puebla R, Moreno JC: Second case of papular-purpuric gloves-and-socks syndrome related to hepatitis B infection. *Br J Dermatol* 145:515-516, 2001.

151. Segui N, Zayas A, Fuertes A, et al: Papular-purpuric "Gloves-and-Socks" syndrome related to rubella virus infection. *Dermatology* 200:89, 2000.

152. Ruzicka T, Kalka K, Diercks K, et al: Papular-purpuric "gloves and socks" syndrome associated with human herpesvirus 6 infection. *Arch Dermatol* 134:242-244, 1998.

153. Ongradi J, Becker K, Horvath A, et al: Simultaneous infection by human herpesvirus 7 and human parvovirus B19 in papular-purpuric gloves-and-socks syndrome. *Arch Dermatol 136:672, 2000.*

154. Ghigliotti G, Mazzarello G, Nigro A, et al: Papular-purpuric gloves and socks syndrome in HIV-positive patients. *J Am Acad Dermatol* 43:916-917, 2000.

155. van Rooijen MM, Brand CU, Ballmer-Weber BK, et al: [Drug-induced papular-purpuric gloves and socks syndrome.] *Hautarzt* 50:280-283, 1999.

156. Bodemer C, de Prost Y: Unilateral laterothoracic exanthem in children: A new disease? *J Am Acad Dermatol* 27:693-696, 1992.

157. Taieb A, Megraud F, Legrain V, et al: Asymmetric periflexural exanthem of childhood. *J Am Acad Dermatol* 29:391-393, 1993.

158. Frieden IJ: Childhood exanthems. *Curr Opin Pediatr* 7:411-414, 1995.

159. Gutzmer R, Herbst RA, Kiehl P, et al: Unilateral laterothoracic exanthem (asymmetrical periflexural exanthem of childhood): Report of an adult patient. *J Am Acad Dermatol* 37:484-485, 1997.

160. Gelmetti C, Grimalt R, Cambiaghi S, et al: Asymmetric periflexural exanthem of childhood: Report of two new cases. *Pediatr Dermatol* 11:42-45, 1994.

161. Harangi F, Varszegi D, Szucs G: Asymmetric periflexural exanthem of childhood and viral examinations. *Pediatr Dermatol* 12:112-115, 1995.

162. McCuaig CC, Russo P, Powell J, et al: Unilateral laterothoracic exanthem. A clinicopathologic study of forty-eight patients. *J Am Acad Dermatol* 34:979-984, 1996.

163. Corazza M, Virgili A: Asymmetric periflexural exanthem in an adult. *Acta Derm Venereol* 77:79-80, 1997.

164. Bauza A, Redondo P, Fernandez J: Asymmetric periflexural exanthem in adults. *Br J Dermatol* 143:224-226, 2000.

165. Chan PKS, To KF, Zawar V, et al: Asymmetric periflexural exanthem in an adult. *Clin Exp Dermatol* 29:320-321, 2004.

166. Coustou D, Leaute-Labreze C, Bioulac-Sage P, et al: Asymmetric periflexural exanthem of childhood: A clinical, pathologic, and epidemiologic prospective study. *Arch Dermatol* 135:799-803, 1999.

167. Coustou D, Masquelier B, Lafon ME, et al: Asymmetric periflexural exanthem of childhood: microbiologic case-control study. *Pediatr Dermatol* 17:169-173, 2000.

168. Pauluzzi P, Festini G, Gelmetti C: Asymmetric periflexural exanthem of childhood in an adult patient with parvovirus B19. *J Eur Acad Dermatol Venereol* 15:372-374, 2001.

169. Cherry JD, Bobinski JE, Horvath FL, et al: Acute hemangioma-like lesions associated with ECHO viral infections. *Pediatrics* 44:498-502, 1969.

170. Guillot B, Dandurand M: Eruptive pseudoangiomatosis arising in adulthood: 9 cases. *Eur J Dermatol* 10:455-458, 2000.

171. Angelo C, Provini A, Ferranti G, et al: Eruptive pseudoangiomatosis. *Pediatr Dermatol* 19:243-245, 2002.

172. Larralde M, Ballona R, Correa N, et al: Eruptive pseudoangiomatosis. *Pediatr Dermatol* 19:76-77, 2002.

173. Navarro V, Molina I, Montesinos E, et al: Eruptive pseudoangiomatosis in an adult. *Int J Dermatol* 39:237-238, 2000.

174. Mazereeuw-Hautier J, Cambon L, Bonafe JL: [Eruptive pseudoangiomatosis in an adult renal transplant recipient.] *Ann Dermatol Venereol* 128:55-56, 2001.

175. Stoebner PE, Templier I, Ligeron C, et al: Familial eruptive pseudoangiomatosis. *Dermatology* 205:306-307, 2002.

176. Prose NS, Tope W, Miller SE, et al: Eruptive pseudoangiomatosis: A unique child-hood exanthem? *J Am Acad Dermatol* 29:857-859, 1993.
177. Calza AM, Saurat JH: Eruptive pseudoangiomatosis: A unique childhood exan-them? *J Am Acad Dermatol* 31:517-518, 1994.
178. Neri I, Patrizi A, Guerrini V, et al: Eruptive pseudoangiomatosis. *Br J Dermatol* 143:435-438, 2000.

Statistics of Interest to the Dermatologist

MARTIN A. WEINSTOCK, MD, PHD, AND MARGARET M. BOYLE, BS
Brown University Dermatoepidemiology Unit, Providence, Rhode Island

Morbidity and Mortality

Health Care Delivery in the United States

Miscellaneous

TABLE 1.—New Cases of Selected Reportable Infectious Diseases in the United States

	1940	1950	1960	1970	1980	1990	2000	2004*
AIDS	—	—	—	—	—	41,595	40,758	39,097†
Anthrax	76	49	23	2	1	0	1	—
Congenital Rubella	—	—	—	77	50	11	9	—
Congenital Syphilis	—	—	—	—	—	3865	529	312
Diphtheria	15,536	5796	918	435	3	—	1	—
Gonorrhea	175,841	286,746	258,933	600,072	1,004,029	690,169	358,995	307,845
Hansen's Disease	—	44	54	129	223	198	91	82
Lyme Disease	—	—	—	—	—	—	17,730	18,523
Measles	291,162	319,124	441,703	47,351	13,506	27,786	86	37‖
Plague	1	3	2	13	18	2	6	3
Rocky Mountain Spotted Fever	457	464	204	380	1163	651	495	1514
Syphilis (primary and secondary)	—	23,939	16,145	21,982	27,204	50,223	5979	7352
Toxic Shock Syndrome	—	—	—	—	—	322	135	119
Tuberculosis‡	102,984§	121,742§	55,494	37,137	27,749	25,701	16,377	11,178
US population (millions)	132	151	179	203	227	249	281	294

Note: Dash indicates that data not available.
*For 52 weeks ending January 1, 2005.
†Last update November 28, 2004.
‡Reporting criteria changed in 1975.
§Data include newly reported active and inactive cases.
‖Of 37 cases reported, 14 were indigenous, and 23 were imported from another country.
(Data from Centers for Disease Control and Prevention: Summary of Notifiable Diseases, United States, 2004. Morb Mortal Wkly Rep 53[51&52]:1213-1220, 2005; Centers for Disease Control and Prevention: Summary of Notifiable Diseases, United States, 2000. Morb Mortal Wkly Rep 49[51&52]:1167-1174, 2001; Centers for Disease Control and Prevention: Annual Summary 1994: Reported morbidity and mortality. Morb Mortal Wkly Rep 43[53]:70-71, 1994; Centers for Disease Control and Prevention: Annual Summary 1984: Reported morbidity and mortality. Morb Mortal Wkly Rep 33:124-129, 1986.)

TABLE 2.—Estimates of HIV/AIDS, 2004

REGION	Adults and Children Living With HIV/AIDS	Adults and Children Newly Affected With HIV	Adult Prevalence (%)*	Adult and Child Deaths Due to HIV/AIDS
Sub-Saharan Africa	23.4-28.4 million	2.7-3.8 million	6.9-8.3	2.1-2.6 million
North Africa and Middle East	230,000-1.5 million	34,000-350,000	0.1-0.7	12,000-72,000
South and Southeast Asia	4.4-10.6 million	480,000-2.0 million	0.4-0.9	300,000-750,000
East Asia	560,000-1.8 million	84,000-830,000	0.1-0.2	25,000-86,000
Oceania	25,000-48,000	2,100-13,000	0.1-0.3	<1,700
Latin America	1.3-2.2 million	170,000-430,000	0.5-0.8	73,000-120,000
Caribbean	270,000-780,000	27,000-140,000	1.5-4.1	24,000-61,000
Eastern Europe and Central Asia	920,000-2.1 million	110,000-480,000	0.5-1.2	39,000-87,000
Western and Central Europe	480,000-760,000	14,000-38,000	0.2-0.3	<8,500
North America	540,000-1.6 million	16,000-120,000	0.3-1.0	8,400-25,000
Total	39.4 million (35.9-44.3 million)	4.9 million (4.3-6.4 million)	1.10% (1.0-1.3%)	3.1 million (2.8-3.5 million)

*The proportion of adults (15-49 years of age) living with HIV/AIDS in 2004, using 2004 population numbers.
(Data from AIDS Epidemic Update, Joint United Nations Programme on HIV/AIDS [UNAIDS] World Health Organization [WHO], December, 2004.)

TABLE 3.—AIDS Cases by Age Group and Exposure Category, and Cumulative Totals Through 2003, United States

	2003		Cumulative Total*	
	No.	(%)	No.	(%)
Adult/adolescent exposure category				
Male-to-male sexual contact	15,859	(35%)	401,392	(45%)
Injecting drug use	7128	(16%)	218,196	(24%)
Male-to-male sexual contact And injection drug use	1685	(4%)	57,998	(6%)
Hemophilia/coagulation disorder	85	(0%)	5448	(1%)
Heterosexual contact	8605	(19%)	111,147	(12%)
Receipt of blood transfusion, blood components, or tissue†	219	(0%)	9295	(1%)
Other/risk factor not reported or identified	11,220	(25%)	89,399	(10%)
Adult/adolescent SUBTOTAL	44,811	(100%)	892,875	(100%)
Pediatric (<13 years old) exposure category				
Hemophilia/coagulation disorder	0	(0%)	234	(3%)
Mother with/at risk for HIV infection	131	(86%)	8549	(91%)
Receipt of blood transfusion, blood components, or tissue†	2	(1%)	387	(4%)
Other/risk not reported or identified	19	(13%)	178	(2%)
Pediatric SUBTOTAL	152	(100%)	9348	(100%)
TOTAL	44,963	(100%)	902,223	(100%)

Note: Total includes 1 person of unknown sex.
*Includes persons with a diagnosis of AIDS, reported from the beginning of the epidemic through 2003.
†Forty-six adults/adolescents and 3 children developed AIDS after receiving blood screened negative for HIV antibodies. Fourteen additional adults developed AIDS after receiving tissue, organs, or artificial insemination from HIV-infected donors. Four of the 14 received tissue or organs from a donor who was negative for HIV antibody at the time of donation.
(Data from Centers for Disease Control and Prevention: *HIV/AIDS Surveillance Rep* 15:32, 2003.)

TABLE 4.—Selected Causes of Death, United States, 1992 and 2002

	Number of Deaths	
Cause of Death	1992	2002
Malignant melanoma	6568	7514
* Infections of the skin	749	1283
Motor vehicle traffic accidents	39,985	44,065
Accident involving animal being ridden	109	118
Accidental drowning and submersion	3524	3447
Lightning	53	66
Homicide and legal intervention	25,488	18,022
All cancer	520,578	557,271
All causes	2,175,613	2,443,387

(Data from National Center for Health Statistics, Division of Vital Statistics, personal communication, March 2004.)

TABLE 5.—Annual Change in Cancer Incidence in the United States

	Average Annual Percent Change	
	1992-2002	1973-1990
Thyroid	+4.3	+0.8
Liver and intrahepatic bile duct	+3.3	+2.3
Melanoma of the skin	+2.4	+4.1
Kidney and renal pelvis	+1.5	+2.2
Testis	+1.1	+2.6
Breast (female)	+0.4	+1.9
Non-Hodgkin lymphoma	+0.1	+3.6
Esophagus	+0.0	+0.8
Urinary bladder	−0.2	+0.7
Lung and bronchus (female)	−0.2	+4.6
Corpus and uterus, NOS	−0.2	−2.1
Pancreas	−0.3	−0.2
Hodgkin lymphoma	−0.3	−0.1
Myeloma	−0.5	+1.1
Brain and ONS	−0.6	+1.5
Colon rectum	−0.8	+0.2
Leukemia	−0.9	+0.1
Ovary	−0.9	+0.5
Oral cavity and pharynx	−1.5	−0.4
Stomach	−1.5	−1.6
Prostate	−2.0	+3.6
Lung and bronchus (male)	−2.2	+0.6
Cervix uteri	−2.8	−2.7
Larynx	−3.0	0.0
All sites	−0.6	+1.2

Note: SEER 13 areas and NCHS public use data file for the total US. Rates are per 100,000 and age-adjusted to the 2000 US standard million population.

(Data from Ries LAG, Eisner MP, Kosary CL, et al (eds): *Seer Cancer Statistics Review: 1975-2002*, National Cancer Institute, Bethesda, Md, 2005; Surveillance, Epidemiology, and End Results (SEER) Program SEER Stat Database: Incidence—SEER 9 Regs, November 2002 Sub (1973-2000), National Cancer Institute, DCCPS, Surveillance Research Program, Cancer Statistics Branch, released April 2003 based on the November 2002 submission.)

TABLE 6.—Melanoma Incidence and Mortality Rates, United States

Year	Incidence*	Mortality†
1975	7.9	2.1
1976	8.1	2.2
1977	8.9	2.3
1978	8.9	2.3
1979	9.5	2.4
1980	10.5	2.3
1981	11.1	2.4
1982	11.2	2.5
1983	11.1	2.5
1984	11.4	2.5
1985	12.7	2.6
1986	13.3	2.6
1987	13.6	2.6
1988	12.8	2.6
1989	13.7	2.7
1990	13.8	2.8
1991	14.6	2.7
1992	14.7	2.7
1993	14.5	2.7
1994	15.6	2.7
1995	16.3	2.7
1996	17.1	2.8
1997	17.5	2.7
1998	17.7	2.8
1999	17.6	2.6
2000	17.7	2.7
2001	19.3	2.7
2002	18.3	2.6

2005 estimate: 59,580 newly diagnosed cases and 7770 deaths

*Surveillance, Epidemiology and End-Results (SEER) Program, (9 registries of the National Cancer Institute).

†National Center for Health Statistics, United States population. Rates per 100,000 per year, and age-adjusted to the 2000 US standard million population. All races.

(Data from American Cancer Society, Inc. Surveillance Research. *Cancer Facts & Figures 2005* 4:2005; Ries LAG, Eisner MP, Kosary CL, et al [eds]: *SEER Cancer Statistics Review: 1975-2002.* National Cancer Institute, Bethesda, Md, 2005.)

TABLE 7.—Melanoma Five-Year Relative Survival

Year	Whites (%)	Blacks (%)
	Year at Diagnosis	
1960-1963	60	—
1970-1973	68	—
1974-1976	81	67
1977-1979	83	50
1980-1982	83	56
1983-1985	85	74
1986-1988	88	67
1989-1991	89	78
1992-1994	89	59
1995-2001	92	78
	Stage at Diagnosis (1995-2001)	
Local	98	93
Regional	64	37
Distant	16	—

Notes: Dash indicates insufficient data. Relative survival is the observed survival divided by the survival expected in a demographically similar subgroup of the general population. Survival estimates among blacks are imprecise due to small numbers of cases observed.

(Data from Ries LAG, Eisner MP, Kosary CL, et al [eds]: *SEER Cancer Statistics Review: 1975-2002*. National Cancer Institute, Bethesda, Md, 2005.)

TABLE 8.—Contact Dermatitis in Belgium: Proportion of Positive Patch Tests to Standard Chemicals in 317 Patients With at Least 1 Positive Reaction (Among 551 Patients Tested in 2004)

Chemical	(%)
Nickel sulphate	36.3
Cobalt chloride	16.7
Fragrance mix	15.8
Balsam of Peru	13.2
Potassium dichromate	11.0
Paraphenylenediamine	10.4
Colophonium	8.9
Formaldehyde	6.0
Wool alcohols	6.0
Thiuram mix	5.4
Paratertiarybutylphenol-formaldehyde resin	5.0
Methyl (chloro) isothiazolinone	4.1
Budesonide	3.2
Neomycin sulphate	2.8
Mercapto mix	2.2
Quaternium-15	2.2
Paraben mix	1.9
Benzocaine	1.6
Epoxy resin	1.6
Primin	1.6
Tixocortol pivalate	1.6
Mercaptobenzothiazole	1.3
Isopropyl-phenylparaphenylenediamine	0.9
Sesquiterpene lactone mix	0.3
Clioquinol	0.0

(Data from Goossens A, University Hospital, Katholieke Universiteit Leuven, Belgium, personal communication, January 2005.)

TABLE 9.—Dermatology Trainees in the United States

Year Residency to Be Completed	Male Residents	Female Residents	Unknown	Total
MD Programs				
2005	143	198	0	341
2006	140	212	1	353
2007	137	214	1	352
DO Programs				
2005	10	12	2	24
2006	7	10	4	21
2007	14	10	5	29

(Data from American Academy of Dermatology, personal communication, January 2005.)

TABLE 10.—Diplomates Certified by The American Board of Dermatology From 1933 to 2004

Decade Totals (Inclusive Dates)	Average Number Certified per Year
1933-1940	69
1941-1950	74
1951-1960	76
1961-1970	112
1971-1980	247
1981-1990	271
1991-2000	295
2001-2004	312
Individual Year Totals	Actual Number Certified
1999	286
2000	283
2001	305
2002	309
2003	307
2004	329
TOTAL 1933 through 2004	12,557

(Data from The American Board of Dermatology, Inc, personal communication, January 2005.)

TABLE 11.—Physicians Certified in Dermatologic Subspecialties

Physicians Certified for Special Qualification in Dermatopathology, 1974-2004

Year	Dermatologists	Pathologists Average Number Certified	Total
1974-1975	108	44	302
1976-1980	54	49	515
1981-1985	37	34	351
1986-1990	11	14	125
1991-1995	20	20	196
1996-2000	14	32	227
		Actual Number Certified	
2001	10	34	44
2002	14	55	69
2003	14	48	62
2004	16	45	61
TOTAL Certified 1974-2004	947	1008	1955

Dermatologists Certified for Special Qualification in
Clinical and Laboratory Dermatological Immunology, 1985-2004

Year	Number Certified
1985	52
1987	16
1989	22
1991	15
1993	5
1997	5
2001	6
TOTAL 1985-2004	121

Dermatologists Certified for Special Qualification in
Pediatric Dermatology, 2004

2004	90

Notes: No special qualification examination for Dermatopathology was administered in 1992, 1994, and 1996. No special qualification examination in Clinical and Laboratory Dermatological Immunology was administered in 1986, 1988, 1990, 1992, 1994, 1995, 1996, 1998, 1999, 2000, 2002, 2003 or 2004. Special qualification in Pediatric Dermatology began in 2004.
(Data from American Board of Dermatology and American Board of Pathology, personal communication, January 2005.)

TABLE 12.—Visits to Non-Federal Office-Based Physicians in the United States, 2002 (Estimates in Thousands)

		Type of Physician			
Diagnosis	Dermatologist		Other		All Physicians
Acne vulgaris	4248	(13.2%)	997	(0.1%)	5245	(0.6%)
Eczematous dermatitis	2353	(7.3%)	5567	(0.7%)	7921	(0.9%)
Warts	1465	(4.5%)	1576	(0.2%)	3040	(0.3%)
Skin cancer	3138	(9.7%)	1093	(0.1%)	4231	(0.5%)
Psoriasis	†1382	†(4.3%)	*	*	†1574	†(0.2%)
Fungal infections	*	*	1733	(0.2%)	2130	(0.2%)
Hair disorders	*	*	*	*	1301	(0.2%)
Actinic keratosis	3420	(10.6%)	*	*	3876	(0.4%)
Benign neoplasm of the skin	3165	(9.8%)	1442	(0.2%)	4606	(0.5%)
All disorders	37,227	(100%)	857,753	(100%)	889,980	(100%)

Note: Percentage of visits for all disorders is in parentheses.
*Figure suppressed due to small sample size.
†Standard error >30% of estimate.
(Data from National Ambulatory Medical Care Survey 2002, National Center for Health Statistics, Centers for Disease Control and Prevention. Personal communication, January 2005.)

TABLE 13.—Health Insurance Coverage of the United States Population, 2003

	Children 1-17 Years (%)	Adults Aged 18-64 Years (%)	Adults Aged 65 Years and Over (%)
Individually purchased insurance	8	7	26
Employer-provided private insurance	58	63	36
Public insurance, any type	29	17	97
Medicaid/State Children's Health Insurance Program	26	13	9
No health insurance	11	18	1

Note: Some individuals have both public and private insurance, so the numbers will not add to 100%.
(Data from the Employee Benefit Research Institute, estimates from the *March Current Population Survey, 1995-2004 supplements.* Washington, DC, personal communication, January 2005.)

TABLE 14.—Nonelderly Population With Selected Sources of Health Insurance, by Family Income, 2003

Yearly Family Income Level	Employment-Based Coverage %	Individually Purchased %	Public %	Uninsured %	Total %
under $5000	12	11	39	41	100
$5000-$9999	12	9	56	27	100
$10,000-$14,999	18	10	40	37	100
$15,000-$19,999	30	9	33	33	100
$20,000-$29,999	44	8	25	29	100
$30,000-$39,999	60	7	17	21	100
$40,000-$49,999	71	6	13	15	100
$50,000 and over	83	5	7	9	100
TOTAL	63	7	17	18	100

Note: Details may not add to totals because individuals may receive coverage from more than one source.
(Data from Fronstin P, "Sources of Coverage and Characteristics of the Uninsured: Analysis of the March 2004 Current Population Survey." *EBRI Issue Brief*, No. 276 [Washington, DC, Employee Benefit Research Institute], December 2004.)

TABLE 15.—Health Maintenance Organization (HMO) Market Penetration in the United States, January 1, 2004

HMO Penetration in Region

Northeast	34%
Mid-Atlantic	30%
South Atlantic	20%
East South Central	12%
West South Central	12%
East North Central	22%
West North Central	23%
Mountain	25%
Pacific	42%

HMO Penetration Top Ten Most Highly Penetrated Metropolitan Statistical Areas

Vallejo-Fairfield, California	64%
Oakland-Fremont-Hayward, California	63%
Sacramento—Arden-Arcade—Roseville, California	62%
Buffalo-Checktowaga-Tonawanda, New York	56%
Los Angeles-Long Beach-Glendale, California	55%
Stockton, California	54%
Rochester, New York	54%
San Jose-Sunnyvale-Santa Clara, California	54%
Madison, Wisconsin	52%
San Diego-Carlsbad-San Marcos, California	52%

(Data from The InterStudy Competitive Edge: *Managed Care Regional Market Analysis Fall 2004* [January 1, 2004], Interstudy Publications, St Paul, Minnesota, personal communication, January 2005.)

TABLE 16.—National Health Expenditure Amounts: Selected Calendar Years

Spending Category	Billions of Dollars (%)				
	1980	1990	2000	2004*	2005*
Total national health expenditures	246	696	1310	1805	1937
Health services and supplies	234	670	1262	1736	1863
Personal health care	215	609	1138	1549	1664
Hospital care	102	254	417	552	589
Professional services	67	217	425	581	624
Physician and clinical services	47	158	289	397	426
Other professional services	4	18	39	52	56
Dental services	13	32	61	79	84
Other personal health care	3	10	37	53	58
Nursing home and home health	20	65	126	161	171
Home health care	2	13	32	45	50
Nursing home care	18	53	94	115	121
Retail outlet sale of medical products	26	73	171	255	281
Prescription drugs	12	40	122	201	224
Other medical products	14	33	49	55	57
Durable medical equipment	4	11	18	21	22
Other non-durable medical products	10	23	31	34	35
Government administration and net cost					
of private health insurance	12	40	81	128	135
Government public health activities	7	20	44	58	64
Investment	12	26	48	69	74
Research†	6	13	29	43	46
Construction	7	14	19	26	28

Note: Numbers may not add to totals because of rounding.
*Projected values. The health spending projections were based on the 2003 version of the National Health Expenditures (NHE) released in January 2005.
†Research and development expenditures of drug companies and other manufacturers and providers of medical equipment and supplies are excluded from research expenditures but are included in the expenditure class in which the product falls, in that they are covered by the payment received for that product.
(Data from Medicare and Medicaid Services, Office of the Actuary, January 2005.)

TABLE 17.—Results of the American Academy of Dermatology Skin Cancer Screening Program, 1985-2004

Year	Number Screened	Suspected Diagnosis		
		Basal Cell Carcinoma	Squamous Cell Carcinoma	Malignant Melanoma
1985	32,000	1056	163	97
1986	41,486	3049	398	262
1987	41,649	2798	302	257
1988	67,124	4457	474	435
1989	78,486	6266	761	593
1990	98,060	7959	1069	872
1991	102,485	8110	1193	1062
1992	98,440	8403	1280	1054
1993	97,553	7067	1068	2465*
1994	86,895	6908	1235	1010
1995	88,934	7503	1317	1353
1996	94,363	8713	1656	1399
1997	99,554	8730	1685	1469
1998	89,536	6687	1308	1078
1999	89,916	5790	1136	635
2000	65,854	5074	1053	653
2001	70,562	5192	1102	642
2002	64,492	4733	1009	692
2003	70,692	4481	1032	489
2004	71,243	4891	1165	760
TOTAL	1,549,324	117,867	20,406	17,277

*Number of cases included melanoma, "rule out melanoma," and lentigo maligna.
(Data from American Academy of Dermatology: *2004 Skin Cancer Screening Program Statistical Summary Report*, March 2005.)

TABLE 18.—Leading Dermatology Journals

Journal	Total Citations in 2003	Number of Articles Published in 2003
Journal of Investigative Dermatology	17,318	345
Journal of the American Academy of Dermatology	14,057	468
British Journal of Dermatology	12,273	363
Archives of Dermatology	11,248	192
Dermatology	3760	168
Contact Dermatitis	3489	79
Acta Dermato-Venereologica	3283	72
International Journal of Dermatology	2839	213
Dermatologic Surgery	2362	171
Archives of Dermatological Research	2186	72
Clinical and Experimental Dermatology	2054	179
Burns	1742	141
American Journal of Dermatopathology	1674	75
Journal of Cutaneous Pathology	1652	101
Cutis	1602	123
Melanoma Research	1408	74
Dermatologic Clinics	1332	66
Mycoses	1325	100
Annals de Dermatologie et de Venereologie	1306	151
Pediatric Dermatology	1303	108
Journal of Dermatology	1281	133
Journal of Dermatological Science	1123	73
Hautarzt	1076	137
Experimental Dermatology	1004	118
European Journal of Dermatology	1000	136

(Data from *Journal Citation Reports on CD-ROM:JCR*, Science ed. Philadelphia, Institute for Scientific Information, 2005.)

CLINICAL DERMATOLOGY

1 Urticarial and Eczematous Disorders

The Etiology of Different Forms of Urticaria in Childhood
Sackesen C, Sekerel BE, Orhan F, et al (Hacettepe Univ, Ankara, Turkey)
Pediatr Dermatol 21:102-108, 2004   1–1

Introduction.—Most cases of urticaria in children appear to be caused by infections rather than allergies. In a prospective study, 54 children with urticaria underwent extensive investigations to determine potential causes of the disorder.

Methods.—Of all the patients (23 girls, 31 boys; age range, 1-19 years), 37 (68%) were classified as having acute urticaria and had symptoms for less than 6 weeks. In 35% of these cases, the episode was recurrent after a symptom-free period of more than 5 weeks. The 17 patients with chronic urticaria had experienced symptoms for more than 6 weeks. Known causes

TABLE 2.—Infectious Symptoms and Documented Infectious Causes in the Different Groups

	Acute Urticaria		Chronic Urticaria
	Single-Episode	Recurrent	
Number	24	13	17
Symptoms suggesting infection	8 (33%)	6 (46%)	5 (29%)
Fever >38.5°C	7	3	3
Sore throat	2	4	2
Dysuria	1	1	—
Positive throat culture	2 (8%)	1 (8%)	—
Positive urine culture	6 (25%)	—	1 (6%)
Positive EBV (nuclear antigen) IgM	1 (4%)	—	1 (6%)
Positive CMV IgM	—	1 (8%)	—
Positive *M. pneumonia* IgM	1 (4%)	—	—
Positive *C. pneumoniae* IgM	3 (12.5%)	1 (8%)	1 (6%)
Positive *H. pylori* IgG	1 (4%)	—	3 (17.6%)
Positive herpes simplex type I IgM	—	1 (8%)	—
Total number of patients with a probable infection	14/24 (58%)	4/13 (31%)	6/17 (35%)

Abbreviations: EBV, Epstein-Barr virus; *CMV*, cytomegalovirus.
(Courtesy of Sackesen C, Sekerel BE, Orhan F, et al: The etiology of different forms of urticaria in childhood. *Pediatr Dermatol* 21(2):102-108, 2004. Reprinted by permission of Blackwell Publishing.)

TABLE 4.—The Etiologies of Physical Urticaria

	Acute Urticuria		Chronic Urticaria
	Single-Episode	Recurrent	
Number	24	13	17
Physical urticaria	6 (25%)	1 (7.6%)	9 (52.9%)
Cold	—	—	1
Pressure	—	—	1
Sun exposure	1	—	2
Cholinergic	5	1	5
Anxiety	2	1	2
Exercise	—	—	—
Hot bath	3	—	3

Note: The ice-cube test was performed on all patients describing cold-induced urticaria and was positive only in 1.

(Courtesy of Sackesen C, Sekerel BE, Orhan F, et al: The etiology of different forms of urticaria in childhood. *Pediatr Dermatol* 21(2):102-108, 2004. Reprinted by permission of Blackwell Publishing.)

of urticaria were examined, and all patients and their first-degree relatives were questioned about a history of atopic disease. Also recorded were symptoms of anaphylaxis and episodes of angioedema. Patients with a suggestive history underwent skin prick testing, and all participants underwent detailed laboratory tests.

Results.—Chronic urticaria was seen more often in adolescent patients, and 70% of those in the chronic urticaria group were boys. In contrast, boys and girls were equally represented in the acute urticaria group. Angioedema was common (41%), occurring in 37.5% of patients with the acute single-episode type of urticaria, in 54% of those with recurrent urticaria, and in 41% of those with chronic disease. Infections accounted for 48% of acute cases (Table 2), whereas physical factors (Table 4) were the leading cause (53%) in chronic urticaria. Tests for autoimmune disorders, performed in patients with chronic urticaria, showed no abnormal findings.

Conclusion.—Acute urticaria has been considered more common in young individuals, whereas chronic urticaria is thought to be more typical in middle-aged women. However, in this pediatric group, chronic urticaria increased significantly in adolescence and primarily affected boys. The frequency of documented infections as a cause of urticaria suggests that management of the disorder in children should include a survey for certain infectious agents.

▶ This study of 54 children with urticaria was performed in a referral center in Ankara, Turkey. As has been shown previously in children, infections were the most common cause of acute urticaria, and physical factors were the leading cause of chronic urticaria. A urinary tract infection caused by *E coli* was the infection diagnosed most often. No symptoms were present in 5 of the 7 children with urinary tract infections. In addition to a detailed history, the management of urticaria in children should include an evaluation for an infectious cause.

S. Raimer, MD

Association Between Chronic Urticaria and Thyroid Autoimmunity: A Prospective Study Involving 99 Patients
Verneuil L, Leconte C, Ballet JJ, et al (Univ Hosp, Caen, France)
Dermatology 208:98-103, 2004   1–2

Background.—The relationship between chronic urticaria and thyroid autoimmunity is unclear. Whether chronic urticaria correlates statistically with thyroid autoimmunity was investigated.

Methods.—The prospective case–control study included 45 patients with chronic urticaria and 30 healthy volunteers. The frequencies of thyroid autoantibodies in the 2 groups were compared. In addition, the frequencies of chronic urticaria were compared in 32 patients with thyroid diseases with thyroid autoantibodies and in 22 with thyroid diseases without thyroid autoantibodies. Thyroid autoantibodies and thyroid hormones were assessed in all groups. Patients with chronic urticaria also underwent testing for antinuclear antibodies, rheumatoid factor, complement, and IgE, in addition to routine laboratory studies.

Findings.—Patients with chronic urticaria had a significantly higher frequency of thyroid autoantibodies than did healthy control subjects, at 26.7% and 3.3%, respectively. Thyroid hormone levels were within normal limits in all patients with thyroid autoantibodies. Chronic urticaria frequency did not differ significantly in patients with thyroid diseases with or without thyroid antibodies; the frequencies were 12.5% and 9.1%, respectively. The rest of the examinations identified only 1 patient with a connective tissue disorder.

Conclusions.—Chronic urticaria is significantly associated with thyroid autoimmunity. Tests that detect thyroid autoantibodies are relevant in patients with chronic urticaria, but extensive laboratory investigations are not necessary.

▶ The significant association between chronic urticaria and thyroid autoimmunity suggests the importance of determination of thyroid autoantibodies in patients with recurrent hives. Significantly, all patients with thyroid autoantibodies in this study had normal thyroid hormone levels.

B. H. Thiers, MD

Hereditary Angioedema Type III, Angioedema Associated With Angiotensin II Receptor Antagonists, and Female Sex
Bork K, Dewald G (Johannes-Gutenberg Univ, Mainz, Germany)
Am J Med 116:644-645, 2004   1–3

Introduction.—A new type of hereditary angioedema, type III, differs from types I and II in its lack of an association with C-1 inhibitor deficiency. A number of drugs, including angiotensin II type 1 receptor antagonists, can cause angioedema as a side effect. The cases of 2 patients who had pre-existing hereditary angioedema type III, symptoms of which were severely exacerbated by treatment with angiotensin II type 1 receptor antagonists, were reported.

Case 1.—Woman, 65, was 1 of 7 women in her family with recurrent angioedema and normal C1-inhibitor and C4. She had experienced episodes of abdominal pain between the ages of 30 and 32 and of facial swelling at the ages of 57 and 61. Six months after starting treatment with losartan, facial swelling occurred again with greater frequency. No further symptoms were noted in the 18-month period after losartan was discontinued.

Case 2.—Woman, 70, was unrelated to patient in Case 1 but had female relatives with recurrent angioedema and normal C1-inhibitor and C4. Episodes of swelling of the tongue and face began occurring at the age of 29. When valsartan (80 mg daily) was started for hypertension at age 69, the angioedema attacks increased in frequency and severity. No further swelling episodes occurred after the drug was discontinued.

Discussion.—These cases suggest that patients with hereditary angioedema type III are at risk for severe exacerbations when treated with angiotensin II receptor antagonists. The 2 conditions may share a pathogenic pathway. Hereditary angioedema type III has been observed only in women, but male carriers may be identified by reactions to angiotensin II receptor antagonists.

▶ Unlike types I and II, type III hereditary angioedema is not associated with deficiency of the C1-inhibitor. Bork and Dewald describe 2 unrelated patients with the type III variant who experienced a severe exacerbation of symptoms associated with administration of angiotensin II type 1 receptor antagonists. They suggest that individuals with this unique reaction to this class of drugs may be carriers of the hereditary angioedema type III mutation, with the genetic predisposition unmasked when these drugs are prescribed. Interestingly, hereditary angioedema type III has thus far been only observed in women, but pedigree analysis suggests that there must be male carriers of the trait.

B. H. Thiers, MD

The Addition of Zafirlukast to Cetirizine Improves the Treatment of Chronic Urticaria in Patients With Positive Autologous Serum Skin Test Results

Bagenstose SE, Levin L, Bernstein JA (Univ of Cincinnati, Ohio)
J Allergy Clin Immunol 113:134-140, 2004   1–4

Introduction.—Studies in both animals and humans suggest that leukotriene antagonists may be beneficial in the treatment of chronic urticaria, but results have not been consistent. A double-blind placebo-controlled trial sought to determine whether leukotriene-modifying agents have a role in the treatment of chronic urticaria.

Methods.—Patients recruited from 7 centers were required to have a history of a suboptimal response to H_1 antagonists. Autologous serum skin tests were performed in all patients. Randomization was to the second generation H_1 antagonist cetirizine (10 mg at bedtime) and the leukotriene D_4 (LTD_4)-receptor antagonist zafirlukast (20 mg twice a day) or to cetirizine and zafirlukast placebo. Both the physician and patient rated hives during the 3-week treatment period with a 10-cm visual analogue scale and an 11-point treatment effectiveness score.

Results.—The combination therapy with zafirlukast yielded a small but significantly greater improvement than cetirizine monotherapy when physician and patient visual analogue scale ratings were compared. Improvement was significantly greater in patients with positive autologous serum skin test (ASST) results at baseline than in those with negative ASST results at baseline. The average physician treatment efffectiveness scores also showed significant improvement in ASST-positive patients compared with ASST-negative patients receiving zafirlukast.

Conclusion.—Addition of the LTD_4-receptor antagonist zafirlukast to standard therapy using the H_1 antagonist cetirizine was beneficial to patients with autoimmune (ASST positive) chronic urticaria who previously had a suboptimal response to cetirizine monotherapy. Zafirlukast had no significant effects in patients with ASST-negative results. Potential responders to zafirlukast might be identified through ASST screening.

▶ Bagenstose et al report that the leukotriene receptor antagonist zafirlukast has modest efficacy as an adjunct to H_1 antagonists in patients with chronic urticaria and that this effect is noted only in patients with a positive ASST result.

B. H. Thiers, MD

How Atopic Is Atopic Dermatitis?

Flohr C, Johansson SG, Wahlgren C-F, et al (Univ of Nottingham, United Kingdom; Karolinska Univ, Solna, Sweden; Karolinska Inst Stockholm)
J Allergy Clin Immunol 114:150-158, 2004   1–5

Introduction.—Atopy has been defined as a personal and/or familial tendency to become sensitized and produce IgE antibodies. Many patients with clinical allergic disease, especially those with atopic dermatitis (AD), have very high serum total IgE levels, yet the role of IgE sensitization in AD is controversial. Articles that considered the relationship between atopy and AD were identified through a MEDLINE search and assessed for evidence of the diagnostic value of measuring IgE antibodies in AD and to determine if knowledge of IgE sensitization increases clinical diagnostic and predictive ability.

Methods.—MEDLINE was searched from its inception until September 2003. There were no restrictions on language of publication, and the online search was supplemented by an extensive hand search of the literature. Because the number of eligible articles was too small for formal meta-analysis, investigators assigned strength of evidence according to predefined quality criteria and ranked studies accordingly.

Results.—Twelve cross-sectional hospital-based studies reported atopy prevalences ranging from 47% to 75%. Lower levels of atopy-AD were reported in 13 cross-sectional population-based studies, in which the range was 7% to 78%. Inclusion of atopy in the diagnostic criteria for AD did not enhance the criteria's sensitivity and specificity in relation to the clinical phenotype of AD. The less rigidly conducted community surveys tended to report low atopy prevalences. Seven of 8 studies that measured both the number of positive skin prick test responses and IgE antibody levels found these positively associated with AD severity. Results of 2 studies supported a relationship between allergen-specific IgE sensitization and allergic airway disease in later life.

Conclusion.—The association between atopy and AD is both more complex and less strong than previous research suggests. Because as many as two thirds of patients with AD have no measurable allergen-specific IgE antibody sensitization, the continued use of the term *atopic dermatitis* is problematic. The treatment response and prognosis of IgE-associated and non-IgE-associated AD is an important inquiry for future research.

▶ The European Academy of Allergy and Clinical Immunology Nomenclature Task Force defines the term atopy as a personal tendency, familial tendency, or both, usually in childhood and adolescence, to become sensitized and produce IgE antibodies.[1] Previous estimates have suggested that up to 80% of AD cases are associated with atopy.[2] Flohr and colleagues, however, found that up to two thirds of persons with AD are not atopic, casting doubt on the role of IgE sensitization in the pathogenesis of the disease.

B. H. Thiers, MD

References

1. Johansson SGO, Hourihane JO, Bousquet J, et al: A revised nomenclature for allergy. An EAACI position statement for the EAACI nomenclature task force. *Allergy* 56:813-824, 2001.
2. Schmid-Grendelmeier P, Simon D, Simon HU, et al: Epidemiology, clinical features, and immunology of the 'intrinsic' (non-IgE-mediated) type of atopic dermatitis (constitutional dermatitis). *Allergy* 56:841-849, 2001.

Role of Toll-like Receptor 4 in Protection by Bacterial Lipopolysaccharide in the Nasal Mucosa of Atopic Children but Not Adults
Tulic MK, Fiset P-O, Manoukian JJ, et al (Montreal Children's Hosp; McGill Univ, Montreal; Centre Hospitalier de l'Université de Montréal; et al)
Lancet 363:1689-1697, 2004   1–6

Introduction.—Exposure to bacterial products in early life could safeguard against the development of atopy. The "hygiene hypothesis" indicates that diminishing exposure to infection or bacterial products is the cause of the increasing incidence of atopy and asthma. Bacterial lipopolysaccharide (LPS) may be a potential mediator of these protective effects. The effect of bacterial LPS on allergic inflammation and expression of cytokines and LPS receptor (toll-like receptor 4; TLR4) in the nasal mucosa of 15 atopic children, 10 atopic adults, and 7 nonatopic adults was examined.

Methods.—Explanted mucosa resected from the inferior turbinate was cultured with allergen with or without LPS 0.1 mg/L for 24 hours in adults and children undergoing tonsillectomy, adenoidectomy, nasal septal surgery, or sinus surgery. Immunocytochemistry and in situ hybridization were employed to phenotype the cells and cytokines.

Findings.—In explants from atopic children, LPS averted allergen-induced T-helper type 2 (Th2) inflammation and upregulated Th1 cytokine reactivity and expression. These responses were blocked by antibody to interleukin 10. In children, but not adults, LPS produced increases of 3 times in T-cell reactivity, 5 times in T-cell proliferation, and 4 times in interleukin 10 expression, compared to mucosa stimulation with allergen alone.

This difference in response was mirrored by LPS-induced increases in TLR4 reactivity in children, but not adults. The TLR4-positive cells contained interleukin 10. LPS enhanced expression of cells positive for both CD3 and TLR4; both TLRA and interleukin 10; and both CD4 and CD25.

Conclusion.—LPS inhibits allergic inflammation in nasal mucosa of atopic children by skewing local immune responses from Th2 to Th1, along with upregulating production of interleukin 10. These responses are mediated by TLR4. The findings emphasize an important difference between adults and children in their ability to respond to bacterial products. These differences may have a role in normal maturation of the immune system.

Relation of CD4+CD25+ Regulatory T-Cell Suppression of Allergen-Driven T-Cell Activation to Atopic Status and Expression of Allergic Disease
Ling EM, Smith T, Nguyen XD, et al (Imperial College London)
Lancet 363:608-615, 2004   1–7

Introduction.—The prevalence of allergic diseases is increasing. These disorders result from activation of T-helper (Th) 2 cells by allergens. Regulatory CD4+CD25+ T cells suppress T-cell activation in vitro and avert organ-specific autoimmunity in animal models of disease. The relationship between the activity of regulatory T cells and disease in humans was evaluated to ascertain whether the amount of inhibition of allergic responses by CD4+CD25+ T cells was associated with atopy and allergic disease.

Methods.—Blood CD4+CD25+ and CD4+CD25− T cells were isolated from 3 groups of donors: nonatopic participants, those who were atopic with no present symptoms, and those with hay fever. The participants were evaluated during and out of the grass-pollen season. The ability of CD25+ T cells from these donors to suppress allergen-stimulated T-cell proliferation and cytokine production in vitro was evaluated.

Results.—CD4+CD25+ T cells from nonatopic donors suppressed proliferation and interleukin 5 production by their own allergen-activated CD4+CD25− T cells. Inhibition of proliferation by CD4+CD25+ T cells from atopic donors was significantly diminished ($P = .0012$). It was reduced even more by CD4+CD25+ cells isolated from patients with hay fever during the pollen season ($P = .0003$). In patients with hay fever, out-of-season suppression remained less than that observed by regulatory cells from nonatopic donors.

Conclusion.—Allergic disease can result from an improper balance between allergen activation of regulatory CD4+CD25+ T cells and effector Th2 cells. This imbalance could result from a deficiency in suppression by regulatory T cells. Strong activation signals could overcome this regulation. Treatment to enhance regulatory T-cells responses in concert with a decrease in Th2 cell activation may be beneficial in the prevention and treatment of allergic diseases.

▶ These 2 articles (Abstracts 1–6 and 1–7) address the accepted premise that atopy is a Th2-dependent event and that control of atopy may be achieved by manipulating the activity of regulatory T lymphocytes. In the first study (Abstract 1–6), Tulic and colleagues sought laboratory evidence to support the so-called "hygiene hypothesis" which postulates that early exposure of the immune system to bacterial components such as LPS may protect against later development of atopic disorders. The investigators used tissue explant cultures derived from nasal mucosa biopsy specimens obtained from well-characterized atopic children and adults and nonatopic control subjects.

The tissues were stimulated with combinations of appropriate allergen, LPS, and neutralizing antibodies in order to characterize the putative effect of LPS on the allergic response. Although, as the authors admit, this culture model has certain limitations, the results obtained strongly suggested that in atopic children but not adults, LPS decreased the allergen-induced production of Th2 cytokines and significantly enhanced the production of Th1 cytokines.

This effect was largely prevented by including antibody to interleukin 10 in the culture. LPS was also shown to enhance the expression of toll-like receptor 4 (the major LPS receptor) in the mucosal T lymphocytes of these patients, suggesting that this receptor may play a central role in regulation of the Th1/Th2 immune response.

In the second study (Abstract 1–7), Ling et al isolated peripheral blood T cells from atopic and nonatopic subjects and from these cells obtained cell populations highly enriched for those bearing the CD4 and CD25 markers. This cell population is not well characterized but appears, in some models, to exert a suppressive effect on certain T-cell responses.

The investigators showed that CD4+CD25+ T cells derived from nonatopic donors suppressed allergen-induced proliferation and production of interleukin 5 (a Th2 cytokine) by autologous CD25− T cells. In contrast, this inhibition was significantly less in similar studies of atopic individuals. These preliminary results suggest that regulation of the Th2 response in healthy subjects may involve CD4+CD25+ T cells and that this function may be diminished in atopic individuals.

G. M. P. Galbraith, MD

Endotoxin Exposure and Eczema in the First Year of Life
Phipatanakul W, Celedón JC, Raby BA, et al (Children's Hosp, Boston; Brigham and Women's Hosp, Boston; Harvard School of Public Health, Boston)
Pediatrics 114:13-18, 2004   1–8

Background.—Eczema is the most common atopic disease of infancy, and 60% of infants with this condition will manifest characteristic lesions during the first year of life. There has been an increase of two- to threefold in the incidence of eczema during the past 30 years in industrialized countries. Early childhood exposure to endotoxin has been proposed as protective against the development of asthma, allergy, and eczema. The Home Allergens and Asthma Study is a prospective high-cohort study of children with a parental history of asthma or allergies in the Boston metropolitan area. The relationship between exposure to indoor allergens in early childhood and the subsequent development of asthma and allergic diseases was assessed.

Methods.—A prospective birth cohort study was conducted of 498 children who lived in metropolitan Boston and had a history of allergy or asthma in at least 1 parent. A subset of 401 living rooms had house dust samples adequate for an analysis of endotoxins.

Results.—Multivariate analyses, after adjustment for sex, income, and season of birth, showed that high endotoxin levels in the living room at 2 to 3 months of age were inversely associated with physician- or nurse-diagnosed eczema in the first year of life. Exposure to a dog in the home at the age of 2 to 3 months was also inversely associated with eczema in the first year of life; however, the confidence interval widened when endotoxin was included in the model. Variables associated with the development of eczema in the first year of life were paternal history of eczema and maternal specific immunoglobulin E positivity to 1 or more allergens.

Conclusions.—Exposure to high levels of endotoxin in early life may be protective against development of eczema in the first year of life in children with a parental history of asthma or allergies. A paternal history of eczema and maternal sensitization to at least 1 allergen was associated with an increased risk of eczema in the first year of life in these children.

▶ This is one of many articles published in recent years attempting to elucidate environmental factors that appear to either promote or protect against the development of eczema and other atopic diseases. In this study, a high level of endotoxins found in house dust appeared to be protective against atopic dermatitis among children with a parental history of asthma or allergies. Consistent with previous studies, having a dog in the household also appeared to be protective, decreasing the odds of developing eczema by approximately 50%. The authors postulate that the presence of a dog increases endotoxin levels in the home.

S. Raimer, MD

Cohort Study of Sibling Effect, Infectious Diseases, and Risk of Atopic Dermatitis During First 18 Months of Life

Benn CS, Melbye M, Wohlfahrt J, et al (Statens Serum Institut, Copenhagen; Projecto de Saúde de Bandim, Bissau, Guinea-Bissau; Karolinska Institutet, Stockholm)
BMJ 328:1223-1226, 2004   1–9

Background.—Having older siblings or pets that can transmit infectious diseases is associated with a decreased risk of allergic disease. It is unclear, however, whether early microbial exposure can actually protect against the development of allergic disease. Thus, the impact of having an infectious disease during the first 6 months of life on the development of atopic dermatitis before age 18 months was investigated.

Methods.—The research subjects were 24,341 mother–child pairs enrolled in a national birth cohort in Denmark. Mothers were interviewed 4 times: twice before giving birth, then again when their children were 6 and 18 months old. Interviews addressed the number of infectious diseases the child had had before 6 months of age, the number of siblings, whether the child attended day care and when, the presence of pets in the household, and whether the child lived on a farm. Information about atopic dermatitis was obtained at the 18-month visit; only children with physician-diagnosed itchy rash or atopic dermatitis that was recurrent and localized to the elbow and knee creases, hands, face, or at least 4 other areas were defined as having atopic dermatitis.

Results.—Of the 24,341 children studied, 13,070 (53.7%) had at least 1 infectious disease before the age of 6 months. At age 18 months, 2638 children (10.8%) had had atopic dermatitis. After data adjustment for sex, number of siblings, season of birth, maternal age, maternal education, and parental history of allergies, having 1 or more infectious diseases before 6 months of age actually increased the incidence of atopic dermatitis in both boys and girls (adjusted incidence rate ratios: 1.04 for boys, 1.13 for girls, 1.08 overall). Conversely, after adjustment was made for the factors already cited and for the presence of infectious disease, the incidence rate ratios for atopic dermatitis decreased with siblings (0.96 per sibling), residence on a farm (0.90), having pets (0.87), and attendance at day care before age 6 months (0.82).

Conclusion.—Infectious disease early in life does not seem to protect against the development of atopic disease by age 18 months. Other factors, however, such as having siblings, living on a far, keeping pets, and attending early day care do appear to offer independent protection against atopic dermatitis.

▶ It has been previously established that the risk of atopic diseases decreases with exposure to siblings, early day care, living on a farm, and contact with pets. Benn et al studied whether infectious diseases early in life protect against the development of atopic diseases and found this not to be the case. Thus, the protective effects described above are apparently mediated independently of clinically apparent infections in the first 6 months of life.

B. H. Thiers, MD

Eczema and Early Solid Feeding in Preterm Infants
Morgan J, Williams P, Norris F, et al (Univ of Surrey, England)
Arch Dis Child 89:309-314, 2004   1–10

Introduction.—Attempts to prevent or delay the development of allergic disorders in infants by maternal exclusion diets during pregnancy and lactation appear to be ineffective. However, existing evidence supports the theory that a delay in the introduction of solid foods during infancy can reduce the risk of eczema. The influence of solid food patterns on the development of eczema was examined in a cohort of preterm infants monitored until 12 months' corrected age (post-term).

Methods.—Parents of reasonably healthy infants born before 37 weeks' gestational age were informed of the study and asked to participate. When consent was given, the mother and infant were visited at home by midwives at regular intervals until the infant was 12 months' post-term. Infants were categorized according to milk feeding practices before the introduction of solid food, and information was collected retrospectively on the timing of the introduction of 12 foods. Families were classified as atopic or nonatopic; also noted was household exposure to furry pets and smoking.

Results.—A total of 257 infants (55% male) from 219 families completed the study. The mean maternal age was 30.8 years, and the mean paternal age was 33.1 years; at recruitment, 14% of mothers and 26.9% of fathers smoked. More than half of the households (57%) had pets, and at least 1 parent had atopy in 53.9% of families. The overall prevalence of eczema at 12 months post-term was 35.8%. Allergic disease was more common in boys (59.3%) than in girls (41.0%). The introduction of 4 or more solid foods at or before 17 weeks post-term was a significant risk factor for development of eczema (odds ratio, 3.49), with or without other atopic symptoms. Other important risk factors were having at least 1 parent with atopy and introducing solid foods before 10 weeks post-term to an infant with parents who did not have atopy.

Conclusion.—The study population was drawn from an affluent part of England where atopic disease was highly prevalent in both parents and infants. Development of eczema did not seem to be related to milk feeding practices (ie, breast, hypoallergenic formula, or cows' milk), the presence of pets in the home, birth weight, or gestational age at birth. However, the early introduction of a variety of solid foods before 17 weeks post-term was associated with a higher risk of eczema.

▶ The authors studied the possible association of the diet of preterm infants delivered at 37 weeks of gestation or less with the presence of eczema at 12 months of age. No difference was noted in the type of milk the infant was fed (ie, breast milk exclusively, hypoallergenic formulas, cows' milk, or a combination of these) and the development of eczema. The introduction of 4 or more solid foods at or before 17 weeks post-term was a significant risk factor for the development of eczema. Thus, this study suggests that a delay in the introduction of solid foods and their introduction 1 at a time may decrease the risk of atopic disease in preterm infants. This was especially true for male infants and for infants with a family history of atopy.

S. Raimer, MD

The Natural Course of Atopic Dermatitis From Birth to Age 7 Years and the Association With Asthma

Illi S, and the Multicenter Allergy Study Group (Charité, Berlin; Univ Children's Hosp, Munich)
J Allergy Clin Immunol 113:925-931, 2004   1–11

Introduction.—The appearance of signs of atopic dermatitis (AD) in childhood is associated with an increased risk of asthma. Little is known, however, about the natural course of AD and factors influencing its prognosis. The German Multicenter Atopy Study provided information on these issues by monitoring newborns with risk factors for atopy at regular intervals until the age of 7 years.

Methods.—Included in the Multicenter Atopy Study were 1314 infants born in 1990 at delivery wards in 5 German cities. The prospective cohort consisted of 499 infants with recognized risk factors for atopy and 815 infants without these risk factors. Follow-up was conducted at the ages of 1, 3, 6, 18, and 24 months, then yearly to age 7. Data on atopic symptoms and diseases, parental smoking habits, and infectious diseases were obtained through parental interviews at follow-up. Serum samples taken at birth and yearly were analyzed for cord blood IgE, total IgE, and specific IgE antibodies to food allergens. Indoor allergen exposure was assessed when the infants were 6 months old. At age 7, a subsample of 800 children had lung functioning measured.

Results.—A total of 1123 children had at least 1 follow-up visit, and 858 (76.4%) had complete data to the age of 7 years. During the first year of life, 13.4% had AD; by age 2 years, the lifetime prevalence had increased to

21.5%. By age 3 years, 43.2% of children with early AD were in complete remission, and 38.3% had an intermittent disease pattern; the remaining 18.7% had symptoms of AD every year. A significant association was found between parental atopy and the manifestation and severity of early AD. Increased total and specific IgE levels at age 2 years demonstrated a strong positive association with early AD, especially with the more severe form. No relationship was noted between early AD and other analyzed factors, including parental smoking, mite and cat allergen exposure, parental education, and number of infectious diseases. Early wheezing and a specific sensitization pattern strongly predicted wheezing at school age, irrespective of AD.

Conclusion.—AD is common in infancy, but children are often free of the disease by age 3 years. Many children with asthma at school age experience wheezing before or with the onset of AD. A distinct phenotype, rather than progression from AD to asthma, may be involved in the acquisition of asthma at age 7 years.

▶ In a study of a large cohort of German children followed from birth to age 7 years, the authors looked at numerous factors that have recently been hypothesized to influence the development of AD and the relationship of AD to childhood asthma. The only predictors found to be significant for a poor prognosis for AD were the severity of the disease, atopic sensitization, early wheezing, and a strong family history of atopic disease. That 44% of children in the study developed wheezing either before or concomitantly with the development of AD was interpreted to be evidence against an "atopic march" (ie, AD has been proposed to develop before asthma and, theoretically, aggressive treatment of the AD might lessen the chances of the development of asthma). The authors suggest that a certain phenotype exists as a coexpression of asthma and AD and that it seems to display a specific pattern of atopic sensitization and a more severe course, which results in significant impairment of lung function.

S. Raimer, MD

Factors Influencing Atopic Dermatitis—A Questionnaire Survey of Schoolchildren's Perceptions
Williams JR, Burr ML, Williams HC (Univ of Wales, Cardiff; Queen's Med Centre, Nottingham, England)
Br J Dermatol 150:1154-1161, 2004   1–12

Introduction.—Certain genotypes in association with environmental influences appear to predispose to the onset of atopic dermatitis (AD), but little is known about the distribution and relative importance of potential exacerbating and relieving factors in those affected by AD. Nineteen such factors were examined in a population of Welsh schoolchildren with AD.

Methods.—A questionnaire was administered with parental consent to all children in years 8 and 9 (age, 12-14 years) at participating schools in Wales. Children with AD were identified by their responses to skin questions included on the International Study of Asthma and Allergies in Childhood

TABLE 1.—Factors Perceived to Exacerbate, Relieve, and Have No Effect on Rash in 225 Atopic Dermatitis (AD) Responders

| | Percentage of AD Responders | | |
Factor	Rash Exacerbated	Rash Relieved	Rash Unaffected
Sweating	41·8	1·3	38·2
Hot weather	40·0	7·6	32·9
Fabrics	39·1	1·3	38·7
Illness	36·0	2·2	40·0
Dust	32·9	0·9	43·6
Sea swimming	29·8	7·1	42·2
Anxiety/stress	28·4	1·8	46·7
Cold weather	28·4	10·7	38·7
Animals	27·6	1·3	48·9
Grass	26·7	1·8	50·2
Soaps/shampoos	25·8	5·8	46·2
Pool swimming	25·3	4·1	46·7
Cleaning products	24·9	2·7	42·2
Moisturisers/makeup	24·9	16·4	35·6
Metals	16·4	1·3	58·7
Sunlight	15·6	7·1	57·3
Medicines, tablets	6·7	13·8	50·7
Steroid creams	6·2	22·2	33·3
Food/drinks	4·9	2·7	57·8

(Courtesy of Williams JR, Burr ML, Williams HC: Factors influencing atopic dermatitis—A questionnaire survey of schoolchildren's perceptions. *Br J Dermatol* 150:1154-1161, 2004. Reprinted by permission of Blackwell Publishing.)

phase III survey. A supplementary questionnaire was then completed by respondents who believed that they had experienced an itchy rash or eczema in the last 12 months. Participants noted whether the 19 factors made their rash better, worse, or had no effect.

Results.—A total of 225 (90%) of the 250 children identified as having AD answered the supplementary questionnaire. Fourteen of 19 factors were reported to worsen symptoms in at least 20% of respondents (Table 1). Common factors causing exacerbations included sweating, hot weather, and fabrics (wool, in particular); cats were named by 20 respondents as aggravating their symptoms. Thirty-seven (16% of AD responders) reported that contact with metals made their rashes worse. Only 6 children listed foods as causing exacerbations. Steroid creams were the agents most frequently acknowledged as providing relief of AD symptoms.

Discussion.—The factors perceived to be responsible for most exacerbations of AD were sweating, fabrics, and hot weather; steroid creams were thought to provide better relief than other remedies. Only a few children listed foods as worsening their symptoms. The type of information obtained in such questionnaires might be explored during clinical consultations and may aid in the management of patients with AD.

▶ Responding to a questionnaire about factors perceived to cause flares of AD, 12- to 14-year-old children in the United Kingdom reported sweating, hot weather, and fabrics, all of which might increase pruritus, to be factors that precipitated flares of their disease. The authors suggest that similar studies should be conducted in different parts of the world to document factors believed to precipitate AD and that practitioners should spend more time with patients addressing factors perceived to cause flares in their disease.

S. Raimer, MD

The Use of Dietary Manipulation by Parents of Children With Atopic Dermatitis

Johnston GA, Bilbao RM, Graham-Brown RAC (Leicester Royal Infirmary, England)

Br J Dermatol 150:1186-1189, 2004   1–13

Introduction.—Parents of children with atopic dermatitis (AD) frequently turn to complementary therapies and dietary manipulation to manage the disease. Structured interviews were conducted with 100 children who had a diagnosis of AD so that current trends in the use of dietary manipulation could be identified.

Methods.—Study participants were interviewed face-to-face over a 3-month period during their attendance at a pediatric outpatient dermatology department. An accompanying parent or guardian responded for infants and toddlers. The mean age of children interviewed was 7.3 years; 60% of patients with AD were boys. Their ethnicity was mixed: 59% were white, and 35% were Indo-Asian.

Results.—Most children had moderate to severe AD: 70% required bandaging, and 76% needed potent topical steroids. Seventy-five reported having tried some form of food exclusion, and 39 of these believed that their AD had improved as a result. Items commonly mentioned by those practicing avoidance were dairy products (48%), eggs (27%), cow's milk (25%), and candy (13%); 20% avoided food additives and colorings. Dietary supplements frequently given to children with AD (41% of the group) included evening primrose oil (59%) and multivitamins (44%). Only 38 patients had restricted foods after consulting a doctor or dietitian.

Conclusion.—The proportion of patients with AD who exclude food from their diet continues to increase. Compared with a previous study from the same practice, unsupervised dietary manipulation rose from 10% to 39%.

▶ One of the authors of this study had previously published a similar study in 1989 that showed that a majority of patients with AD (71%) were avoiding certain foods or food groups in an attempt to improve their AD.[1] The present study shows very similar results. Approximately half of patients or their parents were manipulating their diet without consulting a physician or a dietician. In addition, 41% were using some sort of dietary supplementation. Although it is unlikely that avoiding a few foods would cause harm to a child, it is possible that inadequate intake of an essential element in the diet, such as protein, could occur. Also, patients frequently did not report dietary supplementation without specific inquiry. It does, therefore, seem prudent to ask our patients with AD about dietary manipulation.

S. Raimer, MD

Reference

1. Webber SA, Graham-Brown RAC, Hutchinson PE, et al: Dietary manipulation in childhood atopic dermatitis. *Br J Dermatol* 121:91-98, 1989.

Frequency and Clinical Role of *Staphylococcus aureus* Overinfection in Atopic Dermatitis in Children
Ricci G, Patrizi A, Neri I, et al (Univ of Bologna, Italy)
Pediatr Dermatol 20:389-392, 2003   1–14

Background.—Atopic dermatitis (AD) is frequently associated with asthma and allergic rhinoconjunctivitis. The skin of patients with AD has shown a remarkable susceptibility to colonization with *Staphylococcus aureus*, and the important role of *S aureus* colonization of the skin as a factor in the exacerbation of AD has been well established. A variety of molecules secreted by most strains of *S aureus* have been described. Some strains of *S aureus* produce endotoxins with T-cell superantigen activity, which have the capacity to worsen AD. Thus, some patients may benefit from eradication of *S aureus* by antimicrobial therapy. However, repeated courses of antibiotic therapy may lead to the development of antibiotic-resistant strains of *S aureus*. The frequency of *S aureus* colonization and its effect on the severity of AD in young children with moderate or severe disease were determined.

Methods.—The study group was composed of 81 children, 2 months to 9 years old, with moderate to severe AD. A total of 308 samples from the cutaneous lesions were analyzed.

Results.—*S aureus* was isolated in 52 (64.2%) children. Of these patients, 5 were also colonized by *S pyogenes*, and 1 was also colonized by *Candida albicans*. The total IgE serum level and specific IgE levels were tested in 61 patients to evaluate their allergic status; a diagnosis of extrinsic AD was made in 43 children, and 18 children were diagnosed with intrinsic AD. A higher presence of *S aureus* was observed in allergic (71%) children than in nonallergic children (49%).

Conclusions.—*S aureus* has an important role in the clinical manifestations of atopic dermatitis and specifically in the worsening of eczematous lesions of the face, neck, and perineum in children younger than 1 year.

▶ In these young Italian children with moderate to severe AD, a high percentage were culture-positive for *S aureus*. The disease improved with antimicrobial therapy. Because the presence of *S aureus* in patients with AD almost certainly exacerbates the disease, and frequent treatment with antimicrobial drugs is not ideal because of the development of resistance, periodic baths with low concentrations of Clorox (sodium hypochlorite) to reduce colonization seem advisable.

S. Raimer, MD

Is High Mole Count a Marker of More Than Melanoma Risk? Eczema Diagnosis Is Associated With Melanocytic Nevi in Children
Dellavalle RP, Hester EJ, Stegner DL, et al (Univ of Colorado, Denver; Kaiser Permanente Health Maintenance Organization of Colorado, Denver)
Arch Dermatol 140:577-580, 2004   1–15

Introduction.—Adults with severe eczema are reported to have significantly fewer melanocytic nevi than matched control subjects, perhaps because of exposure to therapy that inhibits growth of melanocytic cells. A nested case-control study examined the relationship between eczema and nevi in children.

Methods.—Participants were enrolled in a randomized, controlled interventional trial of additional sun protection versus standard care in young children. Those in intervention groups received additional sun protection advice and sun protection materials such as hats, sunglasses, and samples of sunscreen. Skin examinations and parental interviews were conducted when the children were approximately 3 years old. Data recorded included eye color, hair color, degree of freckling, and eczema status.

Results.—Only 281 (39%) of 728 enrolled children were examined after 3 years, primarily because parents could not be reached. Children with a history of eczema diagnosis had more nevi than those without (median, 7.5 vs 5.0 nevi), and this association was strongest in children with lightly pigmented skin. The duration of eczema for more or less than 2 years was not associated with the number of nevi.

Discussion.—Unlike adults with eczema, children with the skin disorder had an increased number of nevi. Greater numbers of nevi reflect solar exposure and are associated with an increased risk of melanoma. Eczema might alter the nevus life cycle, increasing numbers transiently in early childhood, but the relationship between the number of nevi and eczema is yet undetermined.

▶ Unlike adult patients with eczema, who have been reported to have fewer melanocytic nevi than do controls, lightly pigmented 3-year-old children in Colorado with a history of eczema were noted in this study to have a mean of 2.5 more nevi than children of the same age with no history of eczema. No differences were found in the number of nevi in children with medium or dark pigmentation, regardless of their history of eczema. The clinical significance of this finding, if any, is uncertain.

S. Raimer, MD

Topical Application of the Immunosuppressant Tacrolimus Accelerates Carcinogenesis in Mouse Skin

Niwa Y, Terashima T, Sumi H (Niwa Inst for Immunology, Tosashimizu, Japan; Osaka City Univ, Japan; Natl Cancer Ctr Hosp East, Kashiwa, Japan)
Br J Dermatol 149:960-967, 2003   1–16

Introduction.—Tacrolimus, used since the late 1980s to prevent rejection of liver and kidney transplants, carries a risk of carcinogenesis of the skin and other organs. This immunosuppressive agent is now being prescribed as a topical treatment for atopic dermatitis (AD), and side effects thus far have been relatively minor. Findings in a mouse model, however, reveal that topical tacrolimus significantly decreases the CD4/CD8 ratio and has tumor-promoting effects.

Methods.—Seven-week-old female CD-1 mice were divided into 6 treatment groups as follows: (1) The tumor initiator 7,12-dimethylbenz[α]anthracene (DMBA) followed by acetone; (2)DMBA fol-

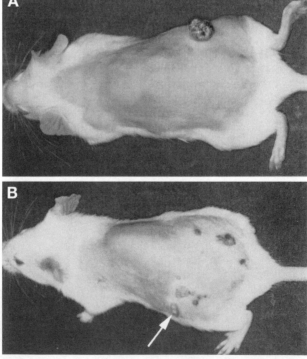

FIGURE 2.—Mice with tumors accelerated by tacrolimus ointment. **A,** A large carcinoma that developed by week 16 in a mouse treated with 7,12-dimethylbenz[α]anthracene (DMBA) plus tacrolimus without 12-O-tetradecanoylphorbol-13-acetate (TPA). **B,** Several tumors (1 carcinoma *arrow*) and several papillomas) that developed by week 17 in a mouse treated with DMBA plus TPA plus tacrolimus. (Courtesy of Niwa Y, Terashima T, Sumi H: Topical application of the immunosuppressant tacrolimus accelerates carcinogenesis in mouse skin. *Br J Dermatol* 149:960-967. 2003. Reprinted by permission of Blackwell Publishing.)

lowed by 12-O-tetradecanoylphorbol-13-acetate (TPA); (3) DMBA followed by acetone plus tacrolimus; (4) DMBA followed by TPA plus tacrolimus; (5) acetone followed by acetone plus tacrolimus; and (6) acetone followed by acetone (control).

All treatments continued for 6 weeks and mice were assessed daily for tumors. Skin tumors were then harvested and prepared for histologic examination.

Results.—Skin tumors developed significantly more often in TPA-treated groups than in the absence of TPA. But 14 weeks after the start of treatment, the mean number of new tumors per mouse per week was 0.47 in group 4, 0.10 in group 2, and 0.01 in group 3, indicating marked synergy between tacrolimus and the DMBA/TPA regimen.

Tacrolimus-treated mice were found to have a significantly reduced CD4/CD8 ratio in axillary and inguinal lymph nodes, supporting a relationship between the immunosuppressive effect of tacrolimus and promotion of tumorigenesis. Most tumors caused by topical tacrolimus were benign papillomas, but 8.5% of all tumors were squamous cell carcinomas (Fig 2; see color plate XIII).

Conclusion.—Patients with AD who receive long-term topical tacrolimus may be at risk for skin carcinogenesis and should undergo careful surveillance for skin lesions. Because AD is not a life-threatening disorder, the benefits of tacrolimus must be weighed against this risk.

▶ This article illustrates some of my own personal discomfort with long-term use of the topical immunosuppressive macrolides, tacrolimus and pimecrolimus. These compounds, which have been approved for the treatment of atopic dermatitis, conceivably could be used on sun-exposed skin for years with unknown consequences in terms of cutaneous carcinogenesis. All dermatologists are familiar with the high incidence of skin cancers in patients treated with systemic cyclosporine, and whether such tumors will develop after long-term topical application of these related drugs is unknown. Certainly, all of us are aware of the consequences of long-term topical steroid use. With these 2 new drugs, we are truly venturing into the unknown. Their claims of a superior safety profile over existing therapies may not be warranted.

B. H. Thiers, MD

Leflunomide as a Novel Treatment Option in Severe Atopic Dermatitis
Schmitt J, Wozel G, Pfeiffer C (Technical Univ Dresden, Germany)
Br J Dermatol 150:1182-1185, 2004   1–17

Background.—T-cell–mediated pathogenesis is increasingly being implicated in the development of atopic dermatitis (AD). Systemic immunosuppressants such as cyclosporine, azathioprine, and mycophenolate mofetil have successfully treated many cases of severe AD, but they are associated with adverse events, many of which are severe. Leflunomide inhibits de novo pyrimidine synthesis and is approved for treating rheumatoid arthritis. The efficacy and safety of leflunomide in 2 patients with severe recalcitrant AD are described.

> *Case Reports.*—The research subjects were 2 men (28 and 44 years old) with long-standing, severe AD that did not respond to other treatments, including systemic immunosuppressants. Each research subject began taking leflunomide at a loading dose of 100 mg/d for 3 days, followed by daily maintenance therapy at 20 mg/d. When they began leflunomide, each patient had almost erythrodermic AD: their eczema area and severity index (EASI) scores were 40.0 or higher, and their visual analog scale (VAS) ratings for itching were 8 or higher. The older patient achieved partial remission of his AD within 4 weeks; at 4 weeks, his EASI score was 4.8, his VAS rating for itching was 5, and his dose was reduced to 10 mg/d. A mild increase in transaminase levels prompted drug discontinuation at week 72; at that time, his EASI score was 4.2, and his VAS rating for itching was 2. His disease remained in control 6 months after drug discontinuation.
>
> The younger patient achieved partial remission of his AD within 7 weeks; his EASI score at 21 weeks was 4.8, and his VAS rating for itching was 2. An exacerbation at 21 weeks was successfully treated with oral prednisolone and tacrolimus ointment, and 5 weeks later, the leflunomide dose was reduced to 10 mg every other day. This dose was maintained until week 69, at which time the dose on alternate days was increased to 20 mg because of breakthrough symptoms. At week 81, his EASI score was 8.4, and his VAS rating for itching was 2. Neither patient experienced severe adverse events.

Conclusion.—Long-term oral leflunomide was effective in these 2 patients with severe recalcitrant AD and may offer a safer alternative to currently available systemic immunosuppressants.

▶ Other immunosuppressive therapies, such as cyclosporine, azathioprine, and mycophenolate mofetil, have been reported, mostly anecdotally, to have a salutary effect on patients with AD. Determining which is the most effective and least toxic of these drugs will require larger, prospective controlled studies.

B. H. Thiers, MD

Prevalence and Relevance of Contact Dermatitis Allergens: A Meta-analysis of 15 Years of Published T.R.U.E. Test Data
Krob HA, Fleischer AB Jr, D'Agostino R Jr, et al (Wake Forest Univ, Winston-Salem, NC)
J Am Acad Dermatol 51:349-353, 2004   1–18

Introduction.—The diagnosis of allergic contact dermatitis (ACD), a frequent cause of visits to dermatology clinics, can be facilitated or confirmed by the patch test procedure. The Thin-layer Rapid Use Epicutaneous (T.R.U.E.) Test, which has become a global standard, contains 23 allergens and allergen mixes reported to be responsible for a large majority of ACD. A MEDLINE search was conducted to measure the overall prevalence and relevance of reactions to the allergens tested by the T.R.U.E. Test.

Methods.—Studies eligible for meta-analysis were published in English from 1966 to June 2000 and used the T.R.U.E. Test in the clinical evaluation of ACD in human subjects. Excluded were studies that did not indicate whether T.R.U.E. Test Panel 1, Panel 2, or both were used and those combining T.R.U.E. Test data with data from other methods. Studies were analyzed for the number of research subjects tested, the number with positive reactions, and the number with relevant reactions.

Results.—The 5 most prevalent allergens were nickel (14.7%), thimerosal (5.0%), cobalt (4.8%), fragrance mix (3.4%), and balsam of Peru (3.0%). The 5 least prevalent allergens were paraben mix (0.5%), black rubber mix (0.6%), quaternium-15 (0.6%), quinoline mix (0.7%), and caine mix (0.7%). Data previously reported from the North American Contact Dermatitis Data Group (NACDG) show the 5 most prevalent allergens to be nickel (14.3%), fragrance mix (14%), neomycin (11.6%), balsam of Peru (10.4%), and thimerosal (10.4%). In NACDG data, the prevalence of allergy to cobalt was 9.2%. With the use of the Significance-Prevalence Index Number, a measure of the clinical importance of contact dermatitis allergens, the top 5 allergens tested by the T.R.U.E. Test are nickel, cobalt, fragrance mix, colophony, and thiuram mix.

Discussion.—The prevalence of common contact allergens as tested by the T.R.U.E. Test is similar to that in articles that reported the use of other patch test methods, but a comparison with NACDG data suggests that this standard patch test system may miss clinically important allergens.

▶ Although more than 3700 allergens have been identified as causing ACD, a relatively small number cause most cases in the United States. The US Food and Drug Administration has approved the use of only 28 allergens for testing, and the T.R.U.E. test uses 23 of them. Clearly, many highly relevant allergens may be missed if the patient is evaluated with the T.R.U.E. test series alone.

B. H. Thiers, MD

Thimerosal Exposure in Infants and Developmental Disorders: A Prospective Cohort Study in the United Kingdom Does Not Support a Causal Association
Heron J, and the ALSPAC Study Team (Univ of Bristol, England)
Pediatrics 114:577-583, 2004   1–19

Background.—Exposure to mercury has been associated with impairment in childhood cognitive development and early motor skills. Thimerosal is a preservative used in several children's vaccines. It contains ethylmercury, an organic compound that is metabolized into mercury. Concern has been raised that this exposure to mercury may be detrimental to young children. This possibility was investigated in a large UK population-based cohort.

Methods.—Population data were obtained from a longitudinal study on childhood health and development that included more than 14,000 children delivered in 1991 and 1992. Their ages at receipt of thimerosal-containing vaccines were recorded. Mercury exposures by 3, 4, and 6 months of age were measured. Cognitive and behavioral development from 6 to 91 months were also assessed.

Findings.—Unexpectedly, the unadjusted results suggested that thimerosal exposure had a beneficial effect. Exposure at 3 months correlated inversely with hyperactivity and conduct problems at 47 months, motor development at 6 and 30 months, sound difficulties at 81 months, as well as speech therapy, special needs, and an inability to function in school (learning difficulty) at 91 months. After adjustment for birth weight, gestation, sex, maternal education, parity, housing tenure, maternal smoking, breastfeeding, and ethnic origins, only 1 result was in the direction hypothesized: poor social behavior at 47 months correlated with thimerosal exposure by 3 months of age. Another 8 parameters supported a beneficial effect.

Conclusions.—Early exposure to thimerosal does not appear to have deleterious effects on neurologic or psychological outcomes in young children. The dangers associated with contaminated multidose vaccine vials far outweigh any potential risk posed by thimerosal.

Thimerosal Exposure in Infants and Developmental Disorders: A Retrospective Cohort Study in the United Kingdom Does Not Support a Causal Association

Andrews N, Miller E, Grant A, et al (Communicable Disease Surveillance Centre, London; Royal Free and Univ College Med School, London; Office for Natl Statistics, London)
Pediatrics 114:584-591, 2004   1–20

Background.—Concerns have been raised about the possible toxicity of thimerosal-containing vaccines. The relationship between the amount of thimerosal that young children receive in diphtheria-tetanus-whole-cell pertussis (DTP) or diphtheria-tetanus (DT) vaccination and subsequent neurodevelopmental disorders was investigated.

Methods.—This retrospective cohort study included 109,863 children, born between 1988 and 1997, who were seen in general practices in the United Kingdom. Children were assessed for general developmental disorders, language or speech delay, tics, attention-deficit disorder, autism, unspecified developmental delays, behavior problems, encopresis, and enuresis. The number of DTP/DT doses received by 3 and 4 months of age and the cumulative age-specific DTP/DT exposure by 6 months of age were determined. Each DTP/DT vaccine dose contained 50 µg of thimerosal.

Findings.—Evidence of a greater risk with increasing doses was found only for tics. The Cox hazard ratio (HR) was 1.5 per dose at 4 months. Increasing doses were significantly, negatively associated with general developmental disorders (HR, 0.87), unspecified developmental delay (HR, 0.8), and attention-deficit disorder (HR, 0.79) at 4 months. The other disorders did not appear to correlate with thimerosal exposure.

Conclusions.—With the possible exception of tics, the neurodevelopmental disorders analyzed were not positively correlated with increasing thimerosal exposure through DTP/DT vaccination at a young age. Increasing exposures to thimerosal seemed to have a protective effect against general developmental disorders, unspecified developmental delay, and attention-deficit disorder.

Thimerosal-Containing Vaccines and Autistic Spectrum Disorder: A Critical Review of Published Original Data

Parker SK, Schwartz B, Todd J, et al (Univ of Colorado, Denver; Ctrs for Disease Control and Prevention, Atlanta, Ga)

Pediatrics 114:793-804, 2004   1–21

Background.—Whether thimerosal-containing vaccines cause autistic spectrum disorders (ASD) and neurodevelopmental disorders (NDDs) has been debated for several years. A systematic literature review was conducted to assess the quality of evidence on the potential correlation between thimerosal-containing vaccines and autism.

Methods.—A literature search of articles published between 1966 and 2004 identified 12 publications meeting selection criteria. All were original articles assessing the relationship between thimerosal-containing vaccines and ASD/NDDs or pharmacokinetics of ethylmercury in vaccines.

Findings.—Ten articles were epidemiologic studies, and 2 were pharmacokinetic studies of ethylmercury. Study design and quality varied significantly. Most of the epidemiologic evidence did not support a correlation between thimerosal-containing vaccines and ASD. The epidemiologic studies that supported such a correlation were of poor quality and not interpretable. The pharmacokinetic studies reported that the half-life of ethylmercury appears to be significantly shorter than that of methylmercury.

Conclusions.—Previous research does not support a correlation between thimerosal-containing vaccines and ASD. The pharmacokinetics of ethylmercury make this relationship less likely.

▶ Although more familiar to dermatologists as a cause of contact dermatitis, thimerosal, when used as a preservative in children's vaccines, has been implicated as a possible cause of autistic and neurodevelopmental disorders. Thimerosal contains ethylmercury, an organic compound that is metabolized into mercury. A related organic mercury-containing compound, methylmercury, can have adverse effects on childhood development, especially with exposure in utero or in the early months of life. Some investigators believe that ethylmercury might have a similar effect, although little evidence supports that claim. Importantly, ethylmercury is more quickly metabolized and eliminated from the body than is methylmercury. The findings of these 3 studies (Abstracts 1–19 to 1–21) are reassuring and do not support a link between thimerosal-containing vaccines and autism or related disorders.

B. H. Thiers, MD

E-Selectin, Thymus- and Activation-Regulated Chemokine/CCL17, and Intercellular Adhesion Molecule-1 Are Constitutively Coexpressed in Dermal Microvessels: A Foundation for a Cutaneous Immunosurveillance System

Chong BF, Murphy J-E, Kupper TS, et al (Brigham and Women's Hosp, Boston; Johns Hopkins School of Medicine, Baltimore, Md)

J Immunol 172:1575-1581, 2004   1–22

Introduction.—The homing of leukocytes from the blood to tissue is an important component of mammalian immune responses. Due to its exposure to the outside environment, the skin needs to recruit leukocytes effectively to ward off potential pathogens. It may be that noninflamed skin uses the same mechanisms as inflamed skin to recruit T cells. Trafficking of T cells to inflamed skin necessitates the interaction of molecules located on the endothelial cells of dermal blood vessels with their counter-receptors on T cells and can be described in a series of distinct steps.

The mechanism directing trafficking of T cells to noninflamed skin is not as well characterized. It may be that basal expression and co-localization of E-selectin, chemokine (eg, CCL17), and ICAM-1 in dermal vessels could act to recruit T cells to noninflamed human skin.

Findings.—Immunohistochemical staining for E-selectin and CD31 revealed E-selectin expression in a restricted subset of dermal vessels in noninflamed human skin from 3 different sites. Confocal multicolor immunofluorescence imaging showed a nonuniform distribution of E-selectin in dermal vessels, along with co-localization of E-selectin with CCL17 and ICAM-1. Coexpression of these molecules on blood vessels in noninflamed skin establishes the basis for a model of a cutaneous immunosurveillance system active in the absence of pathologic inflammation.

Conclusion.—It is probable that skin-homing T cells are recruited to noninflamed skin in a fashion similar to that in inflammatory sites via the coordinate actions of E-selectin, CCL17 (or other chemokines), and ICAM-1, and that these components are constitutively expressed and co-localized on dermal microvessels in noninflamed skin.

▶ The mechanisms by which T cells home to inflamed skin have been well characterized. However, the cellular interactions underlying traffic of T cells through healthy cutaneous tissues has not been examined. These investigators postulated that cutaneous immune surveillance by T lymphocytes may involve cell adhesion factors and cytokines similar to those used in the rapid response to dermal insult. They used immunocytochemical methods to investigate the expression of the adhesion molecules E-selectin and ICAM-1 and the chemokine CCl17 in healthy human skin. These factors are all required for the process of trafficking of memory T cells to areas of skin damage or inflammation.

The results obtained show that these 3 molecules are indeed expressed and co-localize in the healthy human dermis. Interestingly, their distribution is patchy and restricted to a subset of blood vessels in the mid to upper dermis of skin derived from a variety of anatomical sites. It is likely that constitutive expression of these factors represents a mechanism whereby T lymphocytes can patrol the skin in a state of readiness for a cutaneous immune response.

G. M. P. Galbraith, MD

2 Psoriasis and Lichenoid Disorders

In Situ Expression of CD40 and CD40 Ligand in Psoriasis
Ohta Y, Hamada Y (Yokohama Natl Hosp, Japan; Kitasato Univ, Sagamihara, Japan)
Dermatology 209:21-28, 2004   2–1

Introduction.—CD40 is a 50-kD molecule that belongs to the tumor necrosis factor/nerve growth factor receptor superfamily and mediates important molecular events for collaborations between T and B lymphocytes. In human cultured keratinocytes, CD40 is invariably expressed at a constant level and upregulated by γ-interferon in vitro. In vivo, CD40 is consistently expressed in human epidermis, particularly in the basal cell layer. The interaction between CD40 and CD40 ligand (CD40L) provides a signal that augments initiation of cellular immune responses.

Little information regarding the in vivo expression of CD40 and CD40L in cutaneous inflammation has been reported. The potential role of CD40-mediated signals in the pathogenesis of psoriasis was examined.

Methods.—The in situ CD40 and CD40L expression was analyzed immunohistochemically in various stages of psoriatic lesions—fully developed and initial pinpoint.

Results.—In normal skin, faintly positive immunoreactivity for CD40 was observed in the basal keratinocytes and dermal endothelial cells. These had nearly the same intensity as that observed in psoriatic lesional skin. In the dermal infiltrates of psoriatric lesions, CD40 was intensely expressed. Some of these positive cells seemed to be dendritic in shape. CD40 expression was seen in nearly all specimens of psoriatric lesions, but the expression of CD40L was predominantly observed in the initial pinpoint lesions of psoriasis. These appeared to be distributed close to CD40-positive cells.

Conclusion.—CD40L-triggered signals could be involved in the early stage of psoriatic lesion formation.

In Situ Demonstration of CD40 – and CD154-Positive Cells in Psoriatic Lesions and Keratinocyte Production of Chemokines by CD40 Ligation In Vitro

Pasch MC, Timár KK, van Meurs M, et al (Univ of Amsterdam; Erasmus MC Univ, Rotterdam, The Netherlands)
J Pathol 203:839-848, 2004   2–2

Introduction.—Psoriasis is an inflammatory skin disease in which T cells and keratinocytes in the lesions are activated and express activation markers and costimulatory molecules. Ligation of CD40 expressed on activated keratinocytes with CD154 expressed on activated T cells may be involved in the pathogenesis of psoriasis.

The presence of CD40+ and CD154+ cells in psoriatic skin was examined by immunohistochemistry in lesional and nonlesional skin of 10 patients with psoriasis and 5 healthy controls. The influence of CD154-CD40 ligation on the release of chemokines (interleukin-8, RANTES, and MCP-1) and complement components (C3 and factor B) from keratinocytes was also evaluated in vitro.

Findings.—Trials using single- and double-staining revealed that clusters of CD40+ keratinocytes were observed in both lesional and nonlesional skin; CD40+CD1a+ Langerhans cells in lesional, nonlesional, and normal skin; and several CD40+CD83+ cells in lesional skin. The CD1a+ and CD83+ cells consistently expressed CD40 strongly. Many T cells were observed in lesional skin. A small number of T cells expressed CD154. CD154+ T cells were observed in the lesional epidermis of 7 of 10 patients— in 6, in juxtaposition to CD40+ cells, including keratinocytes.

In nonlesional epidermis, CD154+ T cells were observed in 2 patients—in 1, in juxtaposition to CD40+ keratinocytes. In vitro trials revealed that IFN-γ–treated keratinocytes released small amounts of interleukin-8, RANTES, and MCP-1; ligation of these cells with CD154-transfected J558 cells or soluble CD154 greatly augmented the release. This ligation did not augment the release of C3 and factor B.

Conclusion.—CD40+ cells and CD154+ T cells were detected in psoriatic skin lesions. CD40-CD154 ligation on keratinocytes in vitro produced chemokine release.

▶ The cell surface molecule CD40 was first described in lymphoid cells and is known to play a central role in B-T lymphocyte communication through interaction with CD40 ligand (CD40L, also named CD154), which is expressed by activated CD4+ T lymphocytes. In the skin, CD40 is now recognized as a membrane component of several cell types, including Langerhans cells, keratinocytes, fibroblasts, and vascular endothelial cells.

The purpose of these 2 studies (Abstracts 2–1 and 2–2) was to examine the expression of CD40 and its ligand in the lesional skin of psoriatic patients. Ohta and Hamada (Abstract 2–1) used immunocytochemical methods to detect these molecules in both mature psoriatic lesions and the pinpoint lesions representative of newly forming plaques. The results showed that the intensity of expression of CD40 was greater in psoriatic skin than in normal skin and was found primarily in the dermal infiltrates. Interestingly, CD40 ligand was only detected in significant amounts in the perivascular infiltrating cells in pinpoint initial lesions.

Pasch et al (Abstract 2–2) used similar immunohistochemical methods to study these markers in psoriatic lesional and normal skin. In addition, they examined keratinocytes cultured from psoriatic lesions and investigated their activity in co-culture with CD40 ligand–transfected hybridoma cells. These authors also detected an increased expression of CD40 in keratinocytes and Langerhans cells of psoriatic skin and also identified CD40 ligand expression in epidermal T cells of most patient samples, usually in close proximity to the CD40+ cells.

Further investigation showed that co-culture of the CD40+ keratinocytes with CD40 ligand–transfected cells significantly enhanced the release of chemokines, including interleukin-8, by these cells. Together, these studies strongly suggest that expression and ligation of cutaneous CD40+ cells may play a role in the pathogenesis of psoriasis.

G. M. P. Galbraith, MD

Rapid Clearance of Psoriatic Skin Lesions Induced by Topical Cyclopamine: A Preliminary Proof of Concept Study
Taş S, Avci O (Narlidere, Turkey; Izmir, Turkey)
Dermatology 209:126-131, 2004   2–3

Introduction.—The authors reported in a previous study that topical application of cyclopamine, a steroidal alkaloid inhibitor of *hedgehog/smoothened* signaling, induced the differentiation of skin tumor cells displaying arrest of cellular differentiation. No short- or long-term adverse effects were associated with cyclopamine treatment. The effect of topical cyclopamine on psoriatic lesions was examined in 7 patients.

Methods.—A cream preparation containing cyclopamine was applied to 31 psoriatic lesions. In each patient, at least 1 lesion similar in size to the cyclopamine-treated lesion had cream base alone applied. Lesions were assessed for severity before and during treatment, and lesions and surrounding nonlesional skin were excised for histopathologic and immunohistochemical examination.

Results.—At approximately 8 hours after its application, cyclopamine-treated lesions were less erythematous. The time required from treatment initiation to clearance varied among patients, but most lesions markedly regressed by day 2 (Fig 1; see color plate XIII) and cleared by day 4 with uninterrupted therapy. Lesions treated with cream base or a topical corticosteroid showed marginal or insignificant changes over a 4-day period. Clearance was accelerated by combining cyclopamine with clobetasol 17-propionate pretreatment. Cyclopamine-treated lesional skin showed rapid induction of epidermal cell differentiation and reversal of histopathologic

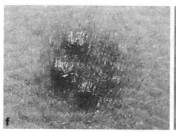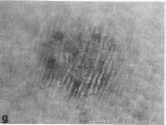

FIGURE 1.—Appearances of psoriatic lesions before and after treatment with topical cyclopamine. f, Psoriatic plaque (approximately 7 × 8 mm) in the antecubital region prior to treatment. g, Same lesion after a day of treatment with cyclopamine cream (approximately 20 μL every 4 h) and nontreated follow-up for 2 days. (Courtesy of Taş S, Avci O: Rapid clearance of psoriatic skin lesions induced by topical cyclopamine: A preliminary proof of concept study. *Dermatology* 209:126-131, 2004. Reproduced with permission of S. Karger AG, Basel.)

signs of disease. There were no indications of adverse effects when the treated sites were examined more than 24 months later.

Conclusion.—The efficacy of cyclopamine and the unusually rapid disappearance of treated lesions are consistent with an intervention involving a primary or proximal causative event related to in the impairment of epidermal differentiation that has pathogenic significance in the formation of psoriatic lesions. Dosages and safety are issues for future research.

▶ Topical cyclopamine is also under study as a potential topical treatment for nonmelanoma skin cancer.

B. H. Thiers, MD

Efficacy of Once-Daily Treatment Regimens With Calcipotriol/Betamethasone Dipropionate Ointment and Calcipotriol Ointment in Psoriasis Vulgaris

Kragballe K, Noerrelund KL, Lui H, et al (Marselisborg Centret, Aarhus, Denmark; LEO Pharma, Ballerup, Denmark; Univ of British Columbia, Vancouver, Canada; et al)
Br J Dermatol 150:1167-1173, 2004   2–4

Introduction.—Calcipotriol and topical corticosteroids have different modes of action in the treatment of psoriasis. The 2 compounds together can improve efficacy and response time, but products available on the market are usually incompatible. Different treatment regimens that used a new combined calcipotriol/corticosteroid product were investigated for their safety and efficacy and were compared with calcipotriol ointment alone.

Methods.—Randomization of the 972 participants with psoriasis vulgaris was to the 2-compound product once daily for 8 weeks followed by calcipotriol ointment once daily for 4 weeks (group 1); the 2-compound product once daily for 4 weeks followed by 8 weeks of treatment with calcipotriol ointment once daily on weekdays and the 2-compound product once daily on weekends (group 2); or to calcipotriol ointment twice daily for

12 weeks (group 3). Outcomes of interest were the percentage reduction in the Psoriasis Area and Severity Index (PASI) and the investigators' global assessments of disease severity.

Results.—The mean reductions in PASI from baseline to the end of 8 weeks of treatment were 73.3% for group 1, 68.2% for group 2, and 64.1% for group 3. In groups 1, 2, and 3, the proportions of patients with absent or very mild disease after 8 weeks of therapy were 55.3%, 47.7%, and 40.7%, respectively. Both analyses found group 1 statistically superior to group 3, but no significant differences were found between groups 2 and 3 in terms of change from baseline. After 12 weeks of treatment, the reduction in PASI did not differ significantly between groups. Pruritus, the most common lesional/perilesional adverse reaction, was most frequent in group 3.

Conclusion.—Both short-term treatment regimens with the newly developed 2-compound product (calcipotriol–betamethasone dipropionate) were safe and effective in patients with psoriasis vulgaris. Optimal effects were reached after 5 weeks and were maintained during the following 3 weeks. Calcipotriol ointment was also effective but less so than the combined product.

▶ When first marketed in the United States, calcipotriene was heavily promoted as an effective nonsteroidal topical treatment for psoriasis. Its main drawback was its slow onset of action. One logical way to circumvent that obstacle would be to combine it with a relatively potent topical steroid. One can only wonder why this took so long. Do I smell a patent expiration?

B. H. Thiers, MD

Costs of Treatment in Patients With Moderate to Severe Plaque Psoriasis: Economic Analysis in a Randomized Controlled Comparison of Methotrexate and Cyclosporine

Opmeer BC, Heydendael VMR, de Borgie CAJM, et al (Univ of Amsterdam)
Arch Dermatol 140:685-690, 2004   2–5

Background.—Clinical decision making about treatment is based mainly on evidence of efficacy, adverse effects, safety, and potential patient discomfort. Total costs associated with treatment may also be taken into account. The costs of methotrexate and cyclosporine for treating psoriasis were compared.

Methods.—Patients with moderate to severe plaque psoriasis and no previous treatment with methotrexate or cyclosporine were included in the cost-minimization analysis. Direct and indirect medical and nonmedical costs associated with 16 weeks of treatment and an additional 36 weeks of follow-up were determined.

Findings.—The mean cumulative costs of 16 weeks of treatment were $1593 for methotrexate and $2114 for cyclosporine; during follow-up, the costs were $2418 and $2306, respectively. The overall difference in cumulative 1-year costs was $409. This represents 10% of the total cost.

Conclusions.—After 1 year, the difference in total costs between these 2 established systemic agents for psoriasis was relatively small. Economic considerations may support but may not be the deciding factor for individual decisions and guidelines for systemic therapy.

▶ The authors appropriately state that the cost of drugs is only 1 element of the total direct and indirect costs associated with the treatment of psoriasis. Other factors to be taken into consideration include effectiveness, adverse effects, safety, convenience, and the ease and comfort of administration. The cost profile in the current study was measured over a period of 1 year. Drugs that may have significant cumulative long-term toxic effects would be more appropriately evaluated over an extended time span so that the potential costs of drug-induced organ dysfunction could be factored into the equation.

B. H. Thiers, MD

Infliximab Induction Therapy for Patients With Severe Plaque-Type Psoriasis: A Randomized, Double-blind, Placebo-controlled Trial
Gottlieb AB, Evans R, Li S, et al (Univ of Medicine and Dentistry of New Jersey, New Brunswick; Centocor Inc, Malvern, Pa; Baylor Univ, Dallas, Tex)
J Am Acad Dermatol 51:534-542, 2004   2–6

Background.—Tumor necrosis factor-α (TNF-α) has been found to be an important mediator in the pathogenesis of psoriasis. Infliximab, a monoclonal antibody, binds specifically to TNF-α and blocks its biological activity. The efficacy and safety of infliximab induction therapy for patients with severe plaque psoriasis were investigated.

Methods.—Two hundred forty-nine patients with severe plaque psoriasis were enrolled in the multicenter, double-blind, placebo-controlled study. The patients were assigned randomly to IV infusions of 3 or 5 mg/kg infliximab or placebo administered at weeks 0, 2, and 6. The primary end point was percentage of patients in each group obtaining a 75% or better improvement in the Psoriasis Area and Severity Index score by week 10. Patients with Physician Global Assessment scores indicating moderate or severe disease at week 26 were eligible for a single infusion of their assigned treatment to assess retreatment safety after 20 weeks of no therapy.

Findings.—By week 10, the proportion of patients achieving a 75% or better improvement were 72% in the 3 mg/kg group, 88% in the 5 mg/kg group, and 6% in the placebo group. Both infliximab groups showed improvement as early as 2 weeks after treatment. One or more adverse events occurred in 63% of the placebo group, 78% of the 3 mg/kg-group, and 79% of the 5 mg/kg-group (Fig 2).

Conclusion.—Infliximab therapy produced rapid, significant improvement in the signs and symptoms of psoriasis. In general, the treatment was tolerated well.

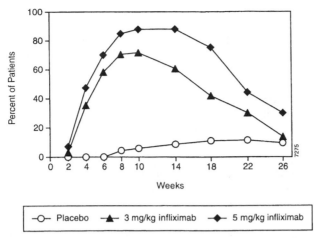

FIGURE 2.—Percent of patients achieving 75% or more improvement in Psoriasis Area and Severity Index score at each assessment point. (Reprinted by permission of the publisher from Gottlieb AB, Evans R, Li S, et al: Infliximab induction therapy for patients with severe plaque-type psoriasis: A randomized, double-blind, placebo-controlled trial. *J Am Acad Dermatol* 51:534-542, 2004. Copyright 2004 by Elsevier.)

▶ The results confirm the previously reported impressive and durable response associated with infliximab therapy. Maximum response was observed 10 weeks after the first infusion, with a gradual tendency to relapse after week 10-14. In patients with rheumatoid arthritis and Crohn's disease, the drug is administered every 8 weeks after the 3-dose induction regimen. A similar regimen might be considered for psoriasis patients, although for some, less frequent administration may be adequate. Despite its impressive efficacy, the side effects associated with infliximab infusions suggest it will likely remain a niche therapy for patients with especially severe disease.

B. H. Thiers, MD

Efficacy and Safety of Leflunomide in the Treatment of Psoriatic Arthritis and Psoriasis: A Multinational, Double-blind, Randomized, Placebo-controlled Clinical Trial

Kaltwasser JP, for the Treatment of Psoriatic Arthritis Study Group (JW Goethe-Universität, Frankfurt, Germany; et al)

Arthritis Rheum 50:1939-1950, 2004   2–7

Introduction.—Patients with psoriatic arthritis (PsA) have limited treatment options. Agents such as methotrexate and cyclosporine may be poorly tolerated or fail to improve symptoms. The multinational, randomized Treatment of Psoriatic Arthritis Study examined the safety and efficacy of leflunomide, an oral pyrimidine synthesis inhibitor, in patients with PsA and psoriasis.

Methods.—Eligible patients were aged 18 to 70, had active PsA and psoriasis with at least 3% skin involvement, and were free of other significant medical conditions. The 24-week trial assigned patients in a double-blind manner to leflunomide or placebo. Active treatment consisted of a 100 mg/d loading dose for 3 days followed by 20 mg/d orally. The primary end point was the proportion in each group classified as responders according to the Psoriatic Arthritis Response Criteria (PsARC). Joint and skin involvement, quality of life, and safety were also reported.

Results.—Of 236 screened patients, 190 met entry criteria and were randomized; 58 treated with leflunomide and 41 treated with placebo completed the study. Lack of efficacy was the main reason for withdrawal. At completion of the trial, 56 (58.9%) patients treated with leflunomide and 27 (29.7%) who received placebo were classified as responders by PsARC. Those in the leflunomide group were also significantly more likely to achieve modified American College of Rheumatology 20% improvement criteria, show improvement in the designated psoriasis target lesions, and have greater changes from baseline in Psoriasis Area and Severity Index scores and quality-of-life assessments. Side effects were common in both treatment groups, but serious adverse events, particularly alanine aminotransferase increases, were more frequent in the leflunomide group (13.5% vs 5.4% with placebo). There were no cases of serious liver toxicity.

Conclusion.—Leflunomide was well-tolerated by a majority of patients with PsA and psoriasis and proved effective in moderating joint and skin symptoms. Compared with biologic agents, orally administered leflunomide is easier to use and less costly.

▶ The clearance rates in psoriasis patients were modest at best. At 24 weeks, 30.4% of patients reached psoriasis area sensitivity index (PASI) 50 and 17.4% reached PASI 75. Although these numbers represented a barely significant improvement over placebo, they also are less than those reported with the newer biologic agents and more traditional oral therapies.

B. H. Thiers, MD

Variation in Calibration of Hand-held Ultraviolet (UV) Meters for Psoralen Plus UVA and Narrow-band UVB Phototherapy
Lloyd JJ (Royal Victoria Infirmary, Newcastle Upon Tyne, England)
Br J Dermatol 150:1162-1166, 2004   2–8

Background.—Handheld ultraviolet (UV) radiometers are routinely used to ensure that patients undergoing psoralen plus UVA (PUVA) or UVB therapy receive reproducible doses of irradiation. Accurate measurements depend on accurate calibration of the instrument, and at present, 7 medical physics departments in the United Kingdom offer radiometer calibration services. The extent of agreement between these 7 centers for calibration of meters used in UVA and narrowband UVB phototherapy was examined.

Methods.—The same UV radiometer with 2 detectors (1 used for PUVA, 1 used for narrowband UVB with a TL-01 lamp) was sent to each of 7 medical physics departments. Each department calibrated each detector and completed a questionnaire about their calibration methods.

Results.—The coefficient of variation for the UVA detector was ±9%, whereas that for the UVB detector was ±30%. Six centers used a spectroradiometer to calibrate the detector, and 1 center used the reference meter method. The spectra from the UVA lamps used at the different centers were very similar, and all centers used TL-01 lamps for calibrating the narrowband UVB detector. However, the fraction of radiation outside the main peak varied among the centers, and overall, only 79% of total UV irradiation was between 280 nm and 315 nm. Even when these variations were taken into account, the coefficient of variation with the UVB detector did not improve. Factors that did possibly affect the calibration accuracy included differences in methodology (eg, only 1 department had formal accreditation for the calibration process) and differences in instrumentation (eg, all centers used deuterium lamp reference standards, but 4 also used quartz halogen reference lamps).

Conclusion.—In the United Kingdom, radiometers used to assess output during PUVA and, especially, narrowband UVB therapy show unacceptably high variability. A calibration accuracy of approximately ±10% seems a reasonable clinical goal and could be achieved if major sources of systematic error were removed.

▶ The lack of reproducibility of meter calibration among the various medical physics departments is frightening. We have run into similar meter calibration problems with technicians servicing our phototherapy machines.

B. H. Thiers, MD

Lichen Striatus: Clinical and Laboratory Features of 115 Children
Patrizi A, Neri I, Fiorentini C, et al (Univ of Bologna, Italy)
Pediatr Dermatol 21:197-204, 2004   2–9

Introduction.—Lichen striatus occurs most often in children between the ages of 6 months and 15 years. Eruptions occur primarily on the limbs and are arranged in bands, mainly along the Blaschko lines. Affected children treated over an 11-year period were reviewed for clinical features of lichen striatus, their response to treatment, associated symptoms or diseases, and follow-up.

Methods.—Patients were seen at a pediatric dermatology unit at the University of Bologna, Italy, between January 1989 and January 2000. The median age of the cohort was 3 years. There were 78 girls and 37 boys, all of whom were white. Except for 2 pairs of siblings with the disorder, patients' family history was negative for lichen striatus. Follow-up data were obtained at periodic examinations or by telephone questionnaire.

Results.—The onset of lichen striatus was generally sudden, and full development was reached within a few days to several weeks. Lesions appeared in the winter in 46 of 115 patients. The most common clinical pattern (89 patients) consisted of pink, red, or flesh-colored, flat-topped, lichenoid papules. In 105 children, papules were grouped in a single linear or curved band. Bands were multiple and approximately parallel in 7 patients, formed a V-shaped pattern over the spine in 2 patients, and coalesced into an oval patch on the forearm in 1 patient. Lesions were limited to a single site in 92 patients; 23 had more than 1 body site affected. Seventy patients had a family or personal history of atopy, but those with and without atopy did not differ in age of onset, extension, or duration of lichen striatus. The mean duration of the disease was 6 months. Spontaneous regression occurred in 105 patients. Thirty-six patients were treated with mild- or medium-strength topical steroids, but this therapy did not appear to change the course of the disease. Only 5 children experienced a relapse, and only 1 had a prolonged course.

Discussion.—The etiology of lichen striatus remains uncertain; however, atopy may be a predisposing factor. It occurs most often in young children, in cold seasons, and with a female predilection. Histopathologic and immunohistochemical features suggest an autoimmune CD8+–mediated response against a mutated keratinocyte clone.

▶ This is the largest published case study of lichen striatus, and it documents well the clinical findings in this condition.

S. Raimer, MD

Patient Satisfaction After the Treatment of Vulvovaginal Erosive Lichen Planus With Topical Clobetasol and Tacrolimus: A Survey Study
Jensen JT, Nird M, LeClair CM (Oregon Health and Science Univ, Portland; Univ of Nevada, Las Vegas)
Am J Obstet Gynecol 190:1759-1765, 2004   2–10

Introduction.—Erosive lichen planus (ELP) is the most common desquamative and erosive dermatosis of the vulva and vagina. The lesions of severe ELP are associated with dyspareunia, pruritus, abnormal discharge, and extreme discomfort, and many cases fail to improve even with high-potency topical corticosteroids. Topical tacrolimus, which has been found safe and effective for a number of steroid-responsive dermatologic conditions, was compared with the topical steroid, clobetasol.

Methods.—The records of all women seen at a vulvar disorder clinic between June 2000 and May 2001 were reviewed to identify those with lichen planus. A survey mailed to women with ELP asked for information on clinical characteristics, sexual function, clinical response, and satisfaction with treatment that consisted of clobetasol 0.05% ointment, tacrolimus 0.1% ointment, or both.

Results.—Seventeen of 19 patients who met inclusion criteria returned the survey. The use of clobetasol ointment was reported by 16 patients and 11 had been treated with tacrolimus. Ten of the 11 who used tacrolimus ointment had been treated with clobetasol. All women reported experiencing sexual pain before their initial examination, and only 2 of 16 reported pain-free intercourse after clobetasol treatment. Switching to tacrolimus brought relief from sexual pain to 2 additional women. The 10 patients who used both therapies found tacrolimus significantly more satisfactory than clobetasol. The median satisfaction scores on a 100-mm visual analog scale were 63 for tacrolimus versus 38 for clobetasol.

Conclusion.—Vulvovaginal ELP causes considerable discomfort in affected women. There was a trend toward symptomatic improvement after the use of both clobetasol and tacrolimus ointments, but patient satisfaction was significantly higher for tacrolimus. No serious adverse events or signs of immune deficiency have been noted in safety studies of tacrolimus (with up to 1 year of follow-up).

▶ A larger, controlled prospective study of tacrolimus treatment would be useful to confirm the retrospective data reported by Jensen and colleagues. As noted by a discussant whose remarks appeared in conjunction with the paper, limitations of this study include the nonrandom subject allocation, potential recall bias, the open label treatment protocol, the small numbers of patients included, and sequential application of the two topical preparations that could have affected interpretation of the treatment results. It was unclear whether any inclusionary or exclusionary criteria were used and important details of the treatment protocols were lacking, as was any comparison between the treatment group and an untreated control group.

B. H. Thiers, MD

Does Treatment of Vulvar Lichen Sclerosus Influence Its Prognosis?
Cooper SM, Gao X-H, Powell JJ, et al (Churchill Hosp, Oxford, England; No 1 Hosp of China Med Univ, Shenyang)
Arch Dermatol 140:702-706, 2004   2–11

Background.—Lichen sclerosus (LS), a chronic inflammatory and scarring disease, can affect any cutaneous site; however, it preferentially affects the anogenital region. The clinical features, symptomatic response to topical steroids, and resolution of clinical signs were documented in a large cohort of women and girls with vulvar LS.

Methods.—The cohort included 253 women and 74 girls with a definitive clinical diagnosis of vulvar LS at 1 center in Oxfordshire, England. The average age of LS onset was 5.4 years among the girls and 55.1 years among the women. The mean follow-up period was 66 months. Topical steroids were given as part of routine care.

Findings.—The first-choice treatment for 50% of the girls and 89% of the women was an ultrapotent topical steroid. Two hundred fifty-five patients had a treatment response. Symptoms improved with treatment in 96% of the patients; 66% became symptom free, and 30% showed partial response. Four percent of the patients had a poor response. Of the 253 patients who had the signs of vulvar LS respond to topical steroids, 23% had a complete response, that is, a return of normal skin texture and color. Sixty-eight percent had a partial response, 7% had a minor response, and 2% had a poor response. Moderate or severe scarring was less common in girls than in women. Squamous cell carcinoma developed in 2.4% of the women.

Conclusions.—Topical treatment with an ultrapotent steroid seems to be effective for women and girls with vulvar LS. This therapy relieves symptoms in most patients, completely reversing the skin changes in about one fifth.

▶ This study, which included a large number of patients, confirms the positive findings from previous limited studies that suggest that topical application of ultrapotent steroids has a favorable symptomatic and prognostic effect in patients with vulvar LS.

B. H. Thiers, MD

3 Bacterial, Mycobacterial, and Fungal Infections

A Prospective, Randomized Pilot Evaluation of Topical Triple Antibiotic Versus Mupirocin for the Prevention of Uncomplicated Soft Tissue Wound Infection

Hood R, Shermock KM, Emerman C (Cleveland Clinic Foundation, Ohio; Metro Health Med Ctr, Cleveland, Ohio)

Am J Emerg Med 22:1-3, 2004   3–1

Introduction.—Both triple antibiotic ointment (TAO) and mupirocin ointment are reported to reduce the rates of infection in patients with soft tissue wounds, but these 2 agents have not been compared for safety and efficacy. There are concerns about sensitization with TAO, an agent that is considerably less expensive than mupirocin. A pilot study examined the difference in infection rates after treatment of uncomplicated soft tissue wounds with TAO and mupirocin.

Methods.—The prospective study excluded patients with puncture wounds, wounds requiring systemic antibiotic treatment, an underlying fracture, antibiotic use within the last 7 days, wounds closed with Dermabond, and wounds already showing signs of infection. Standard wound care and suturing were used in all cases. Fifty patients were randomly assigned to mupirocin (Bactroban) and 49 to TAO (Neosporin), agents with per gram costs of $1.86 and $0.25, respectively.

Results.—Patients returned for a follow-up visit within 7 days of treatment. Rates of self-reported compliance with wound care and dressing changes were similar in the Bactroban and Neosporin groups. Both signs of infection (12% vs 6.1%) and infection (4% vs 0%) were noted more frequently in the Bactroban group, but these differences were not statistically significant, and neither of the 2 cases of infection required treatment. The mean postperiod pain score was higher in the Bactroban group.

Conclusion.—Patients with uncomplicated soft tissue wounds had a low rate of infection after good initial wound management and topical antibiotic treatment. Bactroban, which costs $34.05 more per tube than Neosporin, had no advantage over Neosporin in terms of safety and efficacy. An over-the-counter TAO can be recommended for prophylaxis after uncomplicated soft tissue wounds.

▶ When mupirocin first came to market as a branded drug (Bactroban), its manufacturer carefully performed studies to demonstrate its efficacy in a variety of clinical situations. Although this inferred superiority over other topical antibacterial agents, in reality the manufacturers of these other agents—which long ago had gone generic—had never performed similar tests nor had the financial motivation to do so. The data presented by Hood et al show that, when used to prevent uncomplicated soft tissue wound infections, mupirocin is no more effective than a commonly available triple antibiotic ointment containing neomycin, bacitracin, and polymixin B.

B. H. Thiers, MD

Mupirocin Prophylaxis Against Nosocomial *Staphylococcus aureus* Infections in Nonsurgical Patients: A Randomized Study
Wertheim HFL, Vos MC, Ott A, et al (Erasmus Univ, Rotterdam, The Netherlands; Univ Med Ctr St Radboud, Nijmegen, The Netherlands; Amphia Hosp, Breda, The Netherlands; et al)
Ann Intern Med 140:419-425, 2004   3–2

Background.—Nasal carriage of *Staphylococcus aureus* increases the risk of nosocomial *S aureus* infection. Studies have shown that intranasal application of mupirocin can prevent nosocomial surgical site infections in *S aureus* carriers. Whether intranasal mupirocin prophylaxis can prevent nosocomial *S aureus* infection in nonsurgical nasal *S aureus* carriers was investigated.

Methods.—The subjects were 1602 adults (57% men; mean age, about 57 years) with culture-proven *S aureus* nasal carriage who were hospitalized in nonsurgical departments. One to 3 days after admission, patients were randomly assigned to apply either placebo or 2% mupirocin ointment intranasally twice a day for 5 days. The incidence of nosocomial infection, in-hospital mortality, duration of hospitalization, and time to development of nosocomial *S aureus* infection were compared between the 2 groups. Also, *S aureus* isolates were examined by pulsed-field gel electrophoresis to determine whether the isolates were clonally related.

Results.—The mupirocin and placebo groups were similar in terms of the proportion of patients who had nosocomial *S aureus* infection develop (2.6% vs 2.8%), in-hospital mortality rates (3.0% vs 2.8%), and duration of hospitalization (median, 8 days in both groups). However, the time to the development of nosocomial *S aureus* infection was significantly shorter in the active drug group (12 vs 25 days). Most (77%) of the nosocomial *S aureus* infections were endogenous.

Conclusion.—A strategy involving routine culture for *S aureus* at admission and the subsequent application of intranasal mupirocin in *S aureus* nasal carriers does not prevent nosocomial *S aureus* infection in nonsurgical patients.

▶ Although it has been shown that topically applied mupirocin can eradicate nasal carriage of *S aureus*, whether it can prevent *S aureus* infections in non-surgical, hospitalized patients is uncertain. This large double-blind trial included medically ill, hospitalized patients with positive nasal culture results for *S aureus*. Short-term application of intranasal mupirocin ointment did not prevent *S aureus* infections in these individuals. Whether the drug used in a repetitive dosing regimen would be more effective remains is uncertain.[1]

B. H. Thiers, MD

Reference

1. Chambers HF III, Winston LG: Mupirocin prophylaxis misses by a nose. *Ann Intern Med* 140:484-485, 2004.

Effect of Antibacterial Home Cleaning and Handwashing Products on Infectious Disease Symptoms: A Randomized, Double-Blind Trial
Larson EL, Lin SX, Gomez-Pichardo C, et al (Columbia Univ, New York)
Ann Intern Med 140:321-329, 2004   3–3

Background.—The household use of cleaning and personal hygiene products containing antibacterial ingredients is widespread. However, their effects on the incidence of infectious disease symptoms have not been established. The effect of antibacterial cleaning and hand washing products for consumers on the household occurrence of infectious disease was evaluated.

Methods.—Two hundred thirty-eight households including at least 1 preschool-age child participated in the randomized double-blind trial. A total of 1178 family members, mostly Latino, participated. By random assignment, either antibacterial or non-antibacterial products were given free to the households for general cleaning, laundry, and hand washing. All products used were commercially available, but labels were disguised. Hygiene practices and symptoms of infectious disease were monitored weekly by telephone, by monthly home visits, and in quarterly interviews for 48 weeks.

Findings.—Symptoms recorded were mainly respiratory. During 26.2% of household months, one or more household members had a runny nose; during 23.3%, a cough; and during 10.2%, a sore throat. Fevers were recorded during 11% of household months, vomiting during 2.2%, diarrhea during 2.5%, and boils or conjunctivitis during 0.77%. No significant between-group differences were observed for any symptom or for number of symptoms.

Conclusions.—The antibacterial products tested in this study did not decrease the risk of having symptoms of viral infectious disease. However, the products may have contributed to a decrease in symptoms of bacterial diseases in these households.

▶ The findings indicate that the use of antibacterial products do not reduce the risk of symptoms of viral infections. This may simply reflect the fact that the antibacterial ingredients did not affect the infectious agents responsible for the symptoms or the fact that the greatest risk for exposure and transmission occurs outside the home, where prevention efforts presumably would be more effective. Indeed, studies of several non-home settings, such as day care centers, schools, military training camps, and correctional facilities, have shown that various means of improved hygiene can reduce disease transmission and the effects of disease.[1]

B. H. Thiers, MD

Reference

1. Lachs MS: Beyond Semmelweis: Moving infection control into the community. *Ann Intern Med* 140:397-398, 2004.

Management and Outcome of Children With Skin and Soft Tissue Abscesses Caused by Community-Acquired Methicillin-Resistant *Staphylococcus aureus*
Lee MC, Rios AM, Aten MF, et al (Univ of Texas, Dallas)
Pediatr Infect Dis J 23:123-127, 2004   3–4

Introduction.—Community-acquired methicillin-resistant *Staphylococcus aureus* (CA-MRSA) is an increasingly common infection among children, even in the absence of established risk factors. A prospective, observational study focused on the management and outcome of skin and soft tissue abscesses caused by CA-MRSA in children.

Methods.—A study physician collected data at the patients' initial evaluation, at follow-up evaluations 1 to 6 days later when culture results and susceptibility findings became available, and approximately 1 week after the initial follow-up. Patients' demographics, medical histories, culture results, treatment, symptoms, and outcomes were recorded.

Results.—Sixty-nine children with skin and soft tissues abscesses and culture-proven MRSA were identified during the study period. Initial symptoms included tenderness at the infection site (97%) and erythema (92%); 48% of patients had fevers of 101.0°F or higher, and 91% had abscess fluid positive for gram-positive cocci. Treatment consisted of drainage (96% of patients) and wound packing (65%). Before culture results were known, 52 of 65 children treated as outpatients received cephalexin, 7 were given amoxicillin/clavulanate, 5 were given clindamycin, and 1 was given a combination of trimethoprim–sulfamethoxazole (TMP-SMX) and rifampin. Four children, none of whom received an antibiotic effective against CA-MRSA, were hospitalized at the initial follow-up examination. Culture results led to changes in the antibiotic prescribed in 21 patients: 18 were given

TMP-SMX with rifampin, 2 were given TMP-SMX alone, and 1 was given clindamycin. Three patients (4.3%) had a recurrent MRSA skin infection within 6 months of the initial visit.

Conclusion.—In these previously healthy children with skin and soft tissue abscesses caused by CA-MRSA, an incision and drainage produced clinical improvement in most cases. This result was seen even without administration of an appropriate antibiotic. The initial size of the lesion (>5 cm) was a significant predictor of hospitalization.

▶ The incidence of CA-MRSA infections has increased in many parts of the United States. For non-MRSA soft tissue abscesses, incision and drainage without antibiotics is generally adequate therapy. Lee et al demonstrate that, for MRSA-infected abscesses of less than 5 cm in diameter at the initial evaluation, incision and drainage combined with antibiotics to which the organism is shown by culture to be resistant is as effective as an incision and drainage combined with an antibiotic to which the organism is sensitive. Because increased resistance to antibiotics occurs with frequent antibiotic use and because a limited number of antibiotics are available to which MRSA organisms are susceptible, it would seem prudent to refrain from their use in a situation in which they are unlikely to improve the outcome. All organisms in this study were susceptible to TMP-SMX; this would appear to be the antibiotic of choice for children with lesions greater than 5 cm or for those with multiple lesions in whom antibiotic treatment seems desirable.

S. Raimer, MD

Association Between Carriage of *Streptococcus pneumoniae* and *Staphylococcus aureus* in Children

Regev-Yochay G, Dagan R, Raz M, et al (Tel-Aviv Univ, Israel; Ben Gurion Univ of the Negev, Beer-Sheva, Israel)
JAMA 292:716-720, 2004   3–5

Background.—*Streptococcus pneumoniae* and *Staphylococcus aureus* are common inhabitants of the upper respiratory tract in children and are responsible for common infections in children. *S aureus* is carried by 10% to 35% of children and by approximately 35% of the general adult population. A number of studies have examined the phenomenon of bacterial interference—the suppression of one species by another. However, no studies of potential bacterial interference between *S aureus* and *S pneumoniae* have been performed. Widespread pneumococcal conjugate vaccination may result in epidemiologic changes in the upper respiratory tract flora of children. An interaction between *S pneumoniae* and *S aureus* is of particular significance in light of the recent emergence of community-acquired methicillin-resistant *S aureus*. The prevalence and risk factors of carriage of *S pneumoniae* and *S aureus* in the prevaccination era were examined in young children.

Methods.—This cross-sectional surveillance study examined the nasopharyngeal carriage of *S pneumoniae* and nasal carriage of *S aureus* by

790 children 40 months or younger seen at primary care clinics in central Israel during February 2002. The main outcome measures were carriage rates of *S pneumoniae* (by serotype) and *S aureus* and the risk factors associated with carriage of each pathogen.

Results.—Among the 790 children screened, 43% were found to carry *S pneumoniae*, and 10% carried *S aureus*. *S aureus* carriage among the *S pneumoniae* carriers was 6.5% versus 12.9% in *S pneumoniae* noncarriers. Carriage of *S pneumoniae* among *S aureus* carriers was 27.5% versus 44.8% in *S aureus* noncarriers. Only 2.8% of patients carried both pathogens concomitantly as compared with a 4.3% expected dual carriage. Risk factors for *S pneumoniae* carriage were attendance at day care, having young siblings, and age older than 3 months. These risk factors were negatively associated with *S aureus* carriage.

Conclusions.—Carriage of *S pneumoniae*, specifically carriage of vaccine-type strains, is negatively associated with *S aureus* carriage in children. Further investigation of the implication of these findings is needed.

▶ The data suggest a protective role for *S pneumoniae* carriage against *S aureus carriage*. The authors recommend that future studies of *S pneumoniae* vaccines also investigate concurrent effects on *S aureus* epidemiology.

B. H. Thiers, MD

Safety and Immunogenicity of a Recombinant Multivalent Group A Streptococcal Vaccine in Healthy Adults: Phase 1 Trial

Kotloff KL, Corretti M, Palmer K, et al (Univ of Maryland, Baltimore; ID Biomedical Corp, Bothell, Wash; Univ of Tennessee, Memphis)
JAMA 292:709-715, 2004   3–6

Background.—Group A streptococcal infections and their sequelae are a global health problem and are responsible for a significant burden of disease throughout the world. Efforts to develop a vaccine for prevention of these infections have been going on for more than 70 years. Advances in recent years have allowed previous obstacles associated with the development of a group A streptococcal vaccine to be overcome. A preliminary evaluation of the safety and immunogenicity of ascending doses of a recombinant fusion peptide group A streptococcal vaccine containing N-terminal M protein fragments from serotypes 1, 3, 5, 6, 19, and 24 was administered to healthy volunteers.

Methods.—This open-label, uncontrolled, dose-ascending phase 1 vaccine trial was conducted among 28 healthy adult volunteers 18 to 50 years of age recruited in metropolitan Baltimore from October 5, 1999, to February 26, 2003. Recruitment was by means of newspaper advertisements and posted fliers. The patients were evaluated in the outpatient facility of a vaccine development center. Each volunteer was given 3 spaced IM injections of 50 µg (n = 8), 100 µg (n = 10), or 200 µg (n = 10) of hexavalent group A streptococcal vaccine formulated with aluminum hydroxide into the deltoid muscle of alternating arms. The main outcome measures were assessments of clinical safety, including identification of antibodies that cross-react with host tissues, and immunogenicity, as measured by enzyme-linked immunosorbent assay and assays of opsonophagocytic- and bactericidal-antibody responses.

Results.—The vaccine was well tolerated at 1 year of intensive follow-up. No evidence was found of tissue cross-reactive antibodies or immunologic complications. At the highest dose (200 μg), vaccination provoked significant increases in geometric mean antibody levels to all 6 component M antigens as measured by enzyme-linked immunosorbent assay and to 5 of 6 M types in the opsonophagocytosis assay. In addition, postvaccination increases in serum bactericidal activity of at least 30% were observed in 31 (55%) of 56 assays.

Conclusions.—These findings provided the first evidence in human beings that a hybrid fusion protein is a feasible strategy for evocation of type-specific opsonic antibodies against multiple serotypes of group A streptococcus without eliciting antibodies that cross-react with host tissues. This study represents a major advance in the development of a group A streptococcal vaccine.

▶ The recombinant multivalent group A streptococcal vaccine tested here included protein fragments from 6 pharyngitis-producing strains that have been associated with either outbreaks or a recurrence of rheumatic fever. These strains account for approximately 56% of rheumatic fever episodes and 30% of simple pharyngitis cases in the United States. As such, associated safety issues in the testing of this vaccine warrant careful consideration in light of the potential risk of rheumatic fever. The quite substantial medicolegal and regulatory challenges for group A streptococcal vaccines were discussed in an accompanying editorial.[1]

B. H. Thiers, MD

Reference

1. Pichichero ME: Group A streptococcal vaccines. *JAMA* 292:738-739, 2004.

Streptococcal Intertrigo: An Underrecognized Condition in Children
Honig PJ, Frieden IJ, Kim HJ, et al (Univ of Pennsylvania, Philadelphia; Univ of California, San Francisco; Univ of Virginia, Richmond)
Pediatrics 112:1427-1429, 2003   3–7

Background.—Group A β-hemolytic streptococci (GABHS) cause several widely known skin infections. Less well known is the streptococcal skin infection, GABHS intertrigo, an underrecognized cause of intertriginous eruptions. The typical presentation and clinical course of GABHS intertrigo in 3 patients were described.

TABLE 2.—Distinguishing Features of Candidal and GABHS Intertrigo

	Intertriginous Location	Presence of Satellites	Foul Odor	Typical Treatment
Candidal Intertrigo	Yes	Common	Rare	Topical nystatin or triazole (clotrimazole, econazole)
GABHS Intertrigo	Yes	Rare	Common	Topical mupirocin oral penicillin or cephalexin; topical hydrocortisone 1%

(Courtesy of Honig PJ, Frieden IJ, Kim HJ,at al: Streptococcal intertrigo: An underrecognized condition in children. *Pediatrics* 112:1427-1429, 2003. Copyright 2003. Reproduced with permission.)

Patients and Findings.—The 3 patients were 2 girls and 1 boy, aged 3 months, 5 months, and 5 months, respectively. The condition manifested as intense, fiery-red erythema and maceration in the intertriginous folds of the neck, axillae, or inguinal spaces. Also characteristic were a distinctive foul odor and an absence of satellite lesions. Specific clinical features were identified that help differentiate GABHS intertrigo from other conditions that mimic it (Table 2). In all patients, topical and oral antibiotic treatment with or without concomitant low-potency topical steroid application was successful.

Conclusions.—A variety of common childhood cutaneous infections result from GABHS. Infants and young children may be especially susceptible to GABHS intertrigo, an underrecognized condition in this patient population.

▶ Many β-hemolytic streptococcal infections, including perianal streptococcal disease, are easily diagnosed; however, infection with this organism remains underrecognized as a potential cause of intertriginous eruptions. In addition to antibiotics, compressing macerated areas with a solution containing salts, such as aluminum sulfate and calcium acetate, may hasten the resolution of lesions.

S. Raimer, MD

Effect of a Bacterial Pheromone Peptide on Host Chemokine Degradation in Group A Streptococcal Necrotising Soft-Tissue Infections
Hidalgo-Grass C, Dan-Goor M, Maly A, et al (Hebrew Univ, Jerusalem; Hadassah Med Ctr, Jerusalem; Univ of California, San Diego)
Lancet 363:696-703, 2004   3–8

Introduction.—Necrotizing soft tissue infections caused by group A streptococcus (GAS) are rare (about 0.2 cases per 100,000 individuals). These infections progress rapidly and cause severe necrosis and hydrolysis of soft tissues. The emergence of very widespread and virulent GAS clones indicates that the increased invasiveness may be linked with specific genetic elements acquired by horizontal transmission or phage acquisition. Genetically indistinguishable clones can be isolated from invasive and noninvasive infections, which indicates that host factors may have a role in ascertaining disease outcomes. Large quantities of bacteria and no infiltrating neutrophils have been identified in histopathologic analysis of necrotic tissue. Reported are findings from 2 patients with necrotizing soft tissue infections caused by M14 serotype GAS strains.

Methods.—Reverse transcriptase-polymerase chain reaction, enzyme-linked immunosorbent assay, and dot-blot assays were performed to determine whether GAS induces synthesis of interleukin-8 mRNA yet subsequently degrades the released chemokine protein. Class-specific protease inhibitors were used to characterize the protease that degraded the chemokine. A mouse model of human soft tissue infections was used to assess the pathogenic relevance of GAS chemokine degradation and to examine the therapeutic effect of a GAS predicted 17-amino acid pheromone peptide (SilCR) that downregulates the activity of chemokine protease.

Results.—Two isolates from the necrotic tissue were β-hemolytic GAS strains of an M14 serotype. A trypsin-like protease released by these strains degraded human interleukin-8 and its mouse homologue MIP2. When inoculated subcutaneously in mice, these strains generated a fatal necrotic soft tissue infection with decreased neutrophil recruitment to the site of injection. The M14 GAS strains have a missence mutation in the start codon of *sil*CR, which encodes SilCR. Growth of the M14 strain in the presence of SilCR terminated chemokine proteolysis. When SilCR was injected together with the bacteria, ample neutrophils were recruited to the site of infection, bacteria were cleared without systemic spreading, and the mice survived. The therapeutic effect of SilCR was also obtained in mice who were challenged with M1 and M3 GAS strains, an important cause of invasive infections.

Conclusion.—The unusual decrease in neutrophils in the necrotic tissue of 2 patients with GAS soft tissue infections is partially due to a GAS protease that degrades interleukin-8. In mice, degradation can be controlled via administration of SilCR, which downregulates GAS chemokine protease activity. This downregulation increases neutrophil migration to the site of infection and prevents bacterial spreading and, thus, the development of widespread systemic disease.

▶ Hidalgo-Grass et al show that, in patients with necrotizing GAS soft tissue infections, a protease that degrades interleukin-8 may reduce neutrophils and facilitate the spread of the infection and tissue necrosis. Conversely, in murine studies, administration of a bacterial pheromone peptide (SilCR) that downregulates the protease increases neutrophil migration and prevents bacterial spreading and development of a fulminant lethal systemic infection. This is the first time that a bacterial pheromone has been identified as a potential pathogenicity determinant which, in this instance, acts by regulating protease activity that interferes with host immune function.[1]

B. H. Thiers, MD

Reference

1. Gillespie SH: New tricks from an old dog: Streptococcal necrotising soft-tissue infections. *Lancet* 363:672-673, 2004.

The LRINEC (Laboratory Risk Indicator for Necrotizing Fasciitis) Score: A Tool for Distinguishing Necrotizing Fasciitis From Other Soft Tissue Infections
Wong C-H, Khin L-W, Heng K-S, et al (Singapore Gen Hosp; Changi Gen Hosp, Singapore; Ministry of Health, Singapore)
Crit Care Med 32:1535-1541, 2004   3–9

Background.—For patients with necrotizing fasciitis, early operative debridement is a major determinant of outcome. However, early clinical recognition of this condition is challenging. A novel diagnostic scoring system for distinguishing necrotizing fasciitis from other soft tissue infections, based on laboratory tests routinely performed in assessment of severe soft tissue infections, was presented.

Methods.—The Laboratory Risk Indicator for Necrotizing Fasciitis (LRINEC) score was developed in a cohort of 314 patients and validated in a cohort of 140. The developmental cohort included 89 consecutive patients admitted for necrotizing fasciitis and 225 control subjects selected randomly from patients admitted because of severe cellulitis or abscesses during the same period. Hematologic and biochemical values obtained on admission were converted to categorical variables, and univariate and multivariate logistic regression analyses were done to identify significant predictors.

Findings.—Variables identified as significant predictors were total white blood cell count, hemoglobin, sodium, glucose, serum creatinine, and C-reactive protein. The LRINEC score was derived by converting into integers the regression coefficients of independent predictors in the multiple logistic regression model for diagnosing necrotizing fasciitis. A cut-off value of 6 points yielded positive and negative predictive values of 92% and 96%, respectively. Area under the receiver operating characteristic curves were 0.980 in the developmental cohort and 0.976 in the validation cohort.

Conclusion.—The LRINEC score is a robust indicator useful for identifying clinically early cases of necrotizing fasciitis. The variables used in the score are routinely obtained to assess severe soft tissue infections. Patients with a score of 6 or greater should be evaluated carefully for necrotizing fasciitis.

▶ The authors describe a useful tool, the LRINEC score, which appears to be capable of detecting clinically early cases of necrotizing fasciitis. This severe soft tissue infection is potentially life threatening, and early recognition and aggressive debridement are major prognostic determinants, with any delay in their institution being associated with an increased mortality rate.[1] Unfortunately, differentiation of necrotizing fasciitis from other soft tissue infections can be difficult, with cellulitis or abscesses often considered in the differential diagnosis early in its evolution. If confirmed by future studies, using the LRINEC score may allow for early recognition, prompt treatment, and a lower mortality rate.

B. H. Thiers, MD

Reference

1. Wong CH, Chang HC, Pasupathy S, et al: Necrotizing fasciitis: Clinical presentation, microbiology and determinants of mortality. *J Bone Joint Surg Am* 85-A:1454-1460, 2003.

The Safety and Efficacy of Daptomycin for the Treatment of Complicated Skin and Skin-Structure Infections
Arbeit RD, and the Daptomycin 98-01 and 99-01 Investigators (Paratek Pharmaceuticals, Boston; et al)
Clin Infect Dis 38:1673-1681, 2004   3–10

Background.—Daptomycin is an agent from a new class of antibiotics, the cyclic lipopeptides, that has rapid, concentration-dependent bactericidal activity in vitro against a broad spectrum of gram-positive pathogens. This recently approved drug is fully active against organisms resistant to other available agents, such as oxacillin, vancomycin, and linezolid. Phase 1 and 2 clinical studies have already been reported. The safety and efficacy of daptomycin in the treatment of complicated skin and skin-structure infections were further investigated in 2 blind, multicenter, randomized controlled trials.

Methods.—A total of 1092 patients with complicated skin or skin-structure infections were included in the trials. Patients received 4 mg/kg IV daptomycin every 24 hours for 7 to 14 days, 4 to 12 g IV penicillinase-resistant penicillins per day, or 1 g IV vancomycin every 12 hours.

Findings.—Nine hundred two patients were clinically assessable. The clinical success rate was 83.4% for the daptomycin group and 84.2% for the comparison groups. Among those treated successfully with IV daptomycin, 63% needed only 4 to 7 days of treatment compared with 33% of those treated with the conventional agents. The treatment groups had similar frequencies and distributions of adverse events.

Conclusions.—Daptomycin has shown activity against a wide range of gram-positive organisms, including those resistant to all other currently available drugs. The trials reported above show that daptomycin at a dosage of 4 mg/kg per day is as effective and safe as standard therapy in the treatment of complicated skin or skin-structure infections caused by gram-positive pathogens.

▶ Daptomycin is a new option for treatment of methicillin- and vancomycin-resistant organisms. Although it has activity against a broad range of gram-positive pathogens, it would best be used very selectively as widespread use would tend to encourage the emergence of daptomycin-resistant strains.

B. H. Thiers, MD

Gram-Negative Cellulitis Complicating Cirrhosis
Horowitz Y, Sperber AD, Almog Y (Ben-Gurion Univ, Beer-Sheva, Israel)
Mayo Clin Proc 79:247-250, 2004   3–11

Background.—Patients with cirrhosis are at risk of development of serious bacterial infections. Soft tissue infections occur in up to 11% of patients with cirrhosis, and most of these are due to gram-positive cocci. Four patients with cirrhosis who had fulminant gram-negative cellulitis were described.

> *Case Report.*—Woman, 55, was admitted to the hospital with vomiting, diffuse abdominal pain, and pain in the right leg. She had cirrhosis due to hepatitis C virus infection and coincident hypothyroidism. Hypertension and oliguria developed and the patient was intubated. She was given ofloxacin and clindamycin and transferred to the medical ICU. Chest radiograph results were normal, urine culture was negative, and the patient had only mild ascites. However, her right leg was swollen and multiple hemorrhagic bullae were present.
> Cultures of blood and fluid taken from the bullae were positive for *Escherichia coli.* Despite full supportive treatment, septic shock and multiple organ failure developed, and the patient died. The clinical courses and outcomes for 3 other patients with cirrhosis (2 women and 1 man, 42-73 years of age) were similar.

Conclusion.—Gram-negative enteric pathogens are common in patients with cirrhosis, but skin infections in these patients are typically caused by gram-positive organisms. Because of the high risk of mortality in cirrhotic patients with gram-negative skin infections, early recognition and prompt treatment are crucial. Cutaneous infection with a gram-negative organism should be suspected when patients with cirrhosis develop severe bullous cellulitis. Culture of the bullae contents may assist in the diagnosis. Pending the culture results, these patients should be promptly treated with antibiotics effective against gram-negative bacteria.

▶ Although gram-positive organisms are the most prevalent pathogens in patients with cirrhosis, in cirrhotic patients it is wise to institute therapy with antibiotics that are effective against gram-negative bacteria until culture results are available.

B. H. Thiers, MD

Outbreak of *Pseudomonas aeruginosa* Infections Caused by Commercial Piercing of Upper Ear Cartilage
Keene WE, Markum AC, Samadpour M (Oregon Dept of Human Services, Portland; Klamath County Dept of Public Health, Klamath Falls, Ore; Univ of Washington, Seattle)
JAMA 291:981-985, 2004   3–12

Background.—Sporadic reports of infection developing after ear piercing are not uncommon. Common-source outbreaks of infection after ear piercing, however, have not been documented. In September 2000, an otolaryngologist treated 2 patients with suppurating ear infection who recently had had their upper ear pierced at the same jewelry kiosk. Cultures from wounds in both patients were positive for *Pseudomonas aeruginosa*. Results from the local health department's investigation of this common-source outbreak were described.

Methods.—Health officials inspected the records of the implicated jewelry kiosk to identify people who underwent piercing from August through mid September 2000. Local medical facilities were also contacted. Environmental samples were obtained and submitted for molecular subtyping of isolates. Confirmed infection was defined as any infection that developed at the piercing site within 2 weeks of piercing that grew *P aeruginosa* on culture. Suspected infection was defined as signs and symptoms of external ear infection (eg, drainage of pus or blood) for at least 2 weeks after piercing.

Results.—During the study period, 118 people underwent 186 ear piercings. At least 63 piercings (34%) were made in the upper ear cartilage. *P aeruginosa* grew from specimens obtained from 2 of the 4 kiosk workers; from a "single-use" disinfectant bottle that at least 1 of the workers repeatedly refilled and used to spray the ear, stud, and piercing gun; and from waste water in traps beneath both sinks. In all, 7 piercings (4%) in 7 patients had confirmed *P aeruginosa* infection and 18 (10%) had suspected infection.

All 7 piercings with confirmed infection involved the upper ear cartilage; piercings in the upper ear cartilage were significantly more likely than piercings in the ear lobe to have suspected infection (relative risk, 3.6). Specimens from the 7 cases of confirmed infection were indistinguishable on microrestriction fingerprinting. At least 14 people sought medical attention, including all 7 patients with confirmed infection. These 7 patients were 10 to 19 years old and sought medical advice 2 to 8 days after symptom onset. Most of them were initially treated with cephalosporins or other drugs ineffective against *P aeruginosa*.

Five patients required IV therapy (1 inpatient) or incision and drainage surgery (3 as inpatients, 1 as an outpatient). Active infection took up to 3 months to resolve, and many people had significant disfigurement of the pinna.

Conclusion.—Ear cartilage is much more susceptible to serious *P aeruginosa* infection than is the ear lobe. It is important that infection control training be used, even in nonmedical settings. Physicians treating patients with potential auricular chondritis should include piercing-related *P aeruginosa* infection in the differential diagnosis.

▶ This report illustrates the serious sequelae that can result when infection control techniques are not properly followed and also confirms the previously reported assertion that ear cartilage is more prone to serious infection than is the earlobe.

B. H. Thiers, MD

Macrolide Resistance in *Treponema pallidum* in the United States and Ireland
Lukehart SA, Godornes C, Molini BJ, et al (Univ of Washington, Seattle; St James Hosp, Dublin; San Francisco Dept of Health; et al)
N Engl J Med 351:154-158, 2004   3–13

Background.—Because of its efficacy and convenience, azithromycin is being used increasingly to treat syphilis in North America; however, the Centers for Disease Control and Prevention does not currently recommend it. Several cases of azithromycin failure in the treatment of syphilis have been recognized. One example of clinical failure of this treatment was presented.

> *Case Report.*—Man, 33, with HIV infection was seen in a local emergency department in July 2003 because of a nontender penile ulcer. Azithromycin, 2 g orally, was given. The next day, he independently took an additional 1 g of azithromycin. The day after this additional dose, he came to an STD clinic for follow-up, where the diagnosis of primary syphilis was verified and the treatment was judged to be adequate. However, 3 days later, the patient returned with a persistent ulcer that was found to be dark-field-positive for *Treponema pallidum*. Serum VDRL and *T pallidum* particle-agglutination testing were reactive, and azithromycin treatment was considered a failure. Penicillin G benzathine, 2.4 mU, was given intramuscularly. At the patient's 2-week follow-up visit, the lesion had resolved. At 3 months, a repeat VDRL test was nonreactive. In a specimen of *T pallidum* obtained from this patient, a mutation in the 23S ribosomal RNA gene was identified. Functional azithromycin resistance was confirmed in vivo in a strain of *T pallidum* that contain this mutation. Subsequently, the mutation in the 23S ribosomal RNA gene identified in the *T pallidum* specimen from the current patient was found to occur at a high frequency in clinical specimens obtained from 4 geographically diverse sites.

Conclusion.—Several cases of azithromycin failure in the treatment of syphilis have been observed.

▶ The patients reported in this article, who were seen at selected STD clinics in the United States and Ireland, may not reflect the true prevalence of macrolide resistance of *T pallidum*. In an ongoing multicenter trial of a single 2-g dose of azithromycin for early syphilis, no clinical failures have been observed in approximately 100 study participants who were randomly assigned to receive azithromycin and observed for at least 6 months. In contrast to the patients reported by Lukehart et al, none of the patients in this multicenter trial were infected with HIV. Moreover, the race and demographic characteristics of the trial participants differ considerably from those reported here, and there may, likewise, be substantial geographic differences in the distribution of *T pallidum* strains. Nevertheless, the data presented in this article suggest that the use of azithromycin for treating syphilis should be avoided in geographic regions where macrolide resistance may be relatively high.

B. H. Thiers, MD

Mass Treatment With Single-Dose Azithromycin for Trachoma
Solomon AW, Holland MJ, Alexander NDE, et al (London School of Hygiene and Tropical Medicine; Tumaini Univ, Moshi, Tanzania; Huruma Hosp, Mkuu, Rombo, Tanzania; et al)
N Engl J Med 351:1962-1971, 2004   3–14

Background.—Repeated ocular infection with *Chlamydia trachomatis* can result in trachoma, an important cause of blindness. A quantitative polymerase chain reaction (PCR) assay was used to determine the effect of high-coverage mass distribution of azithromycin on ocular chlamydial infection in a Tanzanian community where trachoma was endemic.

Methods.—Conjunctival swabs were collected from community residents for quantitative PCR assay of *C trachomatis* before treatment and at 2, 6, 12, 18, and 24 months after treatment with azithromycin. At 6, 12, and 18 months, tetracycline eye ointment was given to residents with clinically active trachoma.

Findings.—At baseline, 97.8% of the 978 residents were given an oral dose of azithromycin or, when this therapy was contraindicated, a course of tetracycline eye ointment. The prevalence of infection dropped from 9.5% before mass treatment to 2.1% at 2 months. At 24 months, the prevalence was 0.1%. Overall, the quantitative burdens of ocular *C trachomatis* infection at 2 and 24 months were 13.9% and 0.8% of pretreatment levels, respectively. At each point of assessment after baseline, more than 90% of the total community burden of *C trachomatis* infection occurred in residents who had previously tested positive.

Conclusion.—In this Tanzanian community where trachoma was endemic, the prevalence and intensity of infection declined substantially and remained low for 2 years after mass treatment.

▶ Trachoma remains the leading cause of preventable blindness in the world.[1] The authors demonstrate that one round of very high coverage mass treatment with azithromycin, perhaps aided by subsequent periodic use of tetracycline eye ointment for persons with active disease, can interrupt the transmission of ocular *C trachomatis* infection.

B. H. Thiers, MD

Reference

1. Mariotti SP: New steps toward eliminating blinding trachoma. *N Engl J Med* 351:2004-2007, 2004.

Diagnosis of Tuberculosis in South African Children With a T-Cell-Based Assay: A Prospective Cohort Study
Liebeschuetz S, Bamber S, Ewer K, et al (Ngwelezana Hosp, Empangeni, South Africa; King George V Hosp, Durban, South Africa; Univ of Oxford, England; et al)
Lancet 364:2196-2203, 2004   3–15

Introduction.—Tuberculosis may present with nonspecific symptoms and is a common differential diagnosis in sick children living in areas with a high prevalence of the disease, such as sub-Saharan Africa. Because untreated tuberculosis is rapidly fatal in children with HIV infection, empirical therapy is often administered. A more accurate alternative to the tuberculin skin test (TST), which has low sensitivity in children with active tuberculosis, would improve the diagnostic assessment and prevent inappropriate treatment.

Methods.—A T-cell–based rapid blood test for *Mycobacterium tuberculosis* infection, the enzyme-linked immunospot assay (ELISPOT), was examined for its usefulness in African children with suspected tuberculosis. Children were enrolled from November 2000 through August 2001 at 2 hospitals in kwaZulu-Natal, a region of South Africa with high rates of HIV and tuberculosis. A total of 293 children underwent a full clinical assessment, the TST, and ELISPOT. Test results were compared with final clinical and microbiological diagnoses.

Results.—ELISPOT results were available for 262 children: 57 with confirmed tuberculosis (43 with TST results), 76 with highly probable tuberculosis (73 with TST results), 116 with possible tuberculosis or lost to follow-up (93 with TST results), and 13 without tuberculosis (9 with TST results). The diagnostic sensitivity of ELISPOT (83%) was significantly higher than that of the TST (63%), and this was also true for the subgroup of 116 children for whom both test results were available. In the subgroup with confirmed tuberculosis, the sensitivity of TST was only 35% as compared with the 81% sensitivity of ELISPOT. Combining the tests yielded a sensitivity of 91%. The sensitivity of TST fell significantly in children younger than 3 years (to 51%), with co-infection (36%), or with malnutrition (44%). None of these factors significantly reduced the sensitivity of ELISPOT.

Conclusion.—The diagnostic sensitivity of ELISPOT is superior to that of the TST and is less affected by factors likely to coexist with childhood tuberculosis in developing countries. ELISPOT assays were done in a district hospital laboratory by a pediatrician with only 1 week of training in the test. To have a substantial effect in the developing world, the test must become less expensive, and its technique must be simplified.

▶ An article reviewed in the 2004 YEAR BOOK OF DERMATOLOGY AND DERMATOLOGIC SURGERY showed the ELISPOT assay to be more sensitive and specific than the TST.[1] Although the TST is undoubtedly cheaper, related indirect costs, such as the need for return visits and trained staff to administer and read the tests, must also be considered.

B. H. Thiers, MD

Reference

1. Ewer K, Deeks J, Alvarez L, et al: Comparison of T-cell-based assay with tuberculin skin test for diagnosis of *Mycobacterium tuberculosis* infection in a school tuberculosis outbreak. *Lancet* 361:1168-1173, 2003. (2004 YEAR BOOK OF DERMATOLOGY AND DERMATOLOGIC SURGERY, p 127.)

The Clinical Management and Outcome of Nail Salon–Acquired *Mycobacterium fortuitum* Skin Infection
Winthrop KL, Albridge K, South D, et al (California Dept of Health Services, Berkeley; Santa Cruz County Health Agency, Calif; Santa Cruz Med Clinic, Calif)
Clin Infect Dis 38:38-44, 2004   3–16

Background.—*Mycobacterium fortuitum* and other rapidly growing mycobacteria can cause cutaneous infections, usually in association with trauma or clinical procedures. In 2002, these authors described a large outbreak of severe, lower extremity *M fortuitum* furunculosis among patrons who had received pedicures in a single nail salon whirlpool footbath. Similar outbreaks of furunculosis associated with whirlpool footbaths have occurred since then, but little is known about the natural history and optimal clinical management of these infections. Thus, a subset of patients from the original outbreak was monitored to describe the clinical and diagnostic features of these infections.

Methods.—The authors contacted physicians who had treated patients in the 2002 outbreak (>115 patients) and asked them to enroll all their patients who had been affected. Clinical data on the 61 enrolled patients (60 females; age range, 13-53 years) were analyzed to determine clinical characteristics, disease duration, and response to treatment.

Results.—None of the patients was positive for HIV infection, and 3 were pregnant when they contracted the infection. Patients had 1 to 20 boils at presentation (median, 2 boils), and the disease lasted from 41 to 336 days (mean disease duration, 170 days). In all, 13 patients (21.3%) were not treated, but 48 patients (78.7%) were treated with antibiotics for 2 weeks to 6 months (median, 4 months). The disease resolved in all patients, but 1 initially untreated woman had lymphatic dissemination of the infection and required drainage and antibiotics for a large intrathigh abscess. All isolates tested were susceptible to amikacin, ciprofloxacin, and minocycline. Among the patients with a single boil, the mean disease duration was similar in the treated and untreated groups (147 vs 123 days). Among patients with multiple boils, however, the median duration of the disease was significantly shorter when antibiotic therapy was initiated within 70 days after disease onset.

Conclusion.—Lower extremity *M fortuitum* furunculosis can be self-limiting in healthy hosts, but early antibiotic therapy will benefit patients with multiple boils. Rapidly growing mycobacteria should be considered in the differential diagnosis of patients with difficult-to-treat soft tissue infections, particularly if the patient has a history of using the whirlpool footbaths popular in nail salons.

▶ This article provides further follow-up on the nail salon-acquired *M fortuitum* outbreak reported previously.[1]

B. H. Thiers, MD

Reference

1. Winthrop KL, Abrams M, Yakrus M, et al: An outbreak of mycobacterial furunculosis associated with footbaths at a nail salon. *N Engl J Med* 346:1366-1371, 2002.

Steroid Prophylaxis for Prevention of Nerve Function Impairment in Leprosy: Randomised Placebo Controlled Trial (TRIPOD 1)
Smith WCS, Anderson AM, Withington SG, et al (Univ of Aberdeen, Scotland; Internatl Nepal Fellowship, Pokhera, Nepal)
BMJ 328:1459-1463, 2004   3–17

Introduction.—Nerve function impairment leads to limitations in physical activity and social participation in patients with leprosy. Multidrug treatment for leprosy is aimed primarily at killing *Mycobacterium leprae* and not at preventing progressive damage to peripheral nerves. Because some evidence exists that the addition of steroids might prevent nerve damage, a multicenter, double-blind trial conducted in Bangladesh and Nepal randomly selected patients to placebo or prednisolone, plus multidrug treatment.

Methods.—The study included 636 patients with newly diagnosed multibacillary leprosy. Those in the steroid arm received prednisolone, 20 mg daily for 3 months, with a tapering dose in month 4, in addition to antimycobacterial therapy. Excluded were patients younger than 15 or older than 50 years, women who knew they were pregnant, and those taking long-term medication unrelated to leprosy. Follow-up visits took place at months 1, 2, 3, 4, 6, 9, and 12 after the start of multidrug treatment. The primary outcome measure was signs of acute reaction or new nerve function impairment requiring full-dose prednisolone at 4 months and 1 year.

Results.—At 4 months, prednisolone produced a significant effect in the prevention of reaction and nerve function impairment. A new primary event had been experienced at 4 months by 15% in the placebo group versus 4% in the prednisolone group. The difference was less evident at 12 months (8 months after completion of active treatment) with primary events experienced by 22% of the placebo group and 17% of the prednisolone group. Pre-existing nerve function impairment (at the time of diagnosis) reduced the response to steroid prophylaxis.

Conclusion.—Low-dose prophylactic prednisolone, administered to newly diagnosed patients with leprosy at the start of multidrug treatment, was effective in the short term in reducing signs of reaction and nerve function impairment. However, the beneficial effect of the steroid was not sustained.

▶ A frequent complication of leprosy is irreversible peripheral nerve damage. Such damage usually occurs in reactional states associated with antileprosy treatment and is difficult to treat and reverse. This article shows that low-dose systemic steroids can prevent nerve function impairment and reactions in the short-term, but the effect is not long lasting. Moreover, no benefits were noted in patients with pre-existing nerve function impairment. Any benefits of steroid prophylaxis must be balanced against the potential risk of using such drugs in developing countries where infectious diseases, such as tuberculosis, still predominate.

B. H. Thiers, MD

Clinical and Histological Aspects of Toenail Onychomycosis Caused by *Aspergillus* spp: 34 Cases Treated With Weekly Intermittent Terbinafine
Gianni C, Romano C (S Raffaele Hosp, Milan; Univ of Siena, Italy)
Dermatology 209:104-110, 2004   3–18

Introduction.—*Aspergillus*, the second most common agent of nondermatophytic onychomycosis, does not respond to topical therapy, but systemic treatment with continuous terbinafine or pulsed itraconazole has proven quite effective. This study of patients with toenail onychomycosis caused by *Aspergillus* spp described the clinical appearance of the disorder, the pathogenic role of these organisms, and the efficacy and safety of weekly intermittent terbinafine therapy.

Methods.—In a mycologic study of 2154 patients with onychodystrophy who were seen over a 2-year period, 1288 cases of onychomycosis (57%) were identified. Nondermatophytic onychomycosis caused by *Aspergillus* spp represented 2.6% of all onychomycoses. The 34 affected patients, 12 men and 22 women, ranged in age from 30 to 82 years. Nail samples were taken for confirmation of the diagnosis and were prepared for histologic examination and microscopic examination of cultures.

Results.—All 34 patients were otherwise healthy and not immunosuppressed. The large toenails were most often affected, usually with more that

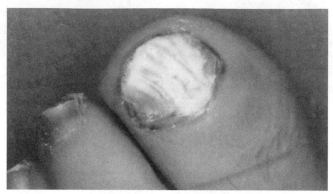

FIGURE 2.—Total chalky deep white nail with paronychia due to *Aspergillus alliaceus*. (Courtesy of Gianni C, Romano C: Clinical and histological aspects of toenail onychomycosis caused by *Aspergillus* spp: 34 cases treated with weekly intermittent terbinafine. *Dermatology* 209:104-110, 2004. Reproduced with permission of S. Karger AG, Basel.)

50% of the surface involved. Clinical features associated with onychomycosis caused by *Aspergillus* spp included a chalky deep white nail (Fig 2; see color plate XIV), rapid involvement of lamina, and painful paronychia without pus. Nails infected with *Aspergillus niger* were often black on one side and white on the other (Fig 5; see color plate XXX), an appearance similar to that observed in culture. Patients were treated with pulsed oral terbi-

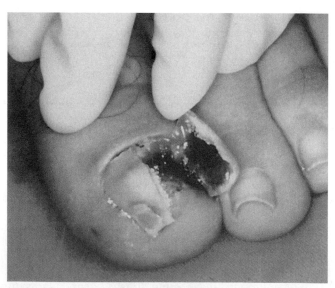

FIGURE 5.—Onychomycosis caused by *Aspergillus niger*: leuconychia and deep dark discoloration. (Courtesy of Gianni C, Romano C: Clinical and histological aspects of toenail onychomycosis caused by *Aspergillus* spp: 34 cases treated with weekly intermittent terbinafine. *Dermatology* 209:104-110, 2004. Reproduced with permission of S. Karger AG, Basel.)

nafine (500 m/d for 1 week each month for 3 months). Four patients discontinued therapy, 2 because of gastrointestinal side effects and 2 because of forgetfulness. No serious adverse events occurred, and blood chemistry findings were normal during therapy. At 12-months' follow-up, 30 patients (88%) had achieved clinical and mycologic recovery.

Conclusion.—Terbinafine was particularly effective in the treatment of nail infections caused by *Aspergillus* spp. The pulsed regimen used in these patients was less costly and demanding than continuous systemic therapy.

▶ Nondermatophytic onychomycoses are said to represent 1.45% to 17.6% of all fungal nail infections. *Scopulariopsis* species are the most commonly implicated, and the genus *Aspergillus* is the second most common. A chalky white nail is one of the distinguishing clinical features of *Aspergillus* nail infections. Rapid extension appears to be the rule, in contrast to the dermatophytic onychomycoses, which spread in a more insidious manner.

B. H. Thiers, MD

Evaluation of In Vitro Resistance in Patients With Onychomycosis Who Fail Antifungal Therapy
Gupta AK, Kohli Y (Univ of Toronto; Hosp for Sick Children, Toronto; Mediprobe Labs Inc, London, Ont, Canada)
Dermatology 207:375-380, 2003   3–19

Background.—The increasing use of antifungals to treat onychomycosis raises concerns about the possible emergence of resistant strains. A retrospective study was done to determine the relationship between in vitro and clinical resistance in strains of *Trichophyton rubrum* cultured from patients with recalcitrant dermatophyte toenail onychomycosis.

Methods.—Dermatophyte strains were obtained from 18 patients with chronic onychomycosis unresponsive to antifungal treatment with itraconazole or terbinafine. Multiple sequential strains from 11 patients were used in the analysis. Susceptibility testing was performed against 4 antifungals—itraconozole, ketoconazole, terbinafine, and ciclopirox—by the broth microdilution method.

Findings.—All strains were susceptible to 3 of the 4 antifungal agents. No direct correlation was found between clinical resistance and in vitro resistance. However, increased minimum inhibitory concentration values for ketoconazole were seen in strains obtained after treatment from 3 patients. Other factors that may have led to treatment failure were found in all but 1 patient.

Conclusion.—Increased resistance in the causative organisms is possible as the use of antifungals to treat various fungal infections increases. However, other factors may also play a role in treatment failure.

▶ Unfortunately, no clear association exists between in vitro resistance to an antifungal agent and clinical response. The authors show that although drug resistance may be a factor in treatment failure, other potential causes may play a more significant role. These may include a reduced immune response against the infecting organism, an underlying dystrophic nail, noncompliance, or environmental factors such as heat and humidity.

B. H. Thiers, MD

4 Viral Infections (Excluding HIV Infection)

Cutting Edge: Prolonged Antigen Presentation After Herpes Virus-1 Skin Infection
Stock AT, Mueller SN, van Lint AL, et al (Univ of Melbourne, Australia; Walter and Eliza Hall Inst of Med Research, Parkville, Australia; Cooperative Research Centre for Vaccine Technology, Brisbane, Australia)
J Immunol 173:2241-2244, 2004   4–1

Introduction.—Recent in vivo trials have reported surprisingly transient levels of antigen (Ag) presentation after infection with certain viruses, bacteria, and parasites. It was possible to detect Ag presentation within hours of infection, yet it appeared to be extinguished variously by 1 or 2 days after its initiation. The loss of Ag presentation in *Listeria monocytogenes* coincided with the emergence of lytic Ag-specific cytotoxic T lymphocytes (CTL) in the lymphoid organ. The kinetics of Ag presentation after skin infection with herpes simplex virus (HSV)-1 were evaluated by means of a murine model.

Methods.—C57BL/6 mice were inoculated with HSV-1 subcutaneously into each hind footpad. The *lacZ*-inducible glycoprotein B (gB)-specific T cell hybridoma HSV-2.3E2 was used to identify gB epitope-bearing APCs in popliteal lymph nodes after HSV-1 footpad infection.

Results.—The period of Ag presentation capable of priming naive CD8+ T cells was comparatively prolonged, persisting for at least 7 days after infection. It continued despite the appearance of localized CTL activity. The Ag presentation was abbreviated to 3 or 4 days post infection by surgical excision of the inoculation site early after infection. The intervention attenuated the size of the primary CTL response, indicating that prolonged presentation is needed to drive maximal CTL expansion.

Conclusion.—In some types of infection, CTL priming can extend well beyond the initial 24 to 48 hours after primary inoculation.

▶ Initiation of a primary cytotoxic T-lymphocyte response to intracellular pathogens is dependent upon recognition by naïve cells of antigenic peptide in the context of MHC I displayed by Ag-presenting cells. It has been shown previously that the period of Ag presentation is relatively short (1 to 2 days) after infection with organisms such as *Listeria* and malaria parasites.

In this study, the investigators examined the kinetics of Ag presentation in a murine model of skin infection with HSV-1. The results obtained showed that Ag presentation and CTL activity persisted for at least 1 week after initial infection. Early excision of the site of infection in the skin severely limited spread of the virus to the dorsal root ganglia and subsequent reemergence of virus in the skin. However, even in the absence of replicating virus, persistence of viral Ag presentation was detectable in the draining lymph nodes for about 4 days.

This prompted the authors to examine the effect of early excision of infection on the expansion of the cytotoxic cell population. The data revealed that a minimum period of 2 hours after infection was necessary to stimulate detectable proliferation of the viral-specific T cells and that although a strong T-cell response was found after site excision 24 hours after infection, this was only half the magnitude of the response after uninterrupted infection. It therefore seems likely that persistence of Ag presentation is—at least in HSV infection—required for an optimal immune response.

G. M. P. Galbraith, MD

Neonatal Genital Herpes Simplex Virus Type 1 Infection After Jewish Ritual Circumcision: Modern Medicine and Religious Tradition
Gesundheit B, Grisaru-Soen G, Greenberg D, et al (Ben Gurion Univ, Beer Sheva, Israel; Tel Aviv Univ, Israel)
Pediatrics 114:e259-e263, 2004   4–2

Background.—In 1 series of neonates undergoing traditional Jewish ritual circumcision, genital neonatal herpes simplex virus type 1 (HSV-1) infection was observed after the procedure. Neonatal genital HSV-1 infection after ritual circumcision was described, and the relationship between genital HSV-1 after circumcision and the practice of the traditional circumcision was investigated.

Methods and Findings.—Eight infants with genital HSV-1 infection after ritual circumcision were included in the analysis. The mean time from circumcision to clinical manifestations was 7.25 days. In all cases, the circumciser had performed an ancient custom of orally suctioning the blood after cutting the foreskin. Currently, this practice is used by only a minority of circumcisers. IV acyclovir therapy was given to 6 infants. Four had recurrent episodes of genital HSV infection. In 1 neonate, HSV encephalitis developed with neurologic sequelae. Of the 4 circumcisers tested for HSV antibodies, all were found to be seropositive.

Conclusions.—Ritual Jewish circumcision that includes the ancient custom of oral suctioning of blood after the foreskin is cut is associated with a serious risk for HSV transmission from the circumciser. This transmission can result in protracted or severe infection in the infant.

▶ In the United States, when a Jewish circumcision is performed, the use of a straw has all but replaced direct oral-genital contact during the ceremony.

B. H. Thiers, MD

Once-Daily Valacyclovir to Reduce the Risk of Transmission of Genital Herpes

Corey L, for the Valacyclovir HSV Transmission Study Group (Univ of Washington, Seattle; et al)
N Engl J Med 350:11-20, 2004   4–3

Background.—Both symptomatic and asymptomatic herpes simplex virus type 2 (HSV-2) infection have been shown to result from sexual transmission. Population-based studies in the United States have indicated that 22% of adults have antibodies to HSV-2 and that an estimated 1.6 million new cases of HSV-2 infection are acquired annually. Worldwide, HSV-2 is the most frequent cause of genital ulcer disease. Transmission of genital herpes to other individuals is the main concern of patients with known genital herpes. Nucleoside analogs against HSV-2 have been shown to suppress shedding of HSV-2 on genital mucosal surfaces and may prevent sexual transmission of HSV. The efficacy of the nucleoside analog valacyclovir against the transmission of HSV-2 was assessed.

Methods.—The study included 1484 immunocompetent, heterosexual, monogamous couples. In each couple, 1 individual had clinically symptomatic genital HSV-2, and the other was susceptible to HSV-2. The partners with HSV-2 infection were randomly assigned to receive either 500 mg of valacyclovir once daily or placebo for 8 months. The susceptible partner was evaluated monthly for clinical signs and symptoms of genital herpes. Source partners were monitored for a recurrence of genital herpes, and 89 were subsequently enrolled in an associated study of HSV-2 mucosal shedding. Both partners in each couple were counseled regarding safer sex and were offered condoms at each visit. The main outcome measure was the reduction in transmission of symptomatic genital herpes.

Results.—Clinically symptomatic HSV-2 infection developed in 4 (0.54%) of 743 susceptible partners in the valacyclovir group compared with its development in 16 (2.2%) of 741 susceptible partners who were given placebo. Acquisition of HSV-2 (including those identified by seroconversion) was observed in 14 (1.9%) of the susceptible partners who received valacyclovir compared with 27 (3.6%) of the partners who received placebo. HSV DNA was detected in samples of genital secretions on 2.9% of the days among the HSV-2–infected source partners who received valacyclovir compared with 10.8% of the days among infected source partners who received placebo. The mean rates of recurrence were 0.11 per month and 0.4 per month for valacyclovir and placebo groups, respectively.

Conclusion.—A once-daily regimen of suppressive therapy with valacyclovir can significantly reduce the risk of transmission of genital herpes among heterosexual, HSV-discordant couples.

▶ These data confirm that a once-daily dose of 500 mg valacyclovir significantly reduces the risk of transmission of genital herpes among heterosexual, HSV-2–discordant couples. However, the observed reduction is not complete; thus, it is important that safe sex practices be maintained to further reduce the risk of transmission. A trial is planned to determine if acyclovir prophylaxis reduces the risk of HIV-1 transmission.[1]

B. H. Thiers, MD

Reference

1. Crumpacker CS: Use of antiviral drugs to prevent herpesvirus transmission. *N Engl J Med* 350:67-68, 2004.

Identification of Potential Candidates for Varicella Vaccination by History: Questionnaire and Seroprevalence Study
MacMahon E, Brown LJ, Bexley S, et al (Guy's and St Thomas' Hosp NHS Trust, London; Guy's, King's, and St Thomas' School of Medicine, London)
BMJ 329:551-552, 2004   4–4

Introduction.—The new guidelines from the UK Joint Commission on Vaccination and Immunization will advise that all workers in health care settings with no history or an uncertain history of chickenpox or shingles at pre-employment evaluation should be tested for varicella zoster virus IgG. Vaccination with the newly licensed varicella vaccine will be advised for workers with a seronegative result. A history of chickenpox has a high positive predictive value for immunity among health care workers in Europe: the seroprevalence rate is 98.5%. The validity of a history of chickenpox is not known in tropical countries, where the mean age of infection is in early adulthood. The Guy's and St Thomas' Hospital NHS Trust in inner London has about 8000 staff and 4700 health care students with increasingly heterogeneous origins. A questionnaire and seroprevalence investigation was performed at the hospital and was evaluated to determine the association between a history of chickenpox, countries of birth and residence, and serologic status.

Methods.—A nurse-administered questionnaire was completed by 747 consecutive staff and students participating in pre-employment screening from September 2001 to July 2002.

Results.—Of 629 tested participants (84%), 6 had equivocal results and were excluded. Participants who denied or who were not sure of past infection were regarded as 1 group. Participants were assigned to "temperate" or "tropical" subgroups according to their country of birth or first residence. Shingles had a positive predictive value of 100%; all 22 participants had IgG-positive findings. Twenty-nine participants in the temperate group had not lived exclusively in temperate zones during their first 12 years and had a decreased risk of having seropositive test results (odds ratio, 0.35 compared with those born and raised in a temperate climate); this was similar to those born and raised in a tropical climate (odds ratio, 0.36). Participants from Sub-Saharan Africa and the Caribbean were disproportionately represented in the seronegative group (29% and 17%, respectively, compared with 18% and 5%, respectively, among all new recruits). In participants with a history of prior infection, the false-positive rate was 9.3% for the tropical group compared with 3.7% for the temperate group ($P = .091$).

Conclusion.—Candidates for varicella vaccination (staff with seronegative findings) will probably be missed if a blanket policy of screening by history alone is implemented. Their number will rise markedly if groups with a significantly higher false-positive rate make up a significant proportion of the health care workforce.

▶ Although a history of varicella is a reliable indicator of past infection in temperate climates, this does not appear to be true for people born and raised in tropical climates. In those areas, seronegative candidates for varicella vaccination will be missed if a blanket policy of screening by history alone is adopted.

B. H. Thiers, MD

Decline in Varicella-Related Hospitalizations and Expenditures for Children and Adults After Introduction of Varicella Vaccine in the United States
Davis MM, Patel MS, Gebremariam A (Univ of Michigan, Ann Arbor)
Pediatrics 114:786-792, 2004   4–5

Introduction.—Immunization against varicella, recommended for all children aged 12 months and older by the American Academy of Pediatrics in 1995, was anticipated to decrease markedly the number of hospitalizations and costs related to severe varicella. The number of cases significantly declined, but some studies failed to report a similar trend in varicella-related hospitalizations. Data from the Nationwide Inpatient Sample, however, indicate that both hospitalizations and varicella-related costs have been reduced.

Methods.—Data from the Nationwide Inpatient Sample were examined for the years 1993 through 2001. For each year, these data reflect hospital stays from between 800 and 1000 institutions sampled to approximate a 20% stratified sample of nonfederal community hospitals. Represented in the sample are various regions of the country, urban/rural locations, and different types of ownership/control, bed size, and teaching status.

Results.—The annual varicella-related hospitalization rate exceeded 0.5 hospitalizations per 10,000 US population from 1993 to 1995, declined to 0.26 per 10,000 by 1999, and fell further to 0.13 per 10,000 by 2001. Decreases occurred in all age groups but were greatest in the group primarily targeted for vaccination, namely 0- to 4-year-old children. Similar declines were seen in varicella-related hospital discharge (VRHD) charges, which fell from $161.1 million in 1993 to $66.3 million in 2001. In contrast, annual hospital charges for all diagnoses increased during the same period from $406.7 billion to $548.8 billion. The proportion of VRHDs with well-recognized complications changed relatively little over the study period. Inflation-adjusted declines in VRHD charges accrued to Medicaid, private insurance, and "other" payers but not to Medicare.

Conclusion.—In contrast to previous studies, which were limited in scope and methodology, this national analysis confirms that childhood varicella immunization in the United States has led to a clinically and statistically significant reduction in varicella-related hospitalizations and costs.

Effectiveness Over Time of Varicella Vaccine
Vázquez M, LaRussa PS, Gershon AA, et al (Yale Univ, New Haven, Conn; Columbia Univ, New York)
JAMA 291:851-855, 2004   4–6

Introduction.—Recent reports of outbreaks of chickenpox in groups with substantial rates of immunization as well as studies of immunized children with breakthrough infections have increased concerns regarding the current recommendations for administration of varicella vaccine. The effectiveness of varicella vaccine over time since vaccination and by age at the time of vaccination was evaluated in a case-control investigation of patients from 20 different group practices.

Methods.—Case subjects were identified by active surveillance of all physician practices. A total of 339 eligible children 13 months of age or older had clinically diagnosed chickenpox and a polymerase chain reaction test result positive for varicella-zoster virus DNA. For every patient, 2 control subjects were matched by age and pediatric practice. The primary outcome measure was the effectiveness of the vaccine, particularly the effects of time since vaccination and age at time of vaccination, adjusted for possible confounders.

Results.—The adjusted overall effectiveness of the vaccine was 87% (95% confidence interval, 81%-91%; $P < .001$). There was a marked difference in the vaccine's effectiveness in the initial year after vaccination (97%) and in years 2 to 8 after vaccination (84%; $P = .003$). The vaccine's effectiveness in year 1 was notably lower if the vaccine was administered at an age younger than age 15 months (73%) versus administration at 15 months or older (99%; $P = .01$). The difference in effectiveness overall for children immunized at age younger than 15 months versus 15 months or older was not significant (81% vs 88%; $P = .17$). Most cases of chickenpox in children who had been vaccinated were mild.

Conclusion.—The effectiveness of varicella vaccine diminishes significantly after 1 year. Most cases of breakthrough disease are mild. If the vaccine is administered at an age younger than 15 months, its effectiveness is lower in the first year after vaccination, compared to administration at an older age.

▶ These 2 articles (Abstracts 4–5 and 4–6) demonstrate the benefits of immunizing children against varicella. Vaccination has resulted in a significant decrease in varicella-related hospitalizations and subsequent charges. The effectiveness of the vaccine in years 2-8 after vaccination is reported to be 84%. During the first year after vaccination there appears to be better protection for that year only if the vaccine is administered at age 15 months or older. Vaccinated individuals who develop varicella seem to have a less contagious disease than unvaccinated individuals who have the infection. It has been postulated that periodic exposure to wild cases of varicella plays a role in boosting the immunity of vaccinated individuals. As varicella becomes less common, monitoring will be necessary to document that immunity is being maintained. Additional vaccinations may be required to provide continuing adequate immunity against the disease.

S. Raimer, MD

Contagiousness of Varicella in Vaccinated Cases: A Household Contact Study
Seward JF, Zhang JX, Maupin TJ, et al (Ctrs for Disease Control and Prevention, Atlanta, Ga; Los Angeles County Dept of Health Services)
JAMA 292:704-708, 2004   4–7

Background.—Approximately 4 million cases of varicella, resulting in 10,600 hospitalizations and 100 deaths, developed annually in the United States before the initiation of a varicella vaccination program. Most of these cases occurred in children, which is indicative of the highly contagious nature of the disease. Compared with unvaccinated cases, vaccinated varicella cases (or breakthrough disease) are usually milder and have fewer lesions and constitutional symptoms. Few data are available on the contagiousness of vaccinated varicella cases. In the current study, secondary attack rates within households, according to the disease history and vaccination status of the primary case and household contacts, were described; in addition, the effectiveness of the varicella vaccine was estimated.

Methods.—This population-based active varicella surveillance project took place in a community of about 320,000 individuals in Los Angeles County during 1997 and 2001. The varicella cases were reported by childcare centers, private and public schools, and health care clinicians. Cases were investigated to collect demographic, clinical, medical, and vaccination data. Information on household contacts' ages, varicella histories, and vaccination status was collected.

Results.—A total of 6316 cases of varicella were reported. Among children and adolescents 1 to 14 years of age, secondary attack rates varied by age and by disease and vaccination status of the primary case and of the exposed household contacts. Among the contacts 1 to 14 years of age exposed to unvaccinated case patients, the secondary attack rates were 71.5% if they were unvaccinated and 15.1% if they were vaccinated. Vaccinated case patients were half as contagious as unvaccinated case patients. However, vaccinated case patients with 50 lesions or more were similarly contagious compared with unvaccinated case patients, whereas vaccinated case patients with fewer than 50 lesions were only one third as contagious. The vaccine effectiveness for prevention of all disease was 78.9% (95% CI, 69.7%-85.3%); for moderate disease, the rates were 92% (for patients with 50-500 lesions) and 100% (for patients with a complication necessitating a visit to a clinician); and for severe disease, the rate was 100%.

Conclusions.—The varicella vaccine was highly effective under conditions of intense exposure for the prevention of moderate and severe disease and about 80% effective in the prevention of all disease. Breakthrough varicella cases in household settings were half as contagious as unvaccinated cases of varicella; however, the level of contagiousness varied with the number of lesions.

▶ Although breakthrough varicella cases in the household setting were less contagious than unvaccinated cases of varicella, the actual contagiousness varied with the number of lesions. Vaccinated cases with less than 50 lesions were one third as contagious as unvaccinated cases, whereas vaccinated cases with 50 or more lesions were as contagious as unvaccinated cases. To further emphasize this, a highly contagious breakthrough case with 150 vesicles was the source case in a recently reported varicella outbreak in New Hampshire.[1]

B. H. Thiers, MD

Reference

1. Galil K, Lee B, Strine T, et al: Outbreak of varicella at a day-care center despite vaccination. *N Engl J Med* 347:1909-1915, 2002.

Case-Control Study of the Effect of Mechanical Trauma on the Risk of Herpes Zoster
Thomas SL, Wheeler JG, Hall AJ (London School of Hygiene and Tropical Medicine; Inst of Public Health, Cambridge, England)
BMJ 328:439-440, 2004   4–8

Background.—Increasing age and depressed cell-mediated immunity increase the risk of herpes zoster. Whether mechanical trauma also increases the risk of herpes zoster at the trauma site was investigated.

Methods.—The research subjects were 243 cases 16 to 91 years old with incident zoster and 483 age- and sex-matched control subjects with no previous zoster. All research subjects were questioned about physical trauma severe enough to cause bruising and any surgical procedures in the 6 months before zoster developed. The occurrences of zoster in the 6 months and 1 month before the interview at any body site and at the site of the case patients' zoster were compared between the 2 groups.

Results.—Case patients and control subjects had a similar frequency of trauma at other body sites during the months preceding the interview. However, 7.0% of case patients had trauma within the previous 6 months at the same site as their rash developed compared with only 1.0% of control subjects who had trauma at the case patients' site of the rash ($P = .0002$; adjusted odds ratio, 8.02). Similarly, 4.5% of case patients had trauma within the previous 1 month at the same site as their rash developed compared with only 0.6% of control subjects who had trauma at the case patients' site of the rash ($P = .002$; adjusted odds ratio, 12.07).

Conclusion.—Mechanical trauma markedly increased the risk of zoster at the trauma site during the subsequent month. It may be possible that trauma to a nerve triggers viral reactivation in its dorsal root ganglion.

▶ Mechanical trauma can certainly reactivate herpes simplex virus infection. This controlled study demonstrates that the same phenomenon appears to occur with varicella-zoster virus infection.

B. H. Thiers, MD

The Risk and Prognosis of Cancer After Hospitalisation for Herpes Zoster: A Population-Based Follow-up Study
Sørensen HT, Olsen JH, Jepsen P, et al (Aarhus Univ, Denmark; Inst of Cancer Epidemiology, Copenhagen; Aalborg Hosp, Denmark)
Br J Cancer 91:1275-1279, 2004   4–9

Background.—Some evidence suggests an association between cancer and herpes zoster, but no large trials have prospectively studied this possibility. These authors used nationwide, population-based registries to examine whether hospitalization for herpes zoster is associated with an increased risk of cancer.

Methods.—The Danish Registry of Patients was used to identify 13,414 patients hospitalized for herpes zoster between 1977 and 1996. Patients were excluded from the analysis if they had a history of cancer or organ transplantation before the diagnosis of herpes zoster, if they died during hospitalization for herpes zoster, or if they had a diagnosis of human immunodeficiency virus at any time during the study. Medical records from the remaining 10,588 patients with hospitalization for herpes zoster were linked with those from the Danish Cancer Registry. A control group of 12,193 patients with cancer who did not have herpes zoster was also selected from the Danish Cancer Registry and matched to the cases by age (10-year groups), sex, type of cancer, and calendar year of diagnosis (5-year periods). The expected number of cancers was calculated based on national incidence rates for primary cancers according to age, sex, and site of cancer.

Results.—The incidence of cancer in patients hospitalized with herpes zoster (1427 cancers) was higher than the expected incidence (1239 cancers) (relative risk [RR] 1.2). The risk of cancer in the cases was highest during the first year after hospitalization for herpes zoster (RR 1.3), particularly for those with hematologic cancers (RR 3.4). Furthermore, the risk of developing hematologic cancer was still elevated 10 years after hospitalization for herpes zoster (RR 1.7). Cases that had cancer develop within the first year after hospitalization for herpes zoster were significantly more likely to have distant metastasis than were controls (prevalence ratio 1.27). Overall mortality rates did not differ significantly between the cases and the controls (mortality ratio 1.02). However, mortality in cases with hematologic cancer was much higher than in cases with other types of cancer (mortality ratios 1.38 vs 0.98).

Conclusion.—The risk of several types of cancer—particularly hematologic cancers—is elevated after hospitalization for herpes zoster, especially during the first year after hospitalization. The cases were also more likely than the controls to have advanced cancer. Survival of cases with hematologic cancer was shorter than survival of cases with other types of cancer. These data suggest herpes zoster may be a marker of cancer, particularly hematologic cancer.

Risk Factors for Postherpetic Neuralgia in Patients With Herpes Zoster
Jung BF, Johnson RW, Griffin DRJ, et al (Univ of Rochester, Minn; Univ of Bristol, England; GlaxoSmithKline, Harlow, Essex, England)
Neurology 62:1545-1551, 2004   4–10

Background.—Many patients with herpes zoster continue to feel pain months after the rash has healed. Risk factors for postherpetic neuralgia (PHN) in patients with herpes zoster were investigated.

Methods.—The medical records of 855 patients 15 to 93 years old with herpes zoster who were enrolled within 72 hours of rash onset were reviewed. Demographic and clinical variables were compared among the 114 patients (13.3%) with PHN (ie, presence of pain at 4 months after rash onset) and the 741 patients (86.7%) without PHN. A subset of the latter group containing 39 patients with subacute herpetic neuralgia (ie, pain that persisted 2-3 months after the rash cleared but resolved before the 4-month visit and before PHN could be diagnosed) was also examined separately.

Results.—Compared with patients without PHN, patients with PHN were significantly older (mean age, 61.6 vs 50.9 years), significantly more likely to be women (64.0% vs 49.8%), and significantly more likely to have had a prodrome (93.9% vs 82.6%), severe acute pain (49.1% vs 21.9%), and severe rash (71.9% vs 43.7%). Multivariate analyses confirmed that older age, female sex, presence of a prodrome, more severe pain, and greater rash severity were significant and independent predictors of PHN. Compared with patients with PHN, patients with subacute herpetic neuralgia were significantly younger (mean age 54.0 vs 61.6 years) and significantly less likely to have severe acute pain (25.6% vs 49.1%). However, patients with subacute herpetic neuralgia were significantly more likely to have severe and widespread rash than patients without PHN.

Conclusion.—Certain factors increase the risk of PHN in patients with herpes zoster. Severe and/or widespread rash can cause subacute herpetic neuralgia that does not progress to PHN, but does result in lingering pain for 2 to 3 months after the rash resolves.

▶ Jung et al (Abstract 4–10) reviewed the familiar risk factors for the development of PHN. Sørensen et al (Abstract 4–9) reported that patients hospitalized for herpes zoster (presumably those with more severe disease) had an increased risk for hematologic cancers and were more likely to have advanced cancer than matched controls.

B. H. Thiers, MD

Systematic Review of Topical Capsaicin for the Treatment of Chronic Pain
Mason L, Moore RA, Derry S, et al (Univ of Oxford, England)
BMJ 328:991-995, 2004   4–11

Background.—Capsaicin is the compound in chili peppers that causes them to taste "hot." The mechanism of action is binding to nociceptors to the skin. This causes an initial excitation of neurons and a period of enhanced sensitivity, which is usually perceived as a burning, itching, or pricking sensation. This uncomfortable sensation is accompanied by cutaneous vasodilation and is thought to be the result of selective stimulation of afferent C fibers and the release of substance P. A refractory period ensues, with reduced sensitivity and, after repeated applications, persistent desensitization, possibly due to the depletion of substance P. The efficacy and safety of topically applied capsaicin for relief of chronic pain from neuropathic or musculoskeletal disorders were investigated.

Methods.—An analysis was conducted of randomized controlled trials comparing topically applied capsaicin with placebo or another treatment in adults with chronic pain. The main outcome measure was dichotomous information for the number of patients with a reduction in pain of approximately 50%. Outcomes were extracted at 4 weeks for musculoskeletal conditions and at 8 weeks for neuropathic conditions. Secondary outcome measures were adverse events and withdrawals due to adverse events. Data were obtained from the Cochrane Library, MEDLINE, Embase, PubMed, an in-house database, and manufacturers of topical capsaicin.

Results.—Six double-blind placebo-controlled trials including 656 patients were pooled for analysis of neuropathic conditions. The relative benefit from topical capsaicin 0.075% compared with placebo was 1.4, and the number needed to treat was 5.7. Three double-blind placebo-controlled trials including 368 patients were pooled for analysis of musculoskeletal conditions. The relative benefit from topical capsaicin 0.025% or plaster compared with placebo was 1.5, and the number needed to treat was 8.1.

Approximately one third of the patients experienced local adverse events with capsaicin, which would not have occurred with placebo.

Conclusion.—Topical capsaicin has moderate to poor efficacy in the treatment of chronic musculoskeletal or neuropathic pain, but it may be useful as a adjunct or sole therapy for a limited number of patients who are unresponsive to or intolerant of other treatments.

Systematic Review of Efficacy of Topical Rubefacients Containing Salicylates for the Treatment of Acute and Chronic Pain
Mason L, Moore RA, Edwards JE, et al (Univ of Oxford, England)
BMJ 328:995-998, 2004   4–12

Background.—Rubefacients may act by counterirritation to relieve pain, while topical non-steroidal antiinflammatory drugs (NSAIDs) inhibit cyclooxygenase, which is responsible for the biosynthesis of prostaglandin, which in turn mediates inflammation. Rubefacients are usually used as adjuvants to other therapies and may be useful in the treatment of patients who cannot tolerate oral analgesics. Most sources have attributed the action of rubefacients to counterirritation, but there is uncertainty as to which drugs fall into the category of rubefacients. Salicylates are particularly difficult to categorize, and the ability of topical salicylates to relieve pain is unclear. The efficacy and safety of topical rubefacients containing salicylates were studied for relief of acute and chronic pain.

Methods.—An analysis was conducted of randomized double-blind trials comparing topical rubefacients with placebo or another active treatment in adults with acute or chronic pain, and reporting dichotomous information, around a 50% reduction in pain, and analyses at 1 week for acute conditions and 2 weeks for chronic conditions. Data extracted included the relative benefit and number needed to treat, analysis of adverse events, and withdrawals. Sources of the data included electronic databases and manufacturers of salicylates.

Results.—The analysis included 3 double-blind placebo-controlled trials with information on 182 patients with acute conditions. Topical salicylates were found to be significantly better than placebo. In an analysis of chronic conditions, 6 double-blind placebo-controlled trials had data on 429 patients with chronic conditions and reported that topical salicylates were significantly better than placebo. However, larger, more valid studies showed no significant effect. Local adverse events and withdrawals were generally rare in these trials.

Conclusions.—Information is limited, but topical rubefacients with salicylates may be efficacious in the treatment of acute pain. Moderate to poor efficacy was suggested in patients with musculoskeletal and arthritic pain. Adverse events were rare in studies of acute pain and were poorly reported in studies of chronic pain. Assessments of efficacy for rubefacients are unreliable due to a lack of good clinical trials.

▶ Topical creams containing capsaicin have been advocated to treat the pain associated with conditions as diverse as postherpetic neuralgia, diabetic neuropathy, osteoarthritis, rheumatoid arthritis, pruritus, psoriasis, mastectomy, bladder disorders, and cluster headaches. A large review published more than 10 years ago found efficacy in some of these conditions but only a marginal benefit in treating postherpetic neuralgia.[1] The first study (Abstract 4–11) is hardly a ringing endorsement of these preparations. Mason and colleagues found that for every 6 patients with neuropathic pain using capsaicin 0.075% for 8 weeks, 1 additional patient would benefit, and for every 8 patients with musculoskeletal pain using capsaicin 0.025% for 4 weeks, 1 additional patient would benefit. The incidence of local adverse effects was rather high.

The second study (Abstract 4–12), conducted by the same group of investigators, found that most trials to assess the efficacy of rubefacients containing salicylates have been limited by small size and inadequate design and validity, making the results tentative. Better trials have showed little difference from placebo. Nevertheless, topical capsaicin and topical salicylates may be useful adjuncts to conventional pain treatment.[2]

B. H. Thiers, MD

References

1. Zhang WY, Li Wan Po A: The effectiveness of topically applied capsaicin. A meta-analysis. *Eur J Clin Pharmacol* 46:517-522, 1994.
2. Tramèr MR: It's not just about rubbing—Topical capsaicin and topical salicylates may be useful as adjuvants to conventional pain treatment. *BMJ* 328:998, 2004.

The Detection of Monkeypox in Humans in the Western Hemisphere
Reed KD, Melski JW, Graham MB, et al (Marshfield Clinic, Wis; Marshfield Clinic Research Foundation, Wis; Med College of Wisconsin, Milwaukee; et al)
N Engl J Med 350:342-350, 2004   4–13

Introduction.—Human cases of monkeypox, first recognized in 1958 as a viral zoonosis of captive primates, had occurred until recently only in the Democratic Republic of Congo. The first documented cases of monkeypox virus among humans in the Western Hemisphere were reported in Wisconsin in 2003. The Wisconsin cases were reviewed for clinical feature and laboratory findings.

Methods.—One patient, a 3-year-old girl, became ill after she was bitten by a prairie dog her family had purchased on May 11, 2003. The animal was observed to have ocular discharge, lymphadenopathy, and papular skin lesions on May 13 and died on May 20. Another patient, a man later found to have sold 2 prairie dogs to the index patient's family, was hospitalized after a prairie dog bite. His symptoms and connection to the index patient's prairie dog helped to establish an epidemiologic link. Blood and tissue samples from these 2 cases, 9 additional cases, and prairie dog 1 were collected for histopathologic and electron-microscopic examinations, microbiological cultures, and molecular assays.

Results.—The 11 human monkeypox cases evaluated occurred in 5 males and 6 females ranging in age from 3 to 43 years. All had experienced a febrile illness with skin eruptions (Fig 2; see color plate XV) after direct contact with ill prairie dogs. The prairie dogs involved in the outbreak appear to have been exposed to at least 1 species of rodent recently imported into the United States from West Africa. Skin-lesion tissue from 4 patients showed immunohistochemical or ultrastructural evidence of poxvirus infection. Cell cultures of 7 tissue samples from patients and a submandibular lymph node from prairie dog 1 yielded monkeypox virus, identified by detection of monkeypox-specific DNA sequences.

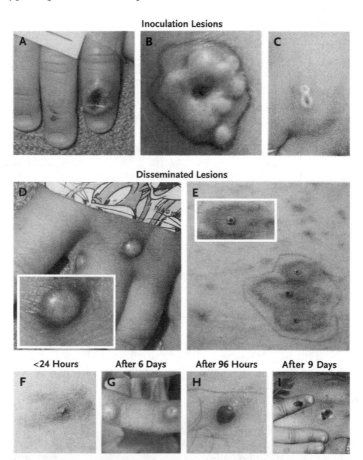

FIGURE 2.—Primary inoculation reactions (Panels A, B, and C), examples of the smallpox-like (Panel D) and umbilicated varicella-like (Panel E) disseminated monkeypox lesions, and the morphological appearance of disseminated lesions over time (Panels F, G, H, and I). Panel A shows a primary inoculation reaction at the site of a prairie dog bite on 1 patient, Panel B a prairie-dog scratch on another patient, and Panel C, a pre-existing cat scratch on still another patient. Panel G shows a disseminated lesion less than 24 hours after its appearance; Panel G, lesions after 6 days; Panel H, a lesion after 96 hours; and Panel I, a lesion after more than 9 days. (Reprinted by permission of *The New England Journal of Medicine* from Reed KD, Melski JW, Graham MB, et al: The detection of monkeypox in humans in the Western Hemisphere. *N Engl J Med* 350:342-350, 2004. Copyright 2004, Massachusetts Medical Society. All rights reserved.)

Four of 11 patients were hospitalized, but there were no deaths and the clinical course was self-limited in all cases. Treatment consisted of antibiotics for 9 patients, IV acyclovir for 1 patient, and valacyclovir for 2 patients.

Conclusion.—Cases of monkeypox among humans and rodents in the Western Hemisphere showed clinical signs and symptoms similar to those described in outbreaks in Africa. The size (72 confirmed or suspected cases) and significance of the current outbreak led the Centers for Disease Control and the Food and Drug Administration to ban the import of all rodents from Africa. State and federal bans curtail further sale and transport of prairie dogs.

▶ Now that smallpox has been eradicated, moneypox may be the most important remaining orthopoxvirus infection. The signs and symptoms noted in this Wisconsin outbreak were similar to those described in outbreaks of the disease in Africa. All patients reported here had contact with a sick pet prairie dog obtained through a common distributor. In this outbreak, there was limited or no spread of the virus through human contact.

B. H. Thiers, MD

Urticaria, Exanthems, and Other Benign Dermatologic Reactions to Smallpox Vaccination in Adults

Greenberg RN, Schosser RH, Plummer EA, et al (Univ of Kentucky, Lexington; DynPort Vaccine Company, Frederick, Md)
Clin Infect Dis 98:958-965, 2004   4–14

Background.—Fears that the smallpox virus may be used in a terrorist attack have prompted the development of new cell-cultured smallpox vaccines (CCSVs). Recently, these authors completed a phase 1 trial of a new CCSV. The development of impressive but benign, self-limiting rashes was noted in some of the vaccinated patients. In this article, urticaria, exanthems, and other benign dermatologic reactions to smallpox vaccination in adults are reported.

Methods and Findings.—The original phase 1 study included 350 adult volunteers, including 250 naive to vaccinia virus vaccine. A new CCSV or a live vaccinia virus vaccine was administered to each participant. Self-limiting rashes occurred in 3.6% of the vaccinia-naive patients and in none of those who had had vaccinia virus vaccine previously. The 9 rashes appeared 6 to 19 days after vaccination. Five different clinical presentations were observed: urticarial rashes resolving within 4 to 15 days occurred in 5 individuals, an exanthem lasting 20 days occurred in 1 (Fig 4), folliculitis occurred in 1, contact dermatitis occurred in 1, and erythematosus papules only on the hands and fingers occurred in 1 participant. In addition, study participants reported pruritus, tingling, and occasional headaches. Antihistamine and acetaminophen therapy provided relief. No fever or significant discomfort was reported.

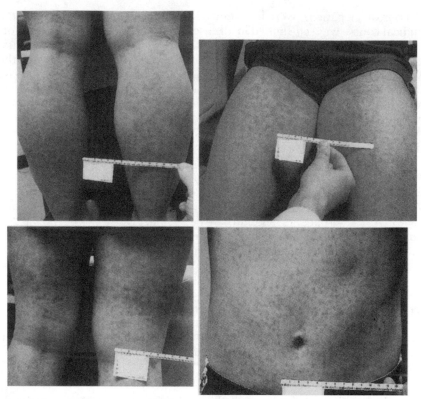

FIGURE 4.—An intense exanthem on the legs and abdomen of a volunteer who received a smallpox vaccination 13 days earlier. The rash resolved 28 days after vaccination. (Courtesy of Greenberg RN, Schosser RH, Plummer EA, et al: Urticaria, exanthems, and other benign dermatologic reactions to smallpox vaccination in adults. *Clin Infect Dis* 38:958-965, 2004. © 2004 by the Infectious Diseases Society of America. All rights reserved. University of Chicago, publisher.)

Conclusions.—Otherwise healthy adults undergoing vaccinia vaccination may experience self-limiting rashes such as urticaria and exanthems. Urticarial rashes can be expected to resolve within 1 week of their appearance. Exanthems, which may be extensive, may persist for more than 3 weeks.

▶ The authors describe the spectrum of self-limited skin reactions that may occur in patients naive to vaccinia virus vaccine. Most urticarial eruptions resolved within 1 week after appearance, whereas the single exanthem was more extensive and persistent, lasting nearly 3 weeks. Additional studies are needed to define the cause of these rashes. Significantly, none of them resembled a primary pox lesion; thus, they probably did not represent generalized vaccinia. Folliculitis after smallpox vaccination of vaccinia-naive recipients has previously been reported and reviewed in the 2004 YEAR BOOK OF DERMATOLOGY AND DERMATOLOGIC SURGERY.[1]

B. H. Thiers, MD

Reference

1. Talbot TR, Bredenberg HK, Smith M, et al: Focal and generalized folliculitis following smallpox vaccination among vaccinia-naive recipients. *JAMA* 289:3290-3294, 2003.

Severe Cutaneous Papillomavirus Disease After Haemopoietic Stem-Cell Transplantation in Patients With Severe Combined Immune Deficiency Caused by Common γc Cytokine Receptor Subunit or JAK-3 Deficiency

Laffort C, Le Deist F, Favre M, et al (Hôpital Necker-Enfants Malades, Paris; Institut Natl de la Santé et de la Recherche Médicale, France; Universita degli Studi di Brescia, Italy; et al)
Lancet 363:2051-2054, 2004   4–15

Background.—Allogeneic hematopoietic stem-cell transplantation (HSCT) is a life-saving treatment for patients with severe combined immune deficiency (SCID). Still, impaired immune functioning in these patients often leads to the development of severe human papillomavirus (HPV) disease. The frequency, characteristics, and risk factors for severe HPV disease after HSCT in patients with SCID were investigated.

Methods.—The medical records of 41 patients with SCID who underwent HSCT between 1971 and 1992 and who were still surviving were examined. All patients had 10 years' follow-up or more.

Results.—In all, 9 patients (7 boys and 2 girls; median age at HSCT, 6.5 months) had severe HPV disease limited to the skin 3 to 15 years (median, 8 years) after HSCT. Transplantation characteristics, immune status, and chimerism did not differ significantly between these 9 patients and the other patients. However, all 9 patients with severe HPV had SCID associated with either a γc or a Janus kinase-3 (JAK-3) deficiency, both of which result in the absence of protein expression. In addition, 4 of these 9 patients had lesions typical of epidermodysplasia verruciformis, a rare genodermatosis. In contrast, none of the patients with other forms of SCID had any signs of HPV disease.

Conclusion.—The only risk factor for severe HPV disease identified in these patients with SCID after HSCT was the molecular type of SCID: only the patients with SCID associated with γc or JAK-3 deficiency developed late-onset severe HPV. In particular, 4 patients had lesions typical of epidermodysplasia verruciformis. These results suggest γc-dependent cytokines may be important in anti-HPV immunity.

▶ The authors identify a specific molecular type of SCID that appears to represent a risk factor for HPV disease. Their data suggest that natural killer cells and γc– or JAK-3–dependent signaling in keratinocytes play an important role in immunity against the infection.

B. H. Thiers, MD

Treatment of Skin Papillomas With Topical α-Lactalbumin–Oleic Acid

Gustafsson L, Leijonhufvud I, Aronsson A, et al (Univ of Lund, Sweden)
N Engl J Med 350:2663-2672, 2004   4–16

Background.—Papillomas are formed by keratinocytes that have been transformed by human papillomavirus. A complex of α-lactalbumin and oleic acid (also called HAMLET, or human α-lactalbumin made lethal to tumor cells) is active against many transformed cells via a mechanism that resembles apoptosis; however, healthy, differentiated cells are unaffected. The efficacy and safety of topical α-lactalbumin–oleic acid on human skin papillomas were investigated.

Methods.—The research subjects were 40 patients (15 males and 25 females; age range, 4-59 years) with cutaneous papillomas resistant to conventional treatment. Patients were randomly assigned to apply either placebo or α-lactalbumin–oleic acid once a day to the lesions for 3 weeks, at which time changes in the volume of each treated lesion were recorded. At this point, 17 patients from each group enrolled in an open-label trial of topical α-lactalbumin–oleic acid for 3 weeks. Patients were monitored for a mean of 2.3 years to characterize lesion clearance.

Results.—During the first phase of the study, in all 20 patients in the α-lactalbumin–oleic acid group, lesion volume was reduced by 75% or greater and in 96% of the lesions (88 of 92 papillomas). In the placebo group, lesion volume was reduced by 75% or greater in only 3 of 20 patients and in only 20% of the lesions (15 of 74 papillomas) ($P < .001$). During the second phase, lesion volume was more than 75% reduced in 87% of patients who received α-lactalbumin–oleic acid during both phases and in 61% of patients who received α-lactalbumin–oleic acid only during phase 2. All but 2 of the patients were available for 2-year follow-up. Of the 38 patients who could be evaluated, 32 patients (84%) were completely free of papillomas, including 76% of patients who received active treatment during both phases and 88% of those who received active treatment only during phase 2. The time to resolution was significantly shorter in patients who used α-lactalbumin–oleic acid for both phases than in patients who used the active drug only during phase 2 (mean, 2.4 vs 9.9 months). Outcomes did not differ significantly between immunocompetent and immunocompromised patients. There were no drug-related adverse events.

Conclusion.—Topical α-lactalbumin–oleic acid can resolve papillomas in vivo, and most patients were still free of lesions at the 2-year follow-up examination. α-Lactalbumin–oleic acid seems to be an effective and safe treatment for papillomas and, perhaps, other cutaneous tumors.

▶ Gustafsson et al introduce a possible new treatment for cutaneous papillomavirus lesions. α-Lactalbumin–oleic acid is a molecular complex from human milk that kills human papillomavirus–transformed cells by a mechanism that resembles apoptosis.[1] Healthy, differentiated cells seem to be resistant to its effects,[2] which seem to be selective for tumor cells and immature cells.

B. H. Thiers, MD

References

1. Svensson M, Hakansson A, Mossberg AK, et al: Conversion of alpha-lactalbumin to a protein inducing apoptosis. *Proc Natl Acad Sci U S A* 97:4221-4226, 2000.
2. Svanborg C, Agerstam H, Aronson A, et al: HAMLET kills tumor cells by an apoptosis-like mechanism: Cellular, molecular, and therapeutic aspects. *Adv Cancer Res* 88:1-29, 2003.

Psychological Impact of Human Papillomavirus Testing in Women WIth Borderline or Mildly Dyskaryotic Cervical Smear Test Results: Cross Sectional Questionnaire Study

Maissi E, Marteau TM, Hankins M, et al (King's College London; Inst of Cancer Research, Sutton, Surrey, England; Univ of Oxford, England)
BMJ 328:1293-1296, 2004   4–17

Introduction.—Testing women for human papillomavirus (HPV) may raise anxiety in those who test positive but may reassure women who have a borderline or mildly dyskaryotic smear but test negative. A cross-sectional questionnaire study examined anxiety, distress, and concern about test results among women who took part in an English pilot study of liquid-based cytology and HPV testing.

Methods.—The study included 867 women who received borderline or mildly dyskaryotic smear test results and were tested for HPV (HPV positive [n = 536]; HPV negative [n = 331]); 143 women with borderline or mildly dyskaryotic smear results who were not tested for HPV; and 366 women with normal smear results. Rating scales determined the outcome measures: anxiety, general distress, concern about the smear results, perceived risk of development of cervical cancer, and the women's understanding of smear results.

Results.—Because the 4 study groups differed in age, educational level, and whether this was their first smear, the analysis controlled for these variables. As expected, the group with normal test results had significantly less anxiety, distress, and concern. The HPV-positive group rated significantly higher on these measures than the other groups taken together. However, women with abnormal smear test results and an HPV-negative finding did not have less anxiety, distress, or concern than women who had abnormal smear test results and who did not undergo HPV testing. In addition, women with abnormal results, whether tested for HPV or not tested, were less likely to know what their results meant than those who received a normal result.

Conclusion.—Women with borderline or mildly dyskaryotic smear test results and negative HPV test results are at lower risk for the development of cervical cancer than those with similar smear test results and HPV positivity. However, both groups experience anxiety upon hearing test results and need to be better informed about the actual prevalence of HPV infection and the significance of smear test results and HPV status.

▶ In patients with borderline or mildly dyskaryotic smear test results, HPV positivity is associated with a measurable increase in anxiety, distress, and concern beyond that associated with the abnormal cytology result. This report emphasizes the importance of patient counseling to put these results into perspective.

B. H. Thiers, MD

Regression of Low-Grade Squamous Intra-epithelial Lesions in Young Women
Moscicki A-B, Shiboski S, Hills NK, et al (Univ of California, San Francisco)
Lancet 364:1678-1683, 2004   4–18

Background.—Low-grade squamous intra-epithelial lesions (LSIL) develop in about one fourth of adolescent and young women after a human papillomavirus (HPV) infection. The rate of LSIL regression in these young patients may be much greater than in older women. The probability of LSIL regression in adolescent and young women was defined, and factors associated with regression were identified.

Methods.—The adolescents and young women included in the analysis were participants in a 10-year study begun in 1980 of the natural history of HPV infection. Patients aged 13 to 22 years attending 1 of 2 family planning clinics between 1990 and 1994 were screened for cervical HPV DNA. One hundred eighty-seven young women tested positive and had no previous history of treatment of squamous intra-epithelial lesions. The median follow-up time from first LSIL diagnosis was 61 months. The median duration of sexual activity at diagnosis was 3.2 years.

Findings.—For the entire cohort, the probability of regression at 12 months was 61%, and at 36 months, it was 91%. Regression of LSIL did not correlate with HPV status at baseline, sexual behavior, contraceptive use, substance or cigarette use, incident sexually transmitted infection, or biopsy. In a multivariate analysis, only HPV status at the current visit correlated with the regression rate, whether the cause of infection was one or more viral types.

Conclusion.—A high rate of LSIL regression was documented in this study of adolescent and young women. This supports management by cytologic observation in this age group. Negative HPV status correlated with regression. Thus, HPV testing may be useful for monitoring LSIL.

▶ The authors recommend serial cytology rather than colposcopy for young women with LSIL. They demonstrate that spontaneous regression often occurs, suggesting that HPV infections can be frequent and transient. Because HPV infections can be manifested clinically as LSIL, the high rate of LSIL in adolescence is not surprising, nor is the high rate of regression in this population.

B. H. Thiers, MD

Treatment of Undifferentiated Vulvar Intraepithelial Neoplasia With 5% Imiquimod Cream: A Prospective Study of 12 Cases
Wendling J, Saiag P, Berville-Levy S, et al (Université Versailles, Boulogne, France)
Arch Dermatol 140:1220-1224, 2004   4–19

Introduction.—The annual incidence of vulvar intraepithelial neoplasia (VIN) has increased during the past 2 decades. Differentiated VIN mainly affects postmenopausal women and does not usually contain human papillomavirus (HPV) DNA sequences. In contrast, undifferentiated VIN predominantly affects women in their 30s and 40s and is associated with high-risk HPV types (mainly HPV-16). The efficacy of 5% imiquimod cream on undifferentiated VIN was examined in a prospective, uncontrolled study.

Methods.—Participants were 12 consecutive patients treated between March 1, 1999, and May 31, 2001. All had histologically confirmed, noninvasive, undifferentiated VIN. Imiquimod cream (each dose of 12.5 mg supplied in individual packets) was to be applied 3 times a week overnight. Patients were asked neither to wash nor have sexual intercourse during the time the cream was in contact with the mucosa. Response was evaluated by physical examination of the vulva and photographs. A complete response required complete resolution, and a partial response was defined as a decrease of 50% or greater in lesion size. Treatment failure was a decrease of less than 50% in lesion size or progression of the lesions.

Results.—The mean patient age was 41 years. Seven of 12 women had multifocal lesions, and the VIN was recurrent in 8. Nine of 10 patients who underwent an additional biopsy for HPV testing were found to have HPV-16; 1 had HPV-33. There were 3 complete responses, 4 partial responses, and 5 failures after mean treatment durations of 3.6, 5.0, and 3.4 months, respectively. None of the lesions progressed to squamous cell carcinoma. Ten patients experienced vulvar discomfort, which led 3 to withdraw from treatment, and 2 patients had flu-like symptoms.

Conclusion.—Conventional treatments of undifferentiated VIN are painful and sometimes mutilating. Imiquimod, which is applied by the patient, could be a valid alternative. In this small series, 5% imiquimod cream was at least 75% effective in 7 of 12 patients. Local tolerance, however, was poor.

▶ The results are inconclusive at best. A randomized study involving a larger number of patients, using different application regimens, and with a lengthy follow-up period, will be necessary to convincingly prove or disprove the efficacy of imiquimod treatment for undifferentiated VIN.

B. H. Thiers, MD

Effect of Antiretroviral Therapy on the Incidence of Genital Warts and Vulvar Neoplasia Among Women With the Human Immunodeficiency Virus

Massad LS, Silverberg MJ, Springer G, et al (Southern Illinois Univ, Springfield, Ill; Johns Hopkins Univ, Baltimore, Md; State Univ of New York, Brooklyn; et al)
Am J Obstet Gynecol 190:1241-1248, 2004   4–20

Background.—Women with HIV often have co-infection with human papillomaviruses (HPVs), which commonly manifest as genital warts and vulvar intraepithelial neoplasia (VIN). The impact of highly active antiretroviral therapy (HAART), used for HIV infection, on genital warts and VIN has not been well documented. The incidence of genital warts and vulvar neoplasia was determined in women with HIV; in addition, the effects of potential predictive factors, especially HAART, on vulvar disease incidence were determined.

Methods.—The multicenter, prospective cohort study included 1562 HIV-seropositive and 469 at risk but seronegative women. All patients were free of warts and VIN at baseline. Every 6 months, the patients underwent CD4 counts, HIV RNA measurement, physical examination, Papanicolaou testing, and biopsies, as indicated.

Findings.—The incidence of warts was 5.01 per 100 person-years in seropositive women and 1.31 per 100 person-years in seronegative women; the incidences of VIN were 4.67 and 1.31 per 100 person-years, respectively. A multivariate analysis indicated that warts correlated with the use of HAART (relative hazard [RH], 0.76), the CD4 count (RH, 0.91 per 100 cell per cm² increase), AIDS (RH, 1.25), abnormal Papanicolaou findings (RH, 2.18), high- or medium-risk HPV types (RH, 1.91), low-risk HPV type (RH, 1.48), smoking (RH, 1.43), having 1 child (RH, 1.54), and age (RH, 0.74 per 10 years). VIN correlated with HAART (RH, 0.65), the CD4 count (RH, 0.92), abnormal Papanicolaou findings (RH, 16.03), high- or medium-risk HPV types (RH, 1.37), and age (RH, 0.85 per 10 years).

Conclusions.—The incidences of warts and VIN in women infected with HIV are high. However, HAART seems to reduce these incidences.

▶ The findings of decreased incidences of warts and VIN in patients receiving HAART are not surprising and likely reflect improved immune functioning among treated patients.

B. H. Thiers, MD

5 HIV Infection

HIV and Hepatitis C Virus RNA in Seronegative Organ and Tissue Donors
Challine D, Pellegrin B, Bouvier-Alias M, et al (Université Paris XII, Créteil)
Lancet 364:1611-1612, 2004   5–1

Introduction.—Nucleic acid testing (NAT) has been introduced to iden-tify HIV RNA and hepatitis C virus (HCV) RNA in pooled blood donations. A large series of organ and tissue donors were evaluated to ascertain whether NAT could identify HIV RNA or HCV RNA and whether this method should be used routinely to improve the safety of transplantation in terms of avoiding the transmission of viruses.

Findings.—Serum samples were evaluated from 3049 consecutive organ and tissue donors, including 2236 brain-dead, heart-beating organ donors, 636 living-tissue donors, and 177 dead cornea donors. Five HCV RNA-positive donors were detected among 2119 HCV-seronegative organ do-nors; 1 HCV RNA-positive donor was identified among 641 HCV-seronegative tissue donors. No HIV-seronegative, HIV RNA-positive donor was detected.

Conclusion.—Routine NAT of organ and tissue donors may increase the safety of transplantation by identifying potentially infectious seronegative donors.

▶ The clinical significance of seronegative HCV viremia and the infectivity of the associated grafts are uncertain. However, a previous article[1] on HCV trans-mission to recipients from a seronegative HCV RNA-positive donor suggests that routine NAT might increase transplantation safety with regard to virus transmission.

B. H. Thiers, MD

Reference

1. Cieslak PR, Hedberg K, Thomas AR, et al: Hepatitis C virus transmission from an antibody-negative organ and tissue donor, United States, 2000-2002. *MMWR Morb Mortal Wkly Rep* 52:273-274, 2003.

Detection of HIV-1 and HCV Infections Among Antibody-Negative Blood Donors by Nucleic Acid–Amplification Testing

Stramer SL, for the National Heart, Lung, and Blood Institute Nucleic Acid Test Study Group (American Red Cross, Gaithersburg, Md; et al)

N Engl J Med 351:760-768, 2004   5–2

Background.—Before 1999, the screening of potential blood donors relied on the use of immunoassays to detect viral antibodies or antigens. In 1999, new screening methods that use nucleic acid amplification for the detection of human immunodeficiency virus type 1 (HIV-1) and hepatitis C virus (HCV) RNA were implemented in the United States on an investigational basis. The use of RNA-based donor screening has facilitated the study of events occurring early in HIV-1 and HCV infection. The relative risk of transmission of HIV-1 and HCV from first-time blood donors and persons who donated blood repeatedly was investigated.

Methods.—An analysis was performed of all antibody-nonreactive blood donations confirmed to be positive for HIV-1 and HCV RNA on nucleic acid–amplification testing of "minipools" (pools of 16 to 24 donations) by the main blood-collection programs in the United States in the first 3 years of nucleic acid screening.

Results.—Of a total of 37,164,054 units screened, only 12 were confirmed to be positive for HIV-1 RNA (1 in 3.1 million donations). Of these 12 donations, only 2 were detected by HIV-1 p24 antigen testing. For HCV, of 39,721,404 units screened, 170 were confirmed to be positive for HCV RNA, or 1 in 230,000 donations—or 1 in 270,000 on the basis of 139 donations confirmed to be positive for HCV RNA with the use of a more sensitive HCV-antibody test. The rates of positive HCV and HIV-nucleic acid–amplification tests were 3.3 and 4.1 times as high, respectively, among first-time donors compared with donors who gave blood repeatedly. Follow up of 67 HCV RNA–positive donors showed that seroconversion occurred a median of 35 days after the index donation, followed by a low rate of resolution of viremia. There were also 3 cases of long-term immunologically silent HCV infection documented.

Conclusions.—Minipool nucleic acid–amplification testing has helped to prevent the transmission of about 5 HIV-1 infections and 56 HCV infections each year in the first 3 years of use. This screening method has reduced the residual risk of transfusion-transmitted HIV-1 and HCV to about 1 in 2 million blood units.

Probability of Viremia With HBV, HCV, HIV, and HTLV Among Tissue Donors in the United States

Zou S, for the Tissue Safety Study Group (American Red Cross, Rockville, Md; et al)
N Engl J Med 351:751-759, 2004   5–3

Background.—Hepatitis B and C virus (HBV and HBC) and human immunodeficiency virus (HIV) have been transmitted by tissue transplantation as well as by blood transfusion. Almost all of these methods of transmission have resulted from the collection of blood during the so-called viremic window period, before infection can be detected by laboratory testing. The probability of collecting blood during this window period has been extensively evaluated. However, similar estimates have not been made for tissue donors. The probability of undetected viremia with HBV, HCV, HIV, and human T-lymphotropic virus (HTLV) among tissue donors was investigated.

Methods.—The rates of prevalence of hepatitis B surface antigen (HBsAg) and antibodies against HIV (anti-HIV), HCV (anti-HCV), and HTLV (anti-HTLV) were determined among 11,391 donors to 5 tissue banks in the United States. Data from this analysis were compared with data from first-time blood donors to generate estimated incidence rates among tissue donors. The probability of viremia undetected by screening at the time of tissue donation was estimated on the basis of incidence estimates and the window periods for these infections.

Results.—The prevalence of confirmed positive tests among tissue donors was 0.093% for anti-HIV, 0.229% for HBsAg, 1.091% for anti-HCV, and 0.068% for anti-HTLV. The incidence rates were estimated to be 30.118, 18.325, 12.380, and 5.586 per 100,000 person-years, respectively. The estimated probability of viremia at donation was 1 in 55,000, 1 in 34,000, 1 in 42,000, and 1 in 128,000, respectively.

Conclusions.—The prevalence of HBV, HCV, HIV, and HTLV infection among tissue donors is lower than that among the general population. However, the estimated probability of undetected viremia at tissue donation is higher among tissue donors than among first-time blood donors. The addition of nucleic acid–amplification testing to the screening of tissue donors can be expected to reduce the risk of these infections among recipients of donated tissues.

▶ Although the incremental benefit in terms of HIV-1 and HCV detection is quite small, nucleic acid-amplification testing (Abstract 5–2) helps assure transfusion recipients that all that is possible is being done to maximize blood safety. The data presented here also show that persistent immunologically silent infection is extremely rare; only 3 seronegative donors with persistent hepatitis C viremia did not seroconvert during the expected time frame. This reinforces the appropriateness of continued reliance on serologic analyses as the primary tools for diagnosis of HIV-1 and HCV infection. The situation is much improved from that which existed 20 years ago, when up to 1 in 100 blood units in the United States transmitted HIV or HCV.[1]

B. H. Thiers, MD

Reference

1. Goodman JL: The safety and availability of blood and tissues—Progress and challenges. N Engl J Med 351:819-822, 2004.

Male Circumcision and Risk of HIV-1 and Other Sexually Transmitted Infections in India
Reynolds SJ, Shepherd ME, Risbud AR, et al (Johns Hopkins Univ, Baltimore, Md; Natl Aids Research Inst, Pune, India)
Lancet 363:1039-1040, 2004   5–4

Background.—Compared with uncircumcised men, circumcised men have a lower risk of HIV-1 infection. Some researchers attribute this reduced risk to the removal of the thinly keratinized mucosa of the inner foreskin and its HIV target cells. Other researchers believe the risk of HIV-1 infection is reduced because circumcised men have fewer risky behaviors than uncircumcised men. Further support for either a behavioral or a biological explanation for the reduced risk of HIV-1 infection in circumcised men was investigated.

Methods.—The subjects were 2298 men with HIV-1 infection attending 3 sexually transmitted disease clinics in India between 1993 and 2000. The risks of HIV-1, HIV-2, syphilis, and gonorrhea were compared between the 2107 uncircumcised men (91.7%) and the 191 circumcised men (8.3%). Data were analyzed by Cox proportional hazard modeling to adjust for differences in sociodemographic and behavioral risk factors between the 2 groups.

Results.—The risk of HIV-1 infection was more than 6 times lower in the circumcised men (adjusted relative risk, 0.15; $P = .0089$). However, circumcision did not protect against HIV-2, syphilis, or gonorrhea (adjusted relative risks, 0.63-0.91; all P values nonsignificant).

Conclusion.—Circumcision protects men against HIV-1 infection but not against other sexually transmitted diseases. The specificity of this relationship supports a biological, rather than a behavioral, explanation for the protective effect of circumcision against HIV-1 infection.

▶ The results suggest that the foreskin has an important role in the biology of sexual transmission of HIV. They clearly do not imply that circumcision is a marker for low-risk behavior, as circumcision had no protective effect against other sexually transmitted diseases.

B. H. Thiers, MD

Dual HIV-1 Infection Associated With Rapid Disease Progression

Gottlieb GS, Nickle DC, Jensen MA, et al (Univ of Washington, Seattle; Univ of Cape Town, South Africa; Univ of Natal, Durban, South Africa; et al)
Lancet 363:619-622, 2004   5–5

Background.—Dual infection with 2 HIV-1 strains has important implications for understanding HIV transmission and for developing an AIDS vaccine. However, the frequency and pathogenic consequences of such dual infection are not well documented. Patients from the multicenter AIDS cohort study, the Seattle primary infection cohort, and the South African female sex worker cohort were analyzed retrospectively for dual infection.

Methods and Findings.—Sixty-four patients were evaluated with the use of heteroduplex mobility assay, viral sequencing, and phylogenetic methods. Outcomes of HIV disease were known in 34 cases. Five patients with AIDS end points had dual HIV-1 infection, of whom 4 had coinfection and 1 had superinfection. All 5 patients had a very rapid progression from seroconversion to clinical AIDS or a CD4+ T-cell count of less than 200 cells per microliter.

Conclusions.—Dual HIV-1 infection appears to correlate with rapid disease progression. Larger studies are needed to determine the effect of dual infection at the population level.

▶ Gottlieb et al show that infection with more than 1 strain of HIV-1 is associated with rapid disease progression. These findings have implications for HIV transmission, treatment, and vaccine development. They postulate that transmission of drug-resistant viruses during primary HIV infection and acquisition of 2 distinct drug-resistant viruses could lead to recombination and the development of multi-drug-resistant strains. The topic of HIV drug resistance has recently been reviewed in detail.[1]

B. H. Thiers, MD

Reference

1. Clavel F, Hance AJ: HIV drug resistance. *N Engl J Med* 350:1023-1035, 2004.

HIV-1 Specific CD8+ T Cells With an Effector Phenotype and Control of Viral Replication

Hess C, Altfeld M, Thomas SY, et al (Massachusetts Gen Hosp, Charlestown, Mass; Harvard Med School, Boston; Univ Hosp Eppendorf, Hamburg, Germany)
Lancet 363:863-866, 2004   5–6

Introduction.—Most individuals infected with HIV-1 cannot control viral replication, despite the presence of virus-specific CD8+ T cells. This may be due to impaired maturation of these virus-specific cells. Individuals with treated acute HIV-1 infection undergoing structured treatment interruption

(STI) can frequently be induced to control viral replication, at least transiently. The maturation phenotypes of immunodominant HIV-1–specific CD8+ T-cell responses were compared in patients with treated acute HIV-1 infection before, during, and after sequential STIs for up to 4.3 years with those observed in HIV-1–infected patients not treated during acute infection.

Methods.—CD45RA and CCR7 were used as markers of lineage differentiation; HLA class I tetramers were used to identify antigen-specific CD8+ T cells. The maturation phenotype of virus-specific CD8+ T cells in individuals who could control viral replication of anti-retroviral therapy was compared with that of those not able to control viral replication.

Results.—In 5 patients with treated acute HIV-1 infection, STI-induced control of viral replication was linked with expansion of virus-specific CD8+ T cells with a fully differentiated effector phenotype. These effector cells were also expanded in treatment-naive chronically infected persons who spontaneously controlled viral replication. Augmented expression of perforin was observed in both settings.

Conclusion.—Full maturation of virus-specific CD8+ T cells is possible in the context of HIV-1 infection, indicating that such maturation may be important in viral control.

▶ It is generally accepted that HIV-specific CD8+ cytotoxic T lymphocytes play a central role in the protective immune response to infection with HIV. The frequent breakdown of this control mechanism has been attributed to a failure of such cells to achieve mature function. This interesting study provides compelling evidence to support this hypothesis.

The authors showed that the population of fully mature viral-specific T cells was strikingly increased in certain patients responding to STI of antiviral therapy and that in those patients whose response subsequently failed, the mature cells diminished to be replaced by pre-terminally differentiated cells. The size of the mature population was significantly inversely correlated with the viral load.

Further studies of patients who experienced long-term control of the infection without therapy showed a similar expanded population of cytotoxic HIV-specific cells. In both groups of patients, the mature cells were shown to be functionally competent in terms of perforin expression.

G. M. P. Galbraith, MD

Persistent GB Virus C Infection and Survival in HIV-Infected Men
Williams CF, Klinzman D, Yamashita TE, et al (Natl Inst of Allergy and Infectious Diseases, Bethesda, Md; Univ of Iowa, Iowa City; Johns Hopkins Univ, Baltimore, Md; et al)
N Engl J Med 350:981-990, 2004   5–7

Background.—GB virus C (GBV-C) replicates in lymphocytes and inhibits replication of HIV in vitro. Some research suggests that GBV-C is associated with a reduced risk of death among HIV-positive patients. However, these studies did not control for differences in the duration of HIV or GBV-C infection.

Methods.—Two hundred seventy-one men participating in he Multicenter Acquired Immunodeficiency Syndrome Cohort Study were evaluated for GBV-C viremia or E2 antibody 12 to 18 months after HIV seroconversion (the early visit). A reverse-transcriptase polymerase chain reaction assay and an enzyme-linked immunosorbent assay were used to evaluate GBV-C viremia and E2 antibodies (ie, antibodies against the GBV-C envelope glycoprotein), respectively. A subgroup of 138 patients were also assessed 5 to 6 years after HIV seroconversion (the late visit).

Methods.—Eighty-five percent of men with HIV seroconversion were found to have GBV-C infection on the basis of findings of E2 antibody (46%) or GBV-C RNA (39%). Only 1 man acquired GBV-C viremia between the early and late visits. However, 9% had GBV-C RNA clearance between these visits. At 12 to 18 months after HIV seroconversion, GBV-C status did not correlate significantly with survival. However, men without GBV-C RNA at the late visit were 2.78 times as likely to die as those with persistent GBV-C viremia. The loss of GBV-C RNA was associated with the worst prognosis and carried a relative hazard of 5.87 for death.

Conclusions.—In this series, GBV-C viremia was significantly associated with a prolonged survival duration among HIV-positive men 5 to 6 years after HIV seroconversion but not at 12 to 18 months. The loss of GBV-C RNA by 5 to 6 years correlated with the poorest prognosis. A better understanding of the interaction between GBV-C and HIV may provide insight into the progression of HIV disease.

▶ Although GBV-C, a close relative of the hepatitis C virus, infects people worldwide, no association between the virus and a known disease state has been demonstrated. Many previously published studies have demonstrated a surprising survival benefit among patients who are coinfected with GBV-C and HIV. It has been postulated that GBV-C increases or augments the innate immune mechanisms that inhibit HIV. A direct antiviral effect has also been postulated. Knowledge of how GBV-C improves the prognosis in HIV-infected patients may lead to better therapies of this increasingly common disease.[1]

B. H. Thiers, MD

Reference

1. Pomerantz RJ, Nunnari G: HIV and GB virus C: Can two viruses be better than one? *N Engl J Med* 350:963-965, 2004.

Inhibition of HIV-1 Replication by GB Virus C Infection Through Increases in RANTES, MIP-1α, MIP-1β, and SDF-1

Xiang J, George SL, Wünschmann S, et al (Univ of Iowa, Iowa City)
Lancet 363:2040-2046, 2004   5–8

Background.—The mortality rate among patients coinfected with HIV and GB virus C (GBV-C) is lower than among HIV-infected patients without GBV-C. HIV gains entry into CD4-positive cells through the chemokine receptors CCR5 or CXCR4. Increased survival rates in HIV-positive patients correlate with high serum levels of ligands for CCR5 and CXCR4, as well as decreased expression of CCR5 on lymphocytes. The effect of GBV-C isolates on HIV-1 strains that use CCR5 or CXCR4 as their coreceptor was investigated, as were the potential mechanisms by which GBV-C may inhibit HIV-1.

Methods.—Peripheral blood mononuclear cells were coinfected with GBV-C and HIV. Replication of HIV was monitored through measures of infectivity and HIV p24 antigen production. Chemokine secretion, chemokine receptor expression, and cellular chemokine mRNA expression were assessed by enzyme-linked immunoassay, flow cytometry, and differential hybridization, respectively.

Findings.—Infection of peripheral blood mononuclear cells with GBV-C resulted in a reduction in replication of clinical and laboratory HIV strains that use CCR5 or CXCR4 as their coreceptor. Inhibition correlated with the GBV-C dose and the timing of infection. The mRNA expression of ligands for CCR5 and CXCR4 was higher in GBV-C–infected cells than in mock-infected cells. Chemokine secretion into culture supernatants was also higher in the GBV-C-infected cells. Incubation with neutralizing antibodies against the relevant chemokines blocked the inhibitory effect of GBV-C on HIV replication. Surface expression of CCR5 was significantly lower in GBV-C-infected cells than in mock-infected cells.

Conclusions.—Infection with GBV-C induces HIV-inhibitory chemokines and decreases expression of the HIV coreceptor CCR5 in vitro. These data help clarify the epidemiologic relationship between GBV-C infection and the longer survival duration in individuals with HIV infection.

▶ HIV uses either of 2 chemokine receptors, CCR5 or CXCR4, for entry into CD4-positive cells. Xiang et al found that coinfection of lymphocytes with GBV-C and HIV inhibits HIV by inducing natural ligands for CCR5 and CXCR4 and by decreasing expression of CCR5 on the surface of lymphocytes. Future HIV disease-modifying vaccines might mimic the way GBV-C causes these changes.

B. H. Thiers, MD

A Randomized Trial of Multivitamin Supplements and HIV Disease Progression and Mortality
Fawzi WW, Msamanga GI, Spiegelman D, et al (Harvard Univ, Boston; Muhimbili Univ, Dar es Salaam, Tanzania)
N Engl J Med 351:23-32, 2004   5–9

Background.—Observational studies suggest micronutrient supplements may slow disease progression in patients with HIV infection. Thus, the effects of micronutrient supplementation on virologic and immunologic variables in HIV-infected pregnant women were prospectively studied.

Methods.—The research subjects were 1078 pregnant women with HIV (mean age, about 24.7 years) living in Dar es Salaam, Tanzania. Patients were randomly assigned to 4 groups to receive daily supplements of either vitamin A alone (preformed vitamin A and beta carotene), multivitamins alone (vitamins B complex, C, and E), vitamin A plus multivitamins, or placebo. Patients were monitored for a median of 71 months to determine a combined end point of HIV disease progression (ie, World Health Organization [WHO] stage 4 disease) or death; CD4+ cell counts and viral loads were also examined and correlated with treatment.

Results.—Vitamin A supplementation alone was not significantly more effective than placebo in improving clinical, virologic, and immunologic variables. With multivitamin monotherapy, however, significantly fewer patients met the combined end point (24.7% vs 31.1% in the placebo group; relative risk [RR], 0.71). Specifically, multivitamins significantly decreased the risks of progression to WHO stage 4 disease (RR, 0.50), death from AIDS-related causes (0.73), and progression to WHO stage 3 or higher disease (RR, 0.72). These risk reductions were stronger during the first 2 years of therapy, but benefits were still significant at 4 years. Multivitamins were also associated with significant improvements in CD4+ cell counts (increase of 48 cells per cubic millimeter), CD8+ cell counts (increase of 43 cells per cubic millimeter), and viral load (decrease of $0.18 \log_{10}$ units) compared with placebo. Oral and gastrointestinal manifestations of HIV disease were also significantly reduced by multivitamin use. Adding vitamin A to multivitamin therapy actually decreased some of the benefits seen with multivitamins alone.

Conclusion.—Among these HIV-infected pregnant women, supplementation with vitamin B complex and vitamins C and E significantly lowered the risk of HIV disease progression compared with placebo. Multivitamins also had positive effects on virologic and immune variables. These results suggest that daily multivitamins may be a low-cost approach to delaying the need for antiretroviral therapy in HIV-infected pregnant women.

▶ This study was done in Tanzania, where many of the patients could be presumed to be nutritionally deprived. It would be interesting to study whether vitamin supplementation would have the same beneficial effect in HIV-infected women in the industrialized world. Previously published data in US men suggest that this might, in fact, be the case.[1-5] However, these findings from observational studies have been challenged.[6,7]

B. H. Thiers, MD

References

1. Abrams B, Duncan D, Hertz-Picciotto I: A prospective study of dietary intake and acquired immune deficiency syndrome in HIV-seropositive homosexual men. *J Acquir Immune Defic Syndr* 6:949-958, 1993.
2. Tang AM, Graham NMH, Kirby AJ, et al: Dietary micronutrient intake and risk progression to acquired immunodeficiency syndrome virus type 1 (HIV-1) infected homosexual men. *Am J Epidemiol* 138:937-951,1993.
3. Tang AM, Graham NMH, Saah AJ: Effects of micronutrient intake on survival in human immunodeficiency virus type 1 infection. *Am J Epidemiol* 143:1244-1256, 1996.
4. Tang AM, Graham NMH, Semba RD, et al: Association between serum vitamin A and E levels and HIV-1 disease progression. *AIDS* 11:613-620, 1997.
5. Tang AM, Graham NMH, Chandra RK, et al: Low serum vitamin B-12 concentrations are associated with faster human immunodeficiency virus type 1 (HIV-1) disease progression. *J Nutr* 127:345-351, 1997.
6. Semba RD, Tang AM: Micronutrients and the pathogenesis of human immunodeficiency virus infection. *Br J Nutr* 81:181-189, 1999.
7. Fawzi WW: Micronutrients and human immunodeficiency virus type 1 disease progression among adults and children. *Clin Infect Dis* 37:112S-116S, 2003.

Clinical Efficacy of Antiretroviral Combination Therapy Based on Protease Inhibitors or Non-nucleoside Analogue Reverse Transcriptase Inhibitors: Indirect Comparison of Controlled Trials

Yazdanpanah Y, Sissoko D, Egger M, et al (Centre Hospitalier de Tourcoing, France; Univ of Bristol, England; Univ of Bern, Switzerland; et al)
BMJ 328:249-253, 2004   5–10

Background.—Industrialized countries in which highly active antiretroviral therapy has been introduced have experienced a dramatic decline in morbidity and mortality among patients infected with human immunodeficiency virus type 1 (HIV-1). Highly active antiretroviral therapy is a combination of 3 drugs, including either a protease inhibitor or a non-nucleoside analogue reverse transcriptase inhibitor (NNRTI) and 2 nucleoside analogue reverse transcriptase inhibitors (NRTIs). The clinical efficacy of triple antiretroviral regimens based on protease inhibitors and NNRTIs was compared in adults positive for antibodies to HIV-1.

Methods.—A systematic review and meta-analysis were conducted that used indirect comparisons of clinical trials that compared 3 drug regimens based on 2 NRTIs and either a protease inhibitor or a NNRTI with 2 drug regimens (2 NRTIs). All of the participants in this study had no previous exposure to protease inhibitors or NNRTIs. Data sources for this study included MEDLINE, the Cochrane controlled trials register, Aidstrials, Aidsdrugs, conference proceedings, and trial registers. The main outcome measure was progression to AIDS or death.

Results.—Fourteen trials involving 6785 patients were identified. Most of the patients had been exposed to an NRTI and had advanced immunodeficiency disease at baseline; of these patients, 1096 progressed to AIDS or died. Half of the trials evaluated protease inhibitor–based triple regimens and half assessed NNRTI-based triple regimens (nevirapine or delavirdine). Triple therapy was found to be more effective than dual therapy. The effect was significant for protease inhibitor–based regimens but was nonsignificant for NNRTI-based regimens. An indirect comparison of these 2 regimens yielded an odds ratio of 0.54 in favor of protease inhibitor–based treatments. Increases in CD4 cell counts were smaller and the suppression of viral replication less pronounced with NNRTI-based regimens.

Conclusions.—There is indirect evidence that protease inhibitor–based triple regimens are superior to regimens based on the NNRTIs nevirapine and delavirdine in patients with advanced immunodeficiency who have been exposed to NRTIs. Large trials with clinical end points are needed to confirm these findings.

▶ Triple drug antiretroviral therapy is currently the gold standard for HIV infected patients. Although no trials have compared the clinical effectiveness of protease inhibitor regimens with NNRTI regimens, indirect comparisons can provide useful information. Such comparisons suggest that protease inhibitor–based triple drug regimens are superior to those with the NNRTIs nevirapine or delavirdine in patients with advanced disease who have previously used nucleoside reverse transcriptase inhibitors. However, as discussed by Lundgren and Phillips in an accompanying editorial, these findings may not be directly applicable to patients starting anti-HIV therapy for the first time, in whom several studies have suggested that the efficacy of NNRTIs is comparable to and perhaps even superior to protease inhibitors.[1-3] Any decision on the "best" treatment for HIV infection must clearly be individualized to each patient.

B. H. Thiers, MD

References

1. Lundgren JD, Phillips AN: Commentary: Indirect comparisons: A novel approach to assessing the effect of anti-HIV drugs. *BMJ* 328:253-254, 2004.
2. Robbins GK, De Gruttola V, Shafer RW, et al: Comparison of sequential three-drug regimens as initial therapy for HIV-1 infection. *N Engl J Med* 349:2293-2303, 2003.
3. Van Leeuwen R, Katlama C, Murphy RL, et al: A randomized trial to study first-line combination therapy with or without a protease inhibitor in HIV-1-infected patients. *AIDS* 17:987-999, 2003.

Stable Partnership and Progression to AIDS or Death in HIV Infected Patients Receiving Highly Active Antiretroviral Therapy: Swiss HIV Cohort Study

Young J, for the Swiss HIV Cohort Study Group (Univ Hosp Basel, Switzerland; et al)

BMJ 328:15-19, 2004   5–11

Background.—Social support (ie, the emotional or tangible support a person has from other people) influences a person's health in many ways. For example, poor social support is associated with a more rapid decline in CD4 cell counts in patients with HIV infection. The effect of having a stable partnership on disease progression in patients with HIV infection receiving highly active antiretroviral therapy (HAART) was prospectively examined.

Methods.—The subjects were 3736 patients with HIV (71% men; median age, 36 years) who began receiving HAART before 2002. Every 6 months, all patients were asked if they had had sexual intercourse with a stable partner during the previous 6 months. Patients were monitored a median of 3.6 years to determine disease progression (ie, increase in clinical Centers for Disease Control and Prevention [CDC] stage) or death. Increases in the CD4 cell count of 100 cells/μL or greater and the attainment of optimal viral suppression (viral load <400 copies/mL) were also examined in light of having a stable partnership.

Results.—During follow-up, most of the patients (2985, or 80%) reported having a stable partnership during at least one 6-month period. At the start of HAART, 52% of patients (545 of 1042 evaluable patients) reported a stable partnership; 5 years later, the proportion had decreased to 46% (190 of 412 patients). After data adjustment, patients with a stable partnership were significantly less likely to progress to AIDS or to die than patients without a stable partnership (hazard ratio 0.79). Patients with a stable partnership were also significantly less likely to die (hazard ratio 0.59) and significantly more likely to have an increase in CD4 cell counts of 100 cells/μL or greater (hazard ratio 1.15). Patients with a stable partnership were also more likely than those without a stable partnership to have optimal viral suppression (hazard ratio 1.06), but the between-group difference was not significant.

Conclusion.—For patients with HIV infection who are receiving HAART, having a stable partnership is associated with a slower rate of progression to AIDS or death, and with a slower decline in CD4 cell counts. Clinicians should be aware that HIV-positive patients receiving HAART who do not have a stable partnership may progress more rapidly to the later stages of the disease.

▶ In the elderly and in people with cardiovascular disease, social support is associated with lower mortality. For patients with HIV infection on HAART, a stable partnership appears to be similarly beneficial.

B. H. Thiers, MD

The Prognostic Importance of Changes in CD4+ Cell Count and HIV-1 RNA Level in Women After Initiating Highly Active Antiretroviral Therapy
Anastos K, Barrón Y, Cohen MH, et al (Montefiore Med Ctr, Bronx, NY; Johns Hopkins Univ, Baltimore, Md; Cook County Hosp, Chicago; et al)
Ann Intern Med 140:256-264, 2004   5–12

Background.—The prognostic value of CD4+ cell counts and HIV-1 RNA concentrations determined after initiation of highly active antiretroviral therapy (HAART) compared with before treatment is unclear. A study to further investigate this question was conducted.

Methods.—A cohort of 1132 patients participated in the Women's Interagency HIV Study. The patients were studied prospectively. Assessment included HIV-1 RNA levels, CD4+ cell counts, and AIDS-defining illness. The median follow-up time was 3.9 years.

Findings.—Compared with women with CD4+ cell counts exceeding 0.35×10^9 cells per liter, women with CD4+ cell counts of less than 0.200×10^9 cells per liter after HAART initiation had a 2.66 (95% CI, 1.42-4.99) relative hazard of death from all causes and a 47.61 (95% CI, 5.69-398.40) relative hazard of death from AIDS. Women with RNA levels of more than 10,000 copies per milliliter had a 3.44 (95% CI, 1.7-7.09) relative hazard of all-cause death compared with women with RNA levels of less than 80 copies per milliliter. Compared with women with CD4+ cell counts exceeding 0.350×10^9 cells per liter, women with post-HAART CD4+ cell counts between 0.2 and 0.35×10^9 cells per liter did not have an increased relative hazard of AIDS-related death or death from any cause. The relative hazard was also not increased in women with post-HAART HIV-1 RNA levels between 80 and 10,000 copies per milliliter compared with those with post-HAART HIV-1 RNA levels of less than 80 copies per milliliter. Post-HAART CD4+ cell count and HIV-1 RNA levels were the only laboratory markers studied that predicted new AIDS-defining illness.

Conclusions.—In this prospective cohort study, post-HAART laboratory markers predicted death and new AIDS-defining illness. The pre-HAART CD4+ cell count and HIV-1 RNA level did not predict clinical outcomes when adjusted for values obtained after HAART initiation. This suggests that even advanced immune suppression can be overcome with HAART that results in CD4+ cell counts exceeding 0.2×10^9 cells/L and RNA levels of less than 10,000 copies per milliliter.

▶ Articles summarized in the 2004 YEAR BOOK OF DERMATOLOGY AND DERMATOLOGIC SURGERY suggested that the initial response to HAART rather than the baseline CD4+ cell count was the most important factor in determining the long-term prognosis in HIV-infected patients.[1,2] The current article confirms that patients with a good CD4+ cell count and HIV-1 RNA response to HAART have a favorable prognosis, despite poor pretreatment values of these markers. Thus, even patients with seemingly overwhelming infection at presentation should be aggressively treated.[3]

B. H. Thiers, MD

References

1. Chene G, Sterne JA, May M, et al: Prognostic importance of initial response in HIV-1 infected patients starting potent antiretroviral therapy: Analysis of prospective studies. *Lancet* 362:679-686, 2003.
2. Porter K, Babiker A, Bhaskaran K, et al: Determinants of survival following HIV-1 seroconversion after the introduction of HAART. *Lancet* 362:1267-1274, 2003.
3. Schooley RT: Starting highly active retroviral therapy for HIV infection: Is it WIHS to wait? *Ann Intern Med* 140:305-306, 2004.

Importance of Cytomegalovirus Viraemia in Risk of Disease Progression and Death in HIV-Infected Patients Receiving Highly Active Antiretroviral Therapy

Deayton JR, Sabin CA, Johnson MA, et al (Univ College, London)
Lancet 363:2116-2121, 2004   5–13

Background.—Several studies indicate that the presence of cytomegalovirus (CMV) in the blood of patients with HIV infection predicts progression to AIDS and death. These studies, however, were performed before highly active antiretroviral therapy (HAART) became available, and HAART has dramatically improved the survival rate and the risk of opportunistic infection in patients with HIV. Thus, the prognostic significance of CMV infection in HIV-infected patients using HAART was investigated.

Methods.—The research subjects were 374 patients with HIV infection (79% men; median age, 36 years) whose CD4+ cell count had ever been less than 100 cells per milliliter. Every 3 months, patients provided blood samples that were tested for CMV by polymerase chain reaction (PCR) analysis. Patients were monitored for a median of 37 months to determine the incidence of new CMV disease, AIDS-defining illness, and death.

Results.—Most patients (94.9%) received HAART at some point during the study, and most patients (84.2%) had CMV-negative findings at baseline. Of 2969 PCR analyses performed, results were consistently negative throughout the follow-up period in 259 patients (69.3%), persistently positive in 15 patients (4.0%), and intermittently positive in 100 patients (26.7%). Only univariate analyses of the effect of CMV status on CMV viremia could be performed because only a few patients reached this end point. These analyses revealed that the most recently measured CMV PCR result was significantly associated with progression to a new CMV event (relative rate, 24.5). In multivariate analyses, the presence of CMV at baseline was a significant and independent risk factor for both progression to an AIDS-defining illness (odds ratio [OR], 1.79) and death (OR, 2.09). When analyses were extended to account for changes in CMV status during the follow-up period, the presence of CMV in blood was even more strongly associated with an increased risk of progression to an AIDS-defining illness (OR, 2.22) and death (OR, 4.14).

Conclusion.—Even with HAART, the presence of CMV in the blood significantly increases the risk of progression to CMV disease, AIDS-defining illness, and death.

▶ The data would seem to suggest that aggressive therapy for CMV infection might reduce disease progression and death in HIV-infected patients. Indeed, a recent study[1] found an improved survival rate in patients with CMV retinitis who received, in addition to HAART, systemic anti-CMV therapy.

B. H. Thiers, MD

Reference

1. Kempen JH, Jabs DA, Wilson LA, et al: Mortality risk for patients with cytomegalovirus retinitis and acquired immune deficiency syndrome. *Clin Infect Dis* 37:1365-1373, 2003.

Single-Dose Perinatal Nevirapine Plus Standard Zidovudine to Prevent Mother-to-Child Transmission of HIV-1 in Thailand
Lallemant M, for the Perinatal HIV Prevention Trial (Thailand) Investigators (Institut de Recherche Pour le Développement, Paris; et al)
N Engl J Med 351:217-228, 2004   5–14

Background.—Zidovudine prophylaxis markedly reduces HIV type 1 transmission rate among infants. However, a large number of babies still become infected. The efficacy of a single dose of oral nevirapine along with zidovudine administered to mothers during labor and to neonates was investigated.

Methods.—The randomized double-blind trial included a total of 1844 Thai women receiving zidovudine in the third trimester of pregnancy between 2001 and 2003. In group 1, mothers and infants both received a single dose of nevirapine. In group 2, mothers and infants received nevirapine and placebo, respectively. In group 3, both mothers and infants received placebo. In addition, the infants were given 1 week of zidovudine treatment. All infants were formula fed.

Findings.—At the first interim analysis, assignment to group 3 was stopped. Among women delivering before the interim analysis, transmission rates were 1.1% in group 1 and 6.3% in group 3. The final transmission rates were 1.9% in group 1 and 2.8% in group 2, which were not significantly different. Nevirapine had effects in subgroups defined by the viral load and CD4 count. Nevirapine produced no serious adverse effects.

Conclusions.—Mother-to-infant HIV transmission can be reduced by administration of a single nevirapine dose to the mother in addition to oral zidovudine prophylaxis beginning at 28 weeks' gestation. This strategy seems to be effective with or without a dose of nevirapine to the infant.

Intrapartum Exposure to Nevirapine and Subsequent Maternal Responses to Nevirapine-Based Antiretroviral Therapy

Jourdain G, for the Perinatal HIV Prevention Trial Group (Harvard Univ, Boston; Institut de Recherche pour le Développement, Paris; Ministry of Public Health, Bangkok, Thailand; et al)

N Engl J Med 351:229-240, 2004
5–15

Background.—Administration of a single intrapartum dose of nevirapine to prevent mother-to-child HIV transmission leads to selection of resistance mutations. Whether clinically significant consequences occur in mothers subsequently treated with a nevirapine-containing regimen has not been determined.

Methods.—In this study, 1844 Thai women receiving zidovudine in the third trimester of pregnancy were assigned randomly to intrapartum nevirapine or placebo. After delivery, 269 women with a CD4 count of less than 250 cells per cubic millimeter were started on a nevirapine-containing antiretroviral regimen. Plasma HIV type 1 RNA was assessed before treatment initiation and 3 and 6 months thereafter.

Findings.—At 6 months, the HIV-1 RNA level was less than 50 copies per milliliter in 49% of women receiving intrapartum nevirapine and in 68% not receiving intrapartum nevirapine. Resistance mutations to nonnucleoside reverse-transcriptase inhibitors were detected in blood samples acquired 10 days postpartum from 32% of women receiving intrapartum nevirapine. The most frequent mutations were K103N, G190A, and Y181C. In the intrapartum nevirapine group, viral suppression was obtained at 6 months in 38% of women with resistance mutations and in 52% of those without resistance mutations. An HIV-1 RNA level equal to or greater than the median of $4.53 \log_{10}$ copies per milliliter before treatment and intrapartum nevirapine treatment correlated independently with virologic failure. After 6 months of treatment, CD4 counts did not differ between groups.

Conclusions.—Women receiving intrapartum nevirapine were less likely to have virologic suppression after 6 months of postpartum therapy with a nevirapine-containing regimen. Strategies are needed to maximize the benefits of antiretroviral prophylaxis against mother-to-child HIV transmission and antiretroviral therapy for mothers.

▶ In a study performed in Thailand, Lallemant et al (Abstract 5–14) demonstrated that adding a single dose of nevirapine to a course of zidovudine starting at 28 weeks' gestation is highly effective in reducing mother-to-child transmission of HIV. One concern regarding the use of antiretroviral agents for the prevention of mother-to-child transmission of HIV is the possibility that these regimens could be ineffective in subsequent pregnancies, in the subsequent management of the infection in mothers, or in infants who become infected despite prophylaxis. In fact, Jourdain et al (Abstract 5–15) found resistance mutations to nucleoside reverse-transcriptase inhibitors (including zidovudine), as well as to nevirapine, even in women who had received only a single dose of this nonnucleoside reverse-transcriptase inhibitor. As stated in an accompaning editorial,[1] additional studies with longer follow-up are needed to quantify the clinical implications of these findings.

B. H. Thiers, MD

Reference

1. Coovadia H: Antiretroviral agents: How best to protect infants from HIV and save their mothers from AIDS. *N Engl J Med* 251:3:289-292, 2004.

A Trial of Three Antiretroviral Regimens in HIV-1–Infected Children
Luzuriaga K, for the PACTG 356 Investigators (Univ of Massachusetts, Worcester; et al)
N Engl J Med 350:2471-2480, 2004   5–16

Introduction.—Because depletion of CD4 T cells and disease progression occur more rapidly in children than in adults infected with HIV-1, early treatment during infancy might be beneficial. Few studies, however, have examined the optimal time for initiation of antiretroviral therapy in infants. This issue was addressed in the Pediatric AIDS Clinical Trials Group Protocol 356 (PACTG 356).

Methods.—The open-label, phase 1-2 PACTG 356 trial enrolled infants at 25 sites in the United States and Puerto Rico between May 1997 and November 1998. Stratification was according to age: 3 months or younger (early therapy) and older than 3 months (delayed therapy). Children were assigned sequentially to 1 of 3 regimens and continued to receive treatment for up to 200 weeks if plasma HIV-1 RNA levels were less than 1000 copies/ mL by 16 weeks.

Results.—Fifty-two children were enrolled, including 31 who had received antiretroviral therapy before study entry. The median age at initiation of therapy was 2.0 months in the early therapy cohort and 7.6 months in the delayed-therapy cohort. Plasma HIV-1 RNA levels fell from a median of 5.3 log copies/mL at baseline to less than 1000 copies/mL at 16 weeks in 32 (62%) infants. At 48 weeks, 50% of infants had plasma HIV-1 RNA levels below 400 copies/mL; at 200 weeks, 44% of infants remained at these levels (60% in the early therapy cohort vs 30% in the delayed-therapy cohort).

Significantly more children treated with stavudine, lamivudine, nevirapine, and nelfinavir had plasma HIV-1 RNA levels of less than 400 copies/ mL at 48 weeks (83%) and 200 weeks (72%) compared with children treated with reverse-transcriptase inhibitors alone. The only treatment-related adverse events of moderate or greater severity occurred in 8 infants receiving a reverse-transcriptase inhibitor regimen. Only 1 child discontinued therapy because of drug-related adverse effects.

Conclusion.—Early (3 months or younger) initiation of therapy appeared to be associated with improved long-term suppression of viral replication in infants with HIV-1 infection. The regimen of stavudine, lamivudine, nevirapine, and nelfinavir appeared to be superior to the 2 reverse-transcriptase inhibitor regimens.

▶ The use of perinatal antiretroviral regimens has markedly reduced mother-to-child transmission of HIV. Some reports have suggested that intensive treatment during the first year of life alone may limit treatment costs and improve outcome. In contrast, the data reported by Luzuriaga et al demonstrate that this is associated with a rapid resumption of viral replication and subsequent CD4 T-cell depletion, negating any long-term benefit of such an approach. These investigators do show that combination therapy with stavudine, lamivudine, nevirapine, and nelfinavir is associated with improved long-term viral suppression. Early initiation of therapy (at 3 months of age or earlier) appears to provide the most significant benefit.

B. H. Thiers, MD

Metabolic Effects of Rosiglitazone in HIV Lipodystrophy: A Randomized, Controlled Trial

Hadigan C, Yawetz S, Thomas A, et al (Massachusetts Gen Hosp, Boston; Brigham and Women's Hosp, Boston)
Ann Intern Med 140:786-794, 2004   5–17

Background.—The treatment of HIV-infected patients with combination antiretroviral drugs is often associated with metabolic abnormalities, including insulin resistance, hypertriglyceridemia, and loss of subcutaneous fat. The identification of the specific mechanisms responsible for these metabolic disturbances has been difficult, but increasing evidence has shown that direct metabolic toxicity from each class of antiretroviral agents may play a role. The loss of subcutaneous fat may be an important mechanism that contributes to the metabolic abnormalities in these patients, and the loss of subcutaneous fat is an important cosmetic concern for patients infected with HIV. Recent studies have suggested that reduced adiponectin levels may be related to disrupted subcutaneous adipogenesis and altered peroxisome proliferator–activated receptor-α signaling. The effects of rosiglitazone, a peroxisome proliferator–activated receptor-agonist, were investigated in HIV-infected men and women with hyperinsulinemia and lipoatrophy.

Methods.—This randomized, double-blind, placebo-controlled 3-month study was conducted in a university hospital and included 28 HIV-infected men and women with hyperinsulinemia and lipoatrophy. Insulin sensitivity was measured by euglycemic hyperinsulinemic clamp testing; subcutaneous leg fat area was measured by CT. Adiponectin, free fatty acid and lipid levels, and safety variables were also tested.

Results.—Rosiglitazone in comparison with placebo improved insulin sensitivity, increased adiponectin levels, and reduced free fatty acid levels. The mean percentage of body fat and subcutaneous leg fat area were significantly increased with rosiglitazone compared with placebo. Mean total cholesterol levels also increased with rosiglitazone compared with placebo.

Conclusions.—This relatively small study would appear to be the first randomized placebo-controlled study to show a statistically significant benefit of peroxisome proliferator–activated receptor-α–agonist therapy for lipoatrophy in HIV-infected patients with insulin resistance.

No Effect of Rosiglitazone for Treatment of HIV-1 Lipoatrophy: Randomised, Double-blind, Placebo-Controlled Trial

Carr A, for the Rosey Investigators (St Vincent's Hosp, Sydney, Australia; AIDS Research Initiative, Sydney, Australia; Univ of New South Wales, Sydney, Australia; et al)

Lancet 363:429-438, 2004   5–18

Background.—At least 50% of HIV-1–infected adults receiving antiretroviral therapy are affected by lipodystrophy, which can be stigmatizing and painful and can lead to suboptimal adherence to antiretroviral treatment. Thiazolidinediones are peroxisome proliferator–activated receptor-gamma agonists that are effective for the treatment of type 2 diabetes and for the treatment of adults with congenital lipodystrophy. Peroxisome proliferator–activated receptor-gamma agonists such as rosiglitazone have been shown to prevent HIV-1 protease inhibitor toxicity to adipocytes in vitro. Whether treatment with rosiglitazone improves lipoatrophy in HIV-1–infected patients receiving antiretroviral therapy was investigated.

Methods.—A total of 108 adults receiving antiretroviral therapy for HIV-1 infection and who were experiencing lipoatrophy were randomly assigned to 4 mg rosiglitazone twice daily (53 patients) or matching placebo (55 patients) for 48 weeks. The study had 80% power to detect a 0.5-kg difference in changes in limb fat with the use of dual-energy x-ray absorptiometry.

Results.—Three study participants, 1 from the rosiglitazone group and 2 from the control group, were lost to follow-up. The mean increase in limb fat was 0.14 kg in the rosiglitazone group and 0.18 kg in the placebo group. Rosiglitazone was found to have no significant benefit in terms of any other measure of lipodystrophy, despite large relative increases in plasma adiponectin levels and in 3 markers of insulin sensitivity. The study drug was discontinued by 6 participants in each group, including 4 who experienced treatment-related side effects. The major adverse events, which may be unique to this population, were asymptomatic hypertriglyceridemia and hypercholesterolemia.

Conclusions.—This study of rosiglitazone in patients receiving antiretroviral therapy for HIV-1 infection did not find improvement in lipoatrophy. The use of less toxic antiretroviral therapy seems to be necessary if lipoatrophy is to be prevented in these patients.

▶ Thiazolidinediones such as rosiglitazone improve insulin sensitivity and stimulate adipogenesis and have been studied for their capability to ameliorate metabolic abnormalities, including lipoatrophy and lipodystrophy, caused by antiretroviral therapy. In the study by Hadigan et al (Abstract 5–17), administration of rosiglitazone improved peripheral fat deposition during 3 months of antiretroviral treatment. However, the small sample size and short duration of treatment limit the generalizability of the findings. In contrast, the 48-week study performed by Carr et al (Abstract 5–18) showed no improvement in lipoatrophy when rosiglitazone was administered to HIV-1-infected adults receiving antiretroviral therapy. Because the morphological changes of HIV-1 lipoatrophy are highly stigmatizing and can cause discomfort, disability, psychological morbidity, and can reduce adherence to or cause discontinuation of otherwise effective antiretroviral therapy, better preventive methods are needed. Moreover, the metabolic changes induced by antiretroviral therapy may contribute to an increased risk of cardiovascular events.[1]

B. H. Thiers, MD

Reference

1. Moyle G, Sutinen J: Managing HIV lipoatrophy. *Lancet* 363:412-414, 2004.

Transcutaneous Immunization Induces Mucosal CTLs and Protective Immunity by Migration of Primed Skin Dendritic Cells
Belyakov IM, Hammond SA, Ahlers JD, et al (NIH, Bethesda, Md; IOMAI Corp, Gaithersburg, Md)
J Clin Invest 113:998-1007, 2004   5–19

Introduction.—The mucosal surface is an important entry point for many infections. The induction of mucosal immune responses and prevention of mucosal transmission are important goals for many vaccines. Skin immunization uses potent bone marrow–derived DCs that reside in the epidermis (ie, Langerhans cells). These cells provide immunosurveillance functions. When activated by microorganisms, they migrate out of the skin to the draining lymph nodes and induce strong effector antigen-specific responses by B and T lymphocytes. The cell-mediated systemic and mucosal responses induced by a transcutaneous immunization (TCI) regimen consisting of an HIV peptide construct with CT or LT or CpG oligodeoxynucleotides as adjuvants were examined.

Findings.—The effect of TCI with an HIV peptide on the induction of mucosal and systemic cytotoxic T lymphocyte (CTL) responses and protective immunity against mucosal challenge with live virus was assessed in female BALB/c or C57BL/6 mice. Robust HIV-specific CTL responses in the spleen and gut mucosa were observed after TCI. The responses depended upon addition of an adjuvant and resulted in protection against mucosal challenge with recombinant vaccina virus encoding HIV gp 160. Adjuvant-activated DCs migrated primarily to draining lymph nodes; however, co-culture with specific T cells and flow cytometry experiments with DCs isolated from Peyer's patches after TCI indicated that activated DCs carrying skin-derived antigen also migrated from the skin to immune-induction sites in gut mucosa and presented antigen directly to resident lymphocytes.

Conclusion.—TCI is safe and effective in inducing strong mucosal antibody and CTL responses.

▶ These investigators used a murine model to investigate the induction of mucosal immunity by TCI. They showed that exposure of abraded mouse skin to a solution containing an HIV peptide resulted in systemic peptide-specific cytotoxic T-lymphocyte activity as measured in spleen cell assays. However, examination of lymphocytes derived from Peyer's patches and lung revealed a similar mucosal cytotoxicity response.

The response was dependent on the addition of adjuvant to the immunizing solution and appeared to be greatest when the solution was applied to the back of the animal. In other experiments, immunized mice were challenged by mucosal infection with recombinant vaccinia virus encoding the HIV peptide. These studies showed that TCI was at least partially protective against infection.

G. M. P. Galbraith, MD

6 Parasitic Infections, Bites, and Infestations

Persistence of *Leishmania* Parasites in Scars After Clinical Cure of American Cutaneous Leishmaniasis: Is There a Sterile Cure?
Mendonça MG, de Brito MEF, Rodrigues EHG, et al (Universidade Federal de Pernambuco, Recife, Brazil)
J Infect Dis 189:1018-1023, 2004   6–1

Background.—In certain infections, such as those caused by herpesvirus, *Mycobacteria*, or *Trypanosoma cruzi*, the pathogen persists long after the patient has been clinically cured of the disease. Whether this is also true for the *Leishmania* parasites in American cutaneous leishmaniasis (ACL) was determined.

Methods.—The research subjects were 32 patients from northern Brazil (66% male, 15-62 years old) who had been treated for ACL and who were clinically cured. All lesions had been healed and had scar formation for 6 months or longer, and patients had no evidence of active disease or relapse. Three punch biopsy samples from the scar site were obtained and analyzed by histopathologic examination, culture, and polymerase chain reaction (PCR).

Results.—Histopathologic examination did not reveal any *Leishmania (Viannia)* parasites in any of the 32 specimens. Culture results were positive from 3 of the scars (9.4%). However, PCR identified DNA specific for *Leishmania (V)* species in 30 of the 32 specimens, including the 3 cases identified by culture. PCR results were positive in 3 scars more than 66 months old, including 1 scar that was 11 years old.

Conclusion.—Of these 32 patients with clinically cured ACL, only 2 had sterile cures. The persistence of *Leishmania (V)* parasites long after a clinical cure of ACL raises several issues regarding the clinical evolution, epidemiology, and control of leishmaniasis, particularly given the increasing incidence of leishmaniasis in patients with AIDS.

▶ *Leishmania* organisms were detected by PCR in the scars of 30 of 32 patients presumed to be clinically cured of ACL. In 3 of these, the parasites could be isolated by culture. The implications of these findings in terms of the evolution and transmission of the disease need further study.

B. H. Thiers, MD

Miltefosine for New World Cutaneous Leishmaniasis
Soto J, Arana BA, Toledo J, et al (Fundación Fader, Bogotá, Colombia; Instituto Colombiano de Medicina Tropical, Medellin, Colombia; Universidad del Valle de Guatemala, Guatemala City; et al)
Clin Infect Dis 38:1266-1272, 2004   6–2

Background.—Miltefosine, an oral agent, yields a better than 95% cure rate in patients with Indian visceral leishmaniasis. In a large-scale, placebo-controlled study, the therapeutic index of miltefosine was investigated in patients with cutaneous leishmaniasis in Colombia and Guatemala.

Methods and Findings.—By random assignment, 49 patients in Colombia received miltefosine, and 24 received placebo. At the Guatemalan site, 40 were assigned to miltefosine and 20 were assigned to placebo. The Colombian site was located in a region where *Leishmania vianna panamensis* is common. The per-protocol cure rates for Colombian patients were 91% in the miltefosine group and 38% in the placebo group. Among the Guatemalan patients, who came from a region where *L v braziliensis* and *L mexicana mexicana* are common, per-protocol cure rates for miltefosine and placebo recipients were 53% and 21%, respectively. Patients tolerated miltefosine treatment well.

Conclusions.—Miltefosine seems to be useful against cutaneous leishmaniasis caused by *L v panamensis* in Colombia. However, it does not seem to be effective against leishmaniasis caused by *L v braziliensis* in Guatemala.

▶ Standard agents for leishmaniasis, including pentavalent antimony, pentamidine, and amphotericin B, are all effective for New World cutaneous leishmaniasis but have disadvantages, including toxic effects and the need for repeated parenteral injections. This study demonstrates the effectiveness of miltefosine against selected *Leishmania* species.

B. H. Thiers, MD

Overdiagnosis of Malaria in Patients With Severe Febrile Illness in Tanzania: A Prospective Study
Reyburn H, Mbatia R, Drakeley C, et al (London School of Hygiene and Tropical Medicine; Kilimanjaro Christian Med Centre, Moshi, Tanzania; Natl Inst of Med Research, Dar es Salaam, Tanzania)
BMJ 329:1212-1215, 2004   6–3

Background.—The majority of the population of sub-Saharan Africa lives in areas of low or moderate malaria transmission. Accuracy of hospital diagnosis depends on the epidemiologic probability of the disease, defined by intensity of malaria transmission and patient age. Diagnosis and outcome in patients treated during a 1-year period for severe or potentially complicated malaria at 10 hospitals in areas with various transmission intensities were analyzed.

Methods.—A total of 4474 patients meeting criteria for severe disease and admitted to 1 of 10 hospitals in northeast Tanzania were included. This group included 2851 children younger than 5 years. Altitude of residence was used as a proxy for transmission intensity.

Findings.—Blood film microscopy showed that 46.1% of the patients had *Plasmodium falciparum*. The proportion of these slide-positive patients declined with increasing age and increasing altitude of residence. Among children aged 5 years or younger who lived at altitudes higher than 600 m, only 31.1% were slide positive, compared with 68.8% of those aged 5 years or younger living at less than 600 m. Sixty-six percent of the 2375 slide-negative patients did not receive antibiotic therapy. Mortality in that group was 7.6%. Case fatality rates were 12.1% for slide-negative patients and 6.9% for slide-positive patients. The strongest predictors of death in slide-negative and slide-positive patients, as well as in both children and adults, were respiratory distress and altered consciousness.

Conclusions.—Malaria is commonly overdiagnosed in Tanzanians with severe febrile illness, especially among residents of areas with low to moderate transmission and among adults. Associated with this overdiagnosis is a failure to treat alternative causes of severe infection. Routine hospital data may overestimate malaria-related mortality by more than 2-fold.

Combination Treatments for Uncomplicated Falciparum Malaria in Kampala, Uganda: Randomised Clinical Trial

Staedke SG, Mpimbaza A, Kamya MR, et al (Univ of California, San Francisco; Univ Med School, Kampala, Uganda)

Lancet 364:1950-1957, 2004   6–4

Background.—Because of *Plasmodium falciparum* resistance, chloroquine monotherapy is ineffective in much of Africa. Research on alternative regimens is limited. The efficacies of chloroquine plus sulfadoxine-pyrimethamine (CSP), amodiaquine plus sulfadoxine-pyrimethamine (ASP), and amodiaquine plus artesunate (AA) were compared in the treatment of uncomplicated malaria in Uganda.

Methods.—A total of 1017 consecutive children, aged 6 months to 10 years, with uncomplicated malaria were screened. Of these, 418 were assigned randomly to chloroquine (25 mg/kg over 3 days) and single doses of sulfadoxine-pyrimethamine (25 mg/kg and 1.25 mg/kg, respectively); amodiaquine (25 mg/kg over 3 days) and sulfadoxine-pyrimethamine; or amodiaquine and artesunate (4 mg/kg daily for 3 days). Ninety-six percent of the patients were assessed for efficacy outcome, and 99% were evaluated for safety.

Findings.—The risk of 28-day clinical treatment failure was 35% with CSP, which was significantly higher than with ASP (9%) or AA (2%). However, the risk of new infection was greater in the AA group. The rate of retreatment over 28 days was 13% for ASP and 12% for AA. In all treatment groups, serious adverse events were uncommon.

Conclusion.—In this study of uncomplicated malaria in Ugandan children, CSP had an unacceptably high risk of treatment failure. Combinations of amodiquine and sulfadoxine-pyrimethamine or artesunate were significantly more effective. Each regimen may be an appropriate alternative for treating this disease in Africa.

Efficacy of the RTS,S/AS02A Vaccine Against *Plasmodium falciparum* Infection and Disease in Young African Children: Randomised Controlled Trial

Alonso PL, Sacarlal J, Aponte JJ, et al (Universitat de Barcelona; Ministerio de Saúde, Maputo, Mozambique; Universidade Eduardo Mondlane, Maputo, Mozambique; et al)
Lancet 364:1411-1420, 2004   6–5

Background.—The availability of a malaria vaccine may contribute greatly to disease control. The efficacy, immunogenicity, and safety of RTS,S/AS02A, a pre-erythrocytic vaccine candidate based on *Plasmodium falciparum* circumsporozoite surface antigen, was investigated.

Methods.—This double-blind, phase IIb, randomized, controlled study was conducted in Mozambique. A total of 2022 children, aged 1 to 4 years, living in 2 different areas were included. All children were assigned randomly to 3 doses of RTS,S/AS02A candidate malaria vaccine or control vaccines.

In cohort 1, consisting of 1605 children, the main end point was time to first clinical episode of *P falciparum* malaria during a 6-month follow-up period. In cohort 2, consisting of 417 children, the efficacy for preventing new infections was determined.

Findings.—One hundred fifteen children in cohort 1 and 50 in cohort 2 were excluded from the final analysis because they did not receive all 3 vaccine doses. In cohort 1, vaccine efficacy (defined as first clinical episode) was 29.9%. After 6 months, the prevalence of *P falciparum* infection was 37% lower in the RTS,S/AS02A recipients than in the placebo recipients. These prevalences were 11.9% and 18.9%, respectively. The efficacy of the vaccine against severe malaria was 57.7%. In cohort 2, the vaccine had a 45% efficacy for extending time to the first infection.

Conclusion.—RTS,S/AS02A vaccination is safe, well tolerated, and immunogenic. The development of a vaccine effective against malaria is possible.

▶ Globally, every other human being is exposed to malaria, a figure that grows and grows.[1] Deaths from malaria total 1 to 3 million per year, with most victims being African children less than 5 years of age. Misdiagnosis is common and treatment resistance is increasing.[2] The 500 million acute malaria episodes that occur each year place a huge burden of suffering, disability, and economic stress on society.[3] The encouraging results presented by Alonso et al (Abstract 6–5) are a small step in reaching the ultimate goal of an effective vaccine against a complex enemy.[4] The field of genomics is also aiding in the fight against this debilitating disease.[5]

B. H. Thiers, MD

References

1. Hay SI, Guerra CA, Tatem AJ, et al: The global distribution and population at risk of malaria: Past, present and future. *Lancet Infect Dis* 4:327-336, 2004.
2. Amexo M, Tolhurst R, Barnish G, et al: Malaria misdiagnosis: Effects on the poor and vulnerable. *Lancet* 364:1896-1898, 2004.
3. Greenwood B: Between hope and a hard place. *Nature* 430:926-927, 2004.
4. Van de Perre P. Dedet J-P: Vaccine efficacy: Winning a battle (not war) against malaria. *Lancet* 364:1380-1383, 2004.
5. Vernick KD, Waters AP: Genomics and malaria control. *N Engl J Med* 351:1901-1904, 2004.

Sustained Clinical Efficacy of Sulfadoxine-Pyrimethamine for Uncomplicated Falciparum Malaria in Malawi After 10 Years as First Line Treatment: Five Year Prospective Study
Plowe CV, Kublin JG, Dzinjalamala FK, et al (Univ of Maryland, Baltimore)
BMJ 328:545-549, 2004   6–6

Background.—In 1993, Malawi changed its first-line antimalarial drug from chloroquine to sulfadoxine-pyrimethamine because of rising rates of resistance to chloroquine. At that time, Malawi was the first African country to make such a change, and the country's decision was controversial. Monitoring of the efficacy of sulfadoxine-pyrimethamine was begun at 1 site in Malawi in 1998. The purpose of this study was to determine the efficacy of sulfadoxine-pyrimethamine for the treatment of falciparum malaria in Malawi from 1998 to 2002.

Methods.—This prospective open-label drug efficacy study was conducted at a health center in a large peri-urban township in Malawi. The study group was composed of patients (mostly children) with uncomplicated *Plasmodium falciparum* malaria, and the parasitologic and therapeutic responses to sulfadoxine-pyrimethamine were assessed. The main outcome measures were therapeutic efficacy and parasitologic resistance to standard sulfadoxine-pyrimethamine treatment at 14 and 28 days of follow-up.

Results.—The efficacy of treatment remained stable, with clinical response rates of 80% or higher throughout the 5 years of the study. Analysis at 28 days of follow-up showed modest but significant trends toward diminishing clinical and parasitologic efficacy over the course of the study period.

Conclusions.—Sulfadoxine-pyrimethamine has defied expectations and has demonstrated good efficacy after 10 years as the first-line antimalarial drug in Malawi. Interim use of sulfadoxine-pyrimethamine may be beneficial in African countries in which chloroquine efficacy is very low and there are no other immediately available alternatives.

▶ When used as first-line treatment for malaria in South America and Southeast Asia, sulfadoxine-pyrimethamine had a short useful therapeutic life because of the rapid development of resistant organisms. Surprisingly, when used in Malawi, resistance was slow to develop, although the declining rate of parasite clearance during the study suggests an imminent decline in efficacy and highlights the need for new effective treatments for the disease. Nevertheless, in African countries where chloroquine has little remaining usefulness, sulfadoxine-pyrimethamine may represent a viable short-term alternative.

B. H. Thiers, MD

Mefloquine Resistance in *Plasmodium falciparum* and Increased *pfmdr1* Gene Copy Number
Price RN, Uhlemann A-C, Brockman A, et al (St George's Hosp, London; John Radcliffe Hosp, Oxford, England; Shoklo Malaria Research Unit, Mae Sod, Tak Province, Thailand; et al)
Lancet 364:438–447, 2004   6–7

Background.—The world's most multidrug-resistant *Plasmodium falciparum* parasites can be found in Thailand. Substantial resistance to mefloquine, introduced in 1984 to treat uncomplicated falciparum malaria, developed within 6 years. Currently, more than 95% of acute infections can be cured by a combination of artesunate with mefloquine. The relationship between polymorphisms in the *P falciparum* multidrug-resistant gene 1 (*pfmdr1*) and responses to mefloquine were assessed in vitro and in vivo.

Methods.—Over 12 years, 618 samples were collected for prospective study from patients with falciparum malaria. A robust real-time polymerase chain reaction (PCR) assay was used to determine *pfmdr1* copy number. In addition, PCR-restriction fragment length polymorphism was used to assess single nucleotide polymorphisms of *pfmdr1*, *P falciparum* chloroquine resistance transporter gene (*pfcrt*), and *P falciparum* Ca^{2+} ATPase gene (*pfATP6*).

Findings.—The most important determinant of in vitro and in vivo resistance to mefloquine and decreased in vitro artesunate sensitivity was an increased copy number of *pfmdr1*. A Cox regression model, controlled for known confounders, demonstrated that an increased *pfmdr1* copy number correlated with attributable hazard ratios of 6.3 for treatment failure after mefloquine monotherapy and 5.4 after artesunate–mefloquine therapy. Single nucleotide polymorphisms in *pfmdr1* correlated with increased mefloquine susceptibility in vitro but not in vivo.

Conclusions.—An increase in the copy number of *pfmdr1* seems to be the best overall predictor of treatment failure with mefloquine. This variable predicts failure even after chemotherapy with the highly effective combination of mefloquine and 3 days of artesunate. Monitoring the *pfmdr1* copy number will be useful in epidemiologic surveys of drug resistance in *P falciparum*, as well as possibly in predicting treatment failure in individuals.

▶ Drug resistance is becoming an increasingly important problem in the treatment of malaria. The findings reported by Price et al suggest that the *pfmdr1* copy number may become a useful tool for population-based surveillance of drug resistance.

B. H. Thiers, MD

Outcomes of Allergy to Insect Stings in Children, With and Without Venom Immunotherapy
Golden DBK, Kagey-Sobotka A, Norman PS, et al (Johns Hopkins Univ, Baltimore, Md)
N Engl J Med 351:668-674, 2004   6–8

Introduction.—There is a perception that children with a systemic allergic reaction to an insect sting will "outgrow" this allergy and thus have no need for venom immunotherapy. Because no long-term studies have confirmed that such children will not have an allergic reaction to insect stings when they are older, more than 500 children were observed for the effects of subsequent stings after an initial reaction.

Methods.—Between 1978 and 1985, allergy to insect stings of varying severity was diagnosed in 1033 children, 365 of whom received venom immunotherapy. All were surveyed by telephone and mail between January 1997 and January 2002 to determine the outcome of stings received since 1987. A total of 512 patients were contacted and responded to the survey. The National Death Index was searched to determine if any of those not contacted had died and to find the cause of any deaths.

Results.—The mean follow-up period for responding patients was 18 years, and the incidence of stings during follow-up was 43%. Those who underwent venom immunotherapy were treated for a mean of 3.5 years. Subsequent systemic reactions were less common in patients who received the immunotherapy (2 of 64, or 3%) than in untreated patients (19 of 111, or 17%). Among untreated patients with moderate to severe systemic allergic reactions, 7 of 22 (32%) had a subsequent systemic allergic reaction. Treated patients with severe allergic reactions had less severe reactions when later stings occurred. Five of the 520 patients who could not be contacted had died, but none of the deaths were known to have been caused by an insect sting.

Conclusion.—Venom immunotherapy during childhood was quite durable in its benefits, significantly reducing the rate of systemic reactions to later stings even 10 to 20 years after treatment. Treated children whose initial reaction was mild had no further allergic reactions to insect stings. A majority of untreated children do outgrow the allergy, but many with moderate to severe reactions remain at risk.

▶ It is commonly believed that children typically outgrow insect-sting allergy, and for this reason it has been thought that venom immunotherapy may not be warranted in children because, with advancing age, reactions would tend to be less severe. Golden and colleagues prove otherwise, showing that for the small percentage of children who have severe sting-induced allergic reactions, there remains a high likelihood that they will have similar severe reactions if they receive subsequent stings. Nevertheless, for those with dermatologic manifestations only, venom immunotherapy may not be warranted.[1]

B. H. Thiers, MD

Reference

1. Gruchalla RS: Immunotherapy in allergy to insect stings in children. *N Engl J Med* 351:707-709, 2004.

Management of Brown Recluse Spider Bites in Primary Care
Mold JW, Thompson DM (Univ of Oklahoma, Oklahoma City)
J Am Board Fam Pract 17:347-352, 2004   6–9

Introduction.—Brown recluse spider bites result in necrotic ulcers with permanent scarring in approximately 20% of cases, and in a few cases trigger serious systemic reactions. The primary toxin causing local and systemic reactions is sphingomyelinase D, which triggers an inflammatory response when incorporated into cell membranes. Treatments of brown recluse bites have included corticosteroids, dapsone, high-dose vitamin C, antihistamines, and electric shock therapy. A lack of randomized, controlled clinical trials promoted this prospective epidemiologic study.

Methods.—Patients were enrolled between May 1995 and October 2002 by family physician members of the Oklahoma Physicians Resource/ Research Network. Data recorded included baseline information, outcomes, and the probability that lesions were caused by a brown recluse spider. After May 1998, patients were offered either nitroglycerine or high-dose vitamin C (both had recently been reported effective) treatment.

Results.—Outcomes were available for 189 of the 262 enrolled participants. Patients were seen at an average of 3.2 days after the bite. The median healing time was 17 days, and only 21% of patients had permanent scarring. Twelve different treatment modalities were used in the group of 174 patients who received a single treatment modality. Both dapsone and corticosteroids were associated with slower healing, and dapsone was associated with an increased probability of scarring. After adjusting for other variables, predictors of more rapid healing included lower severity level, less erythema, less initial necrosis, younger age, no diabetes, and earlier medical attention.

Conclusion.—No treatment approach used in this large series of patients was promising enough to warrant a clinical trial in humans. Patients came from an area inhabited by the brown recluse spider, yet the spider involved was identified by a credible witness or clinician in only 13% of cases.

▶ The lack of convincing evidence that the patients entered into the study did indeed have correctly diagnosed brown recluse spider bites makes the findings suspect at best. An excellent review of brown recluse spider bites has recently been published.[1]

B. H. Thiers, MD

Reference

1. Swanson DL, Vetter RS: Bites of brown recluse spiders and necrotic arachnidism. *N Engl J Med* 352:700-707, 2005.

Crotaline Snake Bite in the Ecuadorian Amazon: Randomised Double Blind Comparative Trial of Three South American Polyspecific Antivenoms
Smalligan R, Cole J, Brito N, et al (Hosp Vozandes del Oriente, Shell, Pastava, Ecuador)
BMJ 329:1129-1133, 2004   6–10

Background.—Crotaline pit viper venom causes vascular endothelial damage, platelet dysfunction, and consumption coagulopathy, resulting in the main lethal effects of intracranial or gastrointestinal bleeding. These disorders and their reversal by certain antivenoms are reflected by whole blood coagulability, which can be assessed at the bedside with the use of a simple, sensitive 20-minute whole blood clotting test. This test was used to compare the efficacies of 3 antivenoms in restoring whole blood coagulability.

Methods.—Two hundred ten of 221 consecutive patients with snake bites between 1997 and 2001 in southeastern Ecuador were recruited for the study. The 3 antivenoms, selected for their preclinical potency against Ecuadorian venoms, were manufactured in Brazil, Colombia, and Ecuador, respectively. Permanent restoration of blood coagulability after 6 and 24 hours was the main outcome measure.

Findings.—In 187 patients, the snakes responsible for the bites were identified. Fifty-eight percent were bitten by *Bothrops atrax*; 36%, *B bilineatus*; and 5%, *B taeniatus, B brazili,* or *Lachesis muta.* Forty-one percent of the patients received Colombian antivenom, and 39% received Brazilian antivenom. Only 20% of the patients received Ecuadorian antivenom because the supply was limited. Two patients died. Local necrosis developed in 10 patients. All the antivenoms restored blood coagulability permanently by 6 or 24 hours in more than 40% of patients; however, the Colombian antivenom was the most effective. An initial 20 mL dose of Colombian antivenom permanently restored blood coagulability in 64% of patients after 6 hours. An initial dose of less than 70 mL was effective at 6 hours in 65% of patients and at 24 hours in 99%. Early anaphylactoid reactions occurred in 53% of patients given the Brazilian antivenom, in 73% given the Colombian, and in

19% given the Ecuadorian. However, only 3 reactions were severe, and no reaction was fatal.

Conclusions.—All 3 antivenoms tested in this study are effective for the treatment of snake bites in southeastern Ecuador. However, the reactogenicity of the Brazilian and Colombian antivenoms is of concern.

▶ I have had the good fortune to visit South America on several occasions. However, I doubt that this article or the accompanying illustration showing a very menacing reptile will be posted on the tourism Web sites of any of these countries!

B. H. Thiers, MD

7 Disorders of the Pilosebaceous Apparatus

The Complete Genome Sequence of *Propionibacterium acnes*, a Commensal of Human Skin
Brüggemann H, Henne A, Hoster F, et al (Georg-August-Univ, Göttingen, Germany; Univ of Ulm, Germany)
Science 305:671-673, 2004   7–1

Introduction.—Several mechanisms are proposed to account for the role of *Propionibacterium acnes* in acne, the most common skin disease. Bacterial enzymes with degradative properties, such as lipases, might damage host tissues and cells. Inflammation could be triggered by immunogenic factors of *P acnes*, such as surface determinants or heat shock proteins. A knowledge of the genome sequence might help in finding alternative targets for acne therapy and other *P acnes*-associated diseases, including corneal ulcers, endocarditis, and sarcoidosis.

Observations.—The genome of *P acnes* strain KPA171202 (No. DSM 16379) consists of a single circular chromosome of 2,560,265 base pairs. A total of 2333 putative genes were predicted and annotated. The genome sequence provided insights into the traits that favor *P acnes* as a major inhabitant of adult human skin. Its capacity to cope with changing oxygen tensions confirms the ability of strains to grow under microaerobic as well as anaerobic conditions. Previous research suggests that free fatty acids, produced by *P acnes* lipase activity on sebum, assist bacterial adherence and colonization of the sebaceous follicle. Examination of the complete genome sequence revealed numerous gene products involved in degrading host molecules, and various immunogenic factors that might play a role in triggering acne inflammation and other *P acnes*-associated diseases were identified. The capability of *P acnes* to survive in a spectrum of environments helps to explain its ubiquity and its potential hazards.

▶ A detailed table in the original article lists selected enzymes and other proteins produced by *P acnes*, and their possible role in degrading host molecules, conferring cell adhesion, and/or mediating inflammation. Knowledge of the genome sequence of *P acnes* should go a long way to understanding how this bacterium triggers inflammation in acne and in other conditions said to be associated with its presence, including corneal ulcers, endocarditis, sarcoidosis, cholesterol gallstones, allergic alveolitis, pulmonary angiitis, and the SAPHO (synovitis, acne, pustulosis, hyperostosis, and osteitis) syndrome.[1,2]

B. H. Thiers, MD

References

1. Yamada T, Eishi Y, Ikeda S, et al: In situ localization of *Propionibacterium acnes* DNA in lymph nodes from sarcoidosis patients by signal amplification with catalysed reporter deposition. *J Pathol* 198:541-547, 2002.
2. Jakab E, Zbinden R, Gubler J, et al: Severe infections caused by *Propionibacterium acnes*: An underestimated pathogen in late postoperative infections. *Yale J Biol Med* 69:477-482, 1996.

Quantitative Documentation of a Premenstrual Flare of Facial Acne in Adult Women

Lucky AW (Dermatology Research Associates, Cincinnati, Ohio)
Arch Dermatol 140:423-424, 2004   7–2

Background.—Flares in facial acne during the luteal phase of the menstrual cycle have been reported. However, no one to date has quantitatively evaluated the presence and degree of such flares. A survey of acne lesion counts in the follicular and luteal phases of the menstrual cycle during 2 full cycles was reported.

Methods.—Forty-one women were enrolled in the study. All were nonpregnant and nonlactating. They were 18 to 44 years of age, in good general health with regular menses, and were receiving no treatment for their acne. Participants available for both late follicular and late luteal phase visits were considered for assessment of premenstrual flare. Twenty-five were available in month 1 and 23 in month 2, for a total of 48 evaluations.

Findings.—Sixty-three percent of the women had a 25% premenstrual increase in the number of inflammatory acne lesions. A 23.2% increase was noted in total acne lesions; 25.3% were inflammatory and 21.2% were comedonal.

Conclusion.—This study is the first to document with acne lesion counts premenstrual acne flares. Almost two thirds of the women assessed had more acne in the late luteal phase than in the late follicular phase of the menstrual cycle.

▶ The author confirms the oft-cited observation that a significant number of adult women experience a premenstrual acne flare.[1]

B. H. Thiers, MD

Reference

1. Stoll S, Shalita AR, Webster GF, et al: The effect of the menstrual cycle on acne. *J Am Acad Dermatol* 45:957-960, 2001.

Comparison of Five Antimicrobial Regimens for Treatment of Mild to Moderate Inflammatory Facial Acne Vulgaris in the Community: Randomised Controlled Trial

Ozolins M, Eady EA, Avery AJ, et al (Queens Med Centre, Nottingham, England; Univ of Leeds, England; Univ of Nottingham, England; et al)
Lancet 364:2188-2195, 2004   7–3

Background.—Acne vulgaris is one of the most common skin diseases, with a prevalence of nearly 100% among adolescents. Acne is increasingly recognized as a primarily inflammatory dermatosis that is also characterized by hyperproliferation and abnormal differentiation of ductal keratinocytes and androgen-mediated seborrhea. Antibiotic therapy has been an important component of acne treatment for 40 years, but acne is not a classic infection and, therefore, direct antiinflammatory activity could be as important (or more important) as inhibition of propionibacterial growth. The efficacy and cost-effectiveness of 5 antimicrobial regimens for mild to moderate facial acne and whether propionibacterial antibiotic resistance has an effect on treatment response were investigated.

Methods.—The study included 649 community participants in a randomized, observer-masked trial. The study participants were assigned to 1 of the following 5 antibacterial regimens: (1) oral oxytetracycline plus topical placebo, (2) oral minocycline plus topical placebo, (3) topical benzoyl peroxide plus oral placebo, (4) topical erythromycin and benzoyl peroxide in a combined formulation plus oral placebo, and (5) topical erythromycin and benzoyl peroxide separately plus oral placebo. The main outcome measures were the patients' self-assessed improvement and reduction in inflammatory lesions at 18 weeks. The analysis was done by intention to treat.

Results.—Moderate or better improvement at 18 weeks was reported in (1) 55% of patients assigned oral oxytetracycline plus topical placebo; (2) 54% of patients assigned to oral minocycline plus topical placebo; (3) 60% of patients assigned topical benzoyl peroxide plus oral placebo; (4) 66% of patients assigned topical erythromycin and benzoyl peroxide in a combined formulation plus oral placebo; and (5) 63% of patients assigned topical erythromycin and benzoyl peroxide separately plus oral placebo. There was moderate improvement in the first 6 weeks. Benzoyl peroxide was the most cost-effective treatment. The efficacy of both tetracyclines was reduced by preexisting tetracycline resistance.

Conclusions.—Topical benzoyl peroxide and benzoyl peroxide/ erythromycin combinations are similar in efficacy to oral oxytetracycline and minocycline in the treatment of acne vulgaris and are not affected by propionibacterial antibiotic resistance.

▶ In this large community-based nonindustry-sponsored study, it was found that moderate or greater improvement of acne was similar among the 5 different treatment regimens, with slightly better results being obtained with benzoyl peroxide/erythromycin combinations. Benzoyl peroxide was the most cost-effective agent and bacterial resistance was not a factor in regimens that included benzoyl peroxide. Because single agents are rarely used for the treatment of acne, and topical agents and systemic antibiotics are frequently used in combination, it is unfortunate that a cohort using both an oral antibiotic (eg, a tetracycline) with either benzoyl peroxide alone or a benzoyl peroxide/erythromycin combination was not included in the study, or that other combinations of topical and oral agents were similarly not evaluated.

An excellent review of acne treatment has recently been published.[1]

S. Raimer, MD

Reference

1. James WD: Acne. *N Engl J Med* 352:1463-1471, 2005.

Antibiotic Use in Relation to the Risk of Breast Cancer
Velicer CM, Heckbert SR, Lampe JW, et al (Univ of Washington, Seattle; Group Health Cooperative, Seattle; Fred Hutchinson Cancer Research Ctr, Seattle; et al)
JAMA 291:827-835, 2004   7–4

Background.—Antibiotic use may be associated with the risk of breast cancer. Antibiotics may affect immune function, inflammation, and metabolism of estrogen and phytochemicals. However, few clinical data have been reported on the possible relationship between antibiotic use and breast cancer risk, which was further investigated by the authors.

Methods.—The case-control study included 2266 women, older than 19 years, with primary invasive breast cancer who were enrolled in a large nonprofit health plan for at least 1 year between 1993 and 2001. A control group consisted of 7953 randomly selected women in the same health plan, frequency-matched by age and length of enrollment. The use of antibiotics was determined from computerized pharmacy records.

Findings.—After adjustment for age and length of health plan enrollment, an increased risk of incident breast cancer correlated with increasing cumulative days of antibiotic use. The odds ratios for breast cancer were 1.00 with 0 days of use, 1.45 with 1 to 50 days, 1.53 with 51 to 100 days, 1.68 with 101 to 500 days, 2.14 with 501 to 1000 days, and 2.07 with 1001 days or more. The risk was increased in all antibiotic classes studied and also in a subanalysis with breast cancer fatality as the outcome. Among women with the greatest levels of tetracycline or macrolide use, breast cancer risk was not increased in those using these agents only for acne or rosacea compared with the risk of those using them exclusively for respiratory tract infections.

Conclusions.—Antibiotic use is associated with an increased risk of incident and fatal breast cancer. It is unknown whether antibiotic use is related causally to breast cancer or whether indication for use, overall weakened immune function, or other factors are relevant. These data underscore the need for prudent long-term antibiotic use.

▶ The findings are of clear concern to dermatologists, who frequently use long-term antibiotic therapy to control acne in women. The authors hypothesize that the effect of antibiotics on intestinal bacteria could change the body's immune system or how the body metabolizes certain foods that may protect against cancer. Subsequent letters to the editor of *JAMA* cited numerous design flaws in the study. An accompanying editorial commented on the overuse of antibiotics, especially for conditions such as colds and other viral illnesses for which they clearly are not indicated.[1]

B. H. Thiers, MD

Reference

1. Ness RB, Cauley JA: Antibiotics and breast cancer—What's the meaning of this? *JAMA* 291:880-881, 2004.

Maintenance Fluconazole Therapy for Recurrent Vulvovaginal Candidiasis
Sobel JD, Wiesenfeld HC, Martens M, et al (Wayne State Univ, Detroit; Univ of Pittsburgh, Pa; Hennepin County Med Ctr, Minneapolis; et al)
N Engl J Med 351:876-883, 2004   7–5

Background.—Recurrent vulvovaginal candidiasis is estimated to occur in 5% to 6% of women during their reproductive years, affecting healthy, immunocompetent women in all segments of society. The condition has several causes, but most women with recurrent infection have no recognizable risk factors. Frequent recurrences of symptomatic vulvovaginitis cause considerable suffering and cost and have a significant adverse effect on the patient's sexual relations. A number of management approaches have been used, but no safe and convenient regimen has yet been found to be effective for the management of recurrent vulvovaginal candidiasis.

Methods.—A group of 387 women with recurrent vulvovaginal candidiasis underwent induction of clinical remission with open-label fluconazole given in three 150-mg doses at 72-hour intervals and were than randomly assigned to treatment with fluconazole (150 mg) or placebo weekly for 6 months, followed by 6 months of observation without therapy. The main outcome measure was the proportion of women in clinical remission at the end of the first 6-month period. Secondary outcome measures were the clinical outcome at 12 months, vaginal mycologic status, and time to recurrence on the basis of Kaplan-Meier analysis.

Results.—Weekly treatment with fluconazole was effective in preventing symptomatic vulvovaginal candidiasis. The proportions of women who were disease free at 6, 9, and 12 months were 90.8%, 73.2%, and 42.9%, respectively, in the fluconazole group versus 35.9%, 27.8%, and 21.9%, respectively, in the placebo group. The median time to clinical recurrence was 10.2 months in the fluconazole group versus 4.0 months in the placebo group. There was no evidence of fluconazole resistance in *Candida albicans* isolates or of superinfection with *C. glabrata*. One patient discontinued fluconazole because of headache.

Conclusions.—The rate of recurrence of symptomatic vulvovaginal candidiasis can be reduced with long-term weekly treatment with fluconazole. However, a long-term cure remains elusive.

▶ The proposed fluconazole regimen might be of benefit to acne patients in whom recurrent vulvovaginal candidiasis develops while on long-term antibiotic therapy. It should be noted, however, that in the current study, patients were prohibited from using antibiotics during the induction phase. Also noteworthy is the high rate of relapse of symptomatic vaginitis shortly after the cessation of suppressive therapy with fluconazole; nevertheless, the number of patients who remained free of infection at 1 year was significantly higher in the fluconazole group than in the placebo group. Although maintenance therapy with fluconazole may be effective, it is clearly not a cure for vulvovaginal candidiasis.[1]

B. H. Thiers, MD

Reference

1. Eschenbach DA: Chronic vulvovaginal candidiasis. *N Engl J Med* 351:851-852, 2004.

Effect of Lactobacillus in Preventing Post-antibiotic Vulvovaginal Candidiasis: A Randomised Controlled Trial
Pirotta M, Gunn J, Chondros P, et al (Carlton, Victoria, Australia; Royal Women's Hosp, Carlton, Victoria, Australia; Univ of Melbourne, Carlton, Victoria, Australia)
BMJ 329:548-551, 2004   7-6

Introduction.—Probiotics are frequently used and recommended for treatment of vulvovaginitis that develops after antibiotic treatment. No published trials have evaluated the value of this approach. The effectiveness of oral or vaginal lactobacillus in preventing vulvovaginitis after antibiotic treatment was evaluated in a randomized, placebo-controlled, double-blind, factorial 2 × 2 trial.

Methods.—Data were available for 235 of 278 nonpregnant women 18 to 50 years of age from 50 general practices and 19 pharmacies who needed a short course of oral antibiotics for a nongynecologic infection. Patients were treated with lactobacillus preparations taken orally, vaginally, or both, from enrollment until 4 days after completion of their antibiotic course. The primary outcome measure was patients' reports of postantibiotic vulvovaginitis. Microbiological evidence of candidiasis was provided by a self-obtained vaginal swab.

Results.—Overall, 23% (55/235) of the cohort had postantibiotic vulvovaginitis. Compared with the odds ratio (OR) for placebo, the OR for developing postantibiotic vulvovaginitis with oral lactobacillus was 1.06 (95% CI, 0.58-1.94) and was 1.38 (95% CI, 0.75-2.54) when vaginal lactobacillus was used. High compliance with antibiotic use and interventions was seen. The trial was terminated after the second interim analysis due to a lack of effect of the interventions. In this cohort, the chances of identifying a significant decrease in vulvovaginitis with oral or vaginal lactobacillus treatment were below 0.032 and 0.0006, respectively.

Conclusion.—Oral or vaginal probiotic treatment with a main constituent of *Lactobacillus rhamnosus* was ineffective in preventing postantibiotic vulvovaginitis candidiasis.

▶ Antibiotic-associated vulvovaginitis is a common problem for women and may affect their compliance with taking prescribed antibiotics (eg, for acne). Many women believe that products containing *Lactobacillus* species will prevent antibiotic-associated vulvovaginitis, but evidence to support this assertion is lacking. Pirotta et al demonstrate that neither oral nor vaginal forms of *Lactobacillus* are effective in preventing antibiotic-associated vulvovaginitis.

B. H. Thiers, MD

The Effect of Isotretinoin on the Pharmacokinetics and Pharmacodynamics of Ethinyl Estradiol and Norethindrone

Hendrix CW, Jackson KA, Whitmore E, et al (Johns Hopkins Univ, Baltimore, Md; GloboMax, LLC, Hanover, Md; Roche Laboratories, Nutley, NJ; et al)
Clin Pharmacol Ther 75:464-475, 2004   7–7

Background.—Several drugs that induce the cytochrome p450 (CYP) 3A4 pathway can reduce concentrations of concomitantly administered hormone contraceptives, resulting in ovulation and contraception failure. Both isotretinoin and ethinyl estradiol are metabolized by the CYP system, primarily CYP3A4. Because of the teratogenic effects of isotretinoin, women of childbearing age who use this drug must avoid becoming pregnant. Whether isotretinoin alters the contraceptive effectiveness of ethinyl estradiol and norethindrone was examined.

Methods.—The research subjects were 26 women 18 to 41 years old with severe, recalcitrant nodular acne. All patients took isotretinoin, 1.0 mg/kg/d, for 16 to 20 weeks. For 1 month before and during and for 1 month after isotretinoin treatment, patients also took ethinyl estradiol and norethindrone tablets (Ortho Novum 7/7/7; Ortho-McNeil Pharmaceuticals, Inc, Raritan, NJ). Blood samples were drawn for pharmacokinetic and pharmacodynamic analyses on days 6 and 20 of the preisotretinoin phase and on days 6 and 20 of the second month of isotretinoin plus oral contraceptive (OC) therapy.

Results.—The addition of isotretinoin to OC treatment caused some significant changes in pharmacokinetic variables compared with the OC alone phase; these changes, however, were small and inconsistent. For example, the maximum plasma concentration of norethindrone decreased significantly from 18.3 ng/mL on day 20 during OC alone to 16.3 ng/mL on day 20 during OC plus isotretinoin. Also, the area under the plasma concentration–time curve from time 0 to 24 hours after drug dosing on day 6 decreased significantly in the combined treatment phase for both ethinyl estradiol (from 1171 to 1022 pg · h/mL, or a 9% decrease) and norethindrone (from 86 to 78 ng · h/mL, or a 9% decrease). Much variability was present in pharmacokinetic variables, and the median coefficients of variation were 44% to 69% for each time point within a phase. The only significant difference in pharmacodynamic variables was a decrease in follicle-stimulating hormone levels on day 20 between the OC alone phase (2.48 mIU/mL) and the OC plus isotretinoin phase (1.72 mIU/mL; a 44% decrease). Much variability was also seen in pharmacodynamic variables, and the median coefficients of variation were 64% to 114% for each time point within a phase. Levels of isotretinoin or its metabolite did not correlate with OC levels. However, OC levels did correlate significantly with progesterone levels. One research subject during the OC only phase and 1 research subject during the OC plus isotretinoin phase had an elevation in progesterone levels consistent with possible ovulation. However, no pregnancies occurred, and there were no serious or unexpected drug-related adverse events.

Conclusion.—Isotretinoin administration caused small decreases in ethinyl estradiol and norethindrone levels (by about 10%), but these effects were small and inconsistent across the study days. The only pharmacodynamic change was a large decrease in follicle-stimulating hormone levels on day 20. Still, the great variability in pharmacokinetic and pharmacodynamic variables, coupled with the teratogenicity of isotretinoin, underscore the need to use birth control methods in addition to OCs when women of childbearing age are taking isotretinoin.

▶ The decrease in both ethinyl estradiol and norethindrone when used in conjunction with isotretinoin was small, although statistically significant, and of uncertain clinical importance. Nevertheless, the findings underscore the need for double contraception in patients of childbearing age undergoing treatment with isotretinoin.

B. H. Thiers, MD

Treatment of Acne Vulgaris With a Pulsed Dye Laser: A Randomized Controlled Trial

Orringer JS, Kang S, Hamilton T, et al (Univ of Michigan, Ann Arbor)
JAMA 291:2834-2839, 2004   7–8

Background.—Some physicians report that phototherapy can improve acne vulgaris. Whether pulsed dye laser treatment is effective for patients with acne vulgaris was examined.

Methods.—The research subjects were 40 patients (24 males and 16 females, 13-31 years old) with acne vulgaris on the face. None had received oral retinoids within the past year; microdermabrasion to the face within 3 months; or other systemic or topical acne therapies, alpha hydroxy acid, or glycolic acid within 1 month. Half of each patient's face remained untreated, while the other half received 1 or 2 nonpurpuric pulses (separated by 2 weeks) from a pulsed dye laser (fluence 3 J/cm^2). Lesion counts were performed at baseline and 12 weeks after beginning therapy. In addition, photographs were taken at these times, and the severity of the acne was graded by dermatologists unaware of the treatment.

Results.—Results did not differ significantly according to the number of pulses received, so the pulse data were pooled. At 12 weeks, the pulsed-treated and untreated sides of the face did not differ significantly in mean papule counts (–4.2 vs –2.2 from baseline; $P = .08$), mean pustule counts (0 vs –1.0; $P = .12$), or mean comedone counts (2.9 vs 1.6; $P = .63$). Photographic assessments also showed no significant differences in the Leeds score between treated skin (from 3.98 at baseline to 3.94 at week 12) and untreated skin (from 3.83 at baseline to 3.79 at week 12).

Conclusion.—One or 2 pulses of a nonpurpuric pulsed dye laser does not improve acne vulgaris of the face.

▶ A study[1] reviewed in the 2004 YEAR BOOK OF DERMATOLOGY AND DERMATOLOGIC SURGERY on the treatment of acne with the pulsed dye laser yielded more favorable results, although the writer of an accompanying editorial appeared to be less impressed.[2] We seem to be moving into an era in which devices as well as drugs will be used to treat more and more conditions previously residing in the province of the "medical" dermatologist. For acne, these include photodynamic therapy and other forms of phototherapy, as well as nonablative therapies.[3,4] Whether these will be superior to existing therapies is a matter of speculation.

B. H. Thiers, MD

References

1. Seaton E, Charakida A, Mouser P, et al: Pulsed-dye laser treatment for inflammatory acne vulgaris: Randomized controlled trial. *Lancet* 362:1347-1352, 2003.
2. Webster GF: Laser treatment of acne. *Lancet* 362:1342, 2003.
3. Hongcharu W, Taylor CR, Chang Y, et al: Topical ALA-photodynamic therapy for the treatment of acne vulgaris. *J Invest Dermatol* 115:183-192, 2000.

4. Ruiz-Esparza J, Gomez JB: Nonablative radiofrequency for active acne vulgaris: The use of deep dermal heat in the treatment of moderate to severe active acne vulgaris (thermotherapy): A report of 22 patients. *Dermatol Surg* 29:333-339, 2003.

Infliximab for Hidradenitis Suppurativa

Sullivan TP, Welsh E, Kerdel FA, et al (Univ of Miami, Fla)
Br J Dermatol 149:1046-1049, 2003   7–9

Background.—Current medical treatments for hidradenitis suppurative (HS), a chronic disease associated with significant morbidity, are only minimally effective. Infliximab is a chimeric monoclonal antibody with a high affinity for tumor necrosis factor-α (TNF-α); it may play an important role in the treatment of disparate inflammatory disorders. The efficacy of infliximab for treating HS was investigated.

Methods and Findings.—This retrospective study included 5 patients, 28 to 57 years old, with HS. Previous treatments included oral and topical antimicrobials, intralesional and oral glucocorticoids, dapsone, clofazimine, isotretinoin, colchicine, and cyclosporine. All patients were given an initial infusion of 5 mg/kg of infliximab. Three patients received a second infusion 4 to 6 weeks after initial therapy. Patients were later contacted and asked to rate their disease activity immediately before and after treatment. Self-reported disease activity scores were significantly reduced after infliximab therapy. These scores correlated with clinical improvement documented by physicians.

Conclusions.—These initial findings suggest that infliximab is a promising HS treatment. Objective and subjective improvement in disease was evident in the 5 patients treated. Additional studies are needed.

▶ This is one of several case reports suggesting the efficacy of infliximab in hidradenitis suppurative, the pathogenesis and treatment of which have recently been reviewed in detail.[1,2] As noted by the authors, the optimal dosing schedule and the duration of remission need to be prospectively studied in a larger group of patients.

B. H. Thiers, MD

References

1. Wiseman MC: Hidradenitis suppurativa: A review. *Dermatol Ther* 17:50-54, 2004.
2. Slade DE, Powell BW, Mortimer PS: Hidradenitis suppurativa: Pathogenesis and management. *Br J Plast Surg* 56:451-461, 2003.

An Open, Randomized, Comparative Study of Oral Finasteride and 5% Topical Minoxidil in Male Androgenetic Alopecia

Arca E, Açikgöz G, Taştan HB, et al (Gülhane Military Med Academy, Etlik-Ankara, Turkey)

Dermatology 209:117-125, 2004   7–10

Introduction.—Androgenetic alopecia (AGA), the most common cause of hair loss in men, can be treated by hair growth promoters such as finasteride, a hormone modifier, and minoxidil, a biological response modifier. Sixty-five men with mild to severe AGA participated in a 12-month study that compared the efficacy of oral finasteride with that of 5% topical minoxidil.

Methods.—Men eligible for the open randomized trial were aged 18 to 50 years and in generally good health. Hair loss was classified as vertex and frontal pattern type II, III, IV, or V according to the modified Norwood-Hamilton scale. Forty participants were assigned to receive 1 mg/d oral finasteride, and 25 were assigned to an application of 5% topical minoxidil solution twice daily. Photographs were taken at baseline and on completion of the trial; efficacy and safety were monitored every 3 months.

Results.—The average patient age was 27.5 years. Randomized groups were similar in age, age at which hair loss began, type of hair loss, and family history. Hair growth had occurred in 80% of patients at the end of finasteride treatment and was classified as dense in 15%, moderate in 30%, and minimal in 35%; 18% showed no change, and 1 patient experienced hair loss. In the minoxidil group, 52% of patients had moderate or minimal hair growth, 20% showed no change, and 28% had hair loss. Side effects were mild overall and disappeared when treatment was stopped. The only clinically significant laboratory changes occurred in the finasteride group, in which serum total testosterone levels were slightly increased and serum free testosterone and serum prostate-specific antigen levels fell slightly compared with baseline values.

Discussion.—Both systemic finasteride and topical minoxidil were effective and safe when used to treat mild to severe AGA. Adverse effects were mild, disappeared when therapy was discontinued, and did not cause any patient to withdraw from the trial. Finasteride was more effective than minoxidil, but a combination of the 2 agents may improve results.

▶ Although the age range of the patients studied was quite wide (18-50 years), the mean age in each group was similar (about 27 years). A larger study that divides the patients into smaller groups based on age and includes the effects of combination minoxidil–finasteride therapy would be welcome.

B. H. Thiers, MD

Decreased Serum Ferritin Is Associated With Alopecia in Women

Kantor J, Kessler LJ, Brooks DG, et al (Univ of Pennsylvania, Philadelphia)
J Invest Dermatol 121:985-988, 2003   7–11

Introduction.—Dermatologists often assess serum iron status in women with hair loss, but there is little objective evidence that alopecia is caused by iron deficiency. Women with 4 different hair loss disorders participated in a study that used analytical methodology to examine the relationship between iron deficiency and hair loss.

Methods.—Thirty women had a diagnosis of telogen effluvium (TE), 52 had androgenetic alopecia (AGA), 17 had alopecia areata (AA), and 7 had alopecia areata totalis/universalis. Eleven women without hair loss and from the same referral base and source population as the patients with hair loss served as control subjects. Patient and control groups were compared for mean age, mean hemoglobin levels, and mean serum ferritin levels.

Results.—Because patients and control subjects did not differ significantly in age, differences in ferritin levels were not considered to be secondary to age variations. The mean hemoglobin levels were similar in all 4 hair loss groups and in the control group, but mean ferritin levels in patients with AGA or AA were statistically significantly lower than levels in women without hair loss. A secondary analysis of women 40 years or younger showed ferritin levels to be significantly lower in patients with AA, TE, and AGA than in control subjects. Younger women with TE had lower hemoglobin levels than younger control subjects.

Conclusion.—In this small series, both hemoglobin and ferritin levels were decreased in some women with alopecia. The findings suggest that an iron deficiency may be involved in the mechanism of some types of hair loss and should be corrected before the start of clinical trials of treatments for alopecia in women.

▶ The serum ferritin level is a measure of body iron stores. Kantor et al postulate a relationship between decreased ferritin levels and AGA and AA (but not alopecia totalis/universalis or TE). Previous studies on the subject have yielded contradictory results.

B. H. Thiers, MD

Melatonin Increases Anagen Hair Rate in Women With Androgenic Alopecia or Diffuse Alopecia: Results of a Pilot Randomized Controlled Trial

Fischer TW, Burmeister G, Schmid HW, et al (Friedrich-Schiller-Univ, Jena, Germany; ASATONA AG, Zug, Switzerland)
Br J Dermatol 150:341-345, 2004   7–12

Background.—Melatonin has been found to have a beneficial effect on hair growth in animals, but its effect on hair growth in humans is unknown. Whether topically applied melatonin affects anagen and telogen hair rate in women with androgenetic or diffuse hair loss was investigated.

Methods.—Forty women were enrolled in the double-blind, randomized, placebo-controlled trial. All had androgenetic or diffuse alopecia. The patients received an application of 0.1% melatonin or placebo solution to the scalp once a day for 6 months. Trichograms were obtained to assess anagen and telogen hair rate. In addition, blood samples were obtained during the study period to monitor the effects of therapy on physiologic melatonin levels.

Findings.—Compared with placebo, melatonin resulted in a significantly increased anagen hair rate in occipital hair in women with androgenetic hair loss. Melatonin significantly increased frontal hair in women with diffuse alopecia. Occipital hair samples of patients with diffuse alopecia and frontal hair counts of patients with androgenetic alopecia also showed increased anagen hair, although the differences were nonsignificant. Increases in plasma melatonin concentrations were associated with topical melatonin treatment, but these levels did not exceed the physiologic night peak.

Conclusion.—This pilot study is the first to demonstrate the effect of topical melatonin on hair growth in humans. Its mode of action is unknown. Melatonin's effects may be linked to induction of an anagen phase.

▶ The effects on human hair growth of sex hormones such as testosterone and dihydrotestosterone have been extensively investigated. Other hormones may have an effect as well. Melatonin has been reported to have a positive effect on hair growth in some animals, and in vitro studies have shown a positive effect of melatonin on hair matrix cell proliferation and hair growth. The findings of Fischer et al suggest an analogous mode of action in humans, ie, induction of an early anagen phase after loss of telogen hairs.

B. H. Thiers, MD

Finasteride Treatment of Patterned Hair Loss in Normoandrogenic Postmenopausal Women
Trüeb RM, and the Swiss Trichology Study Group (Univ Hosp of Zurich, Switzerland)
Dermatology 209:202-207, 2004   7–13

Introduction.—Individuals with androgenetic alopecia, also known as pattern hair loss, experience a progressive decline in scalp hair density. Dihydrotestosterone, the primary androgen implicated in the pathogenesis of androgenetic alopecia, is formed by peripheral conversion of testosterone by the enzyme 5α-reductase. A specific inhibitor of type 2 5α-reductase, finasteride, increases hair growth and slows the progression of hair loss in men. The efficacy of oral finasteride was evaluated in women with pattern hair loss.

Methods.—Study participants were 5 postmenopausal women without clinical or laboratory signs of hyperandrogenism. Off-label use of finasteride was offered after previous treatments had failed. The women took 2.5 or 5 mg/d oral finasteride for up to 18 months. Photographs obtained at baseline

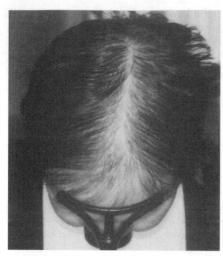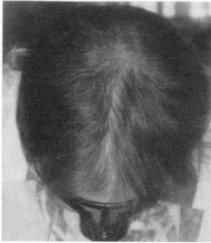

FIGURE 1.—Patient 1. At baseline and at 6 months of oral finasteride 2.5 mg/d; great improvement. (Courtesy of Trüeb RM, and the Swiss Trichology Study Group. *Dermatology* 209:202-207, 2004. Reproduced with permission of S. Karger AG, Basel.)

and at months 6, 12, and 18 were evaluated by dermatologists using a 7-point scale.

Results.—Patients ranged in age from 52 to 69 years. All had scalp hair loss, and none showed any sign of virilization. After treatment with finasteride, 2 patients were judged to have a great improvement (Fig 1; see color plate XV), 1 had moderate or slight improvement, and 2 had a slight improvement or no change. All patients reported a slowing of hair loss as early as 6 months after beginning treatment. Four patients expressed satisfaction with the appearance of their hair compared with baseline. Treatment with finasteride was well tolerated.

Conclusion.—A previous large trial of finasteride in women with pattern hair loss showed no benefits, but the dosage was only 1 mg/d. At significantly higher doses (≥2.5 mg/d), oral finasteride was effective in these postmenopausal women with normal androgen levels.

▶ A previous article[1] did not find any improvement in female pattern alopecia in postmenopausal women treated with 1 mg/d finasteride. Trüeb et al report positive results in postmenopausal women given higher doses of the drug. In contrast, Carmina and Lobo[2] found no benefit with 5 mg/d finasteride in the treatment of alopecia in hyperandrogenic women.

B. H. Thiers, MD

References

1. Price VH, Robert JL, Hordinsky M, et al: Lack of efficacy of finasteride in postmenopausal women with androgenetic alopecia. *J Am Acad Dermatol* 43:768-776, 2000.
2. Carmina E, Lobo RA: Treatment of hyperandrogenic alopecia in women. *Fertil Steril* 79:91-95, 2003.

Finasteride Versus Cyproterone Acetate–Estrogen Regimens in the Treatment of Hirsutism

Beigi A, Sobhi A, Zarrinkoub F (Tehran Univ of Med Sciences, Iran)

Int J Gynaecol Obstet 87:29-33, 2004   7–14

Introduction.—Hirsutism affects 5% to 10% of women and results from increased androgen production, excessive androgen action at the target level, or both. Potentially beneficial agents include finasteride, an inhibitor of type 2 5α-reductase activity, and cyproterone acetate (CPA), which appears to act by binding to the androgen receptor and reducing androgen biosynthesis. Forty women with hirsutism were recruited for a 9-month trial of finasteride and CPA plus ethinyl estradiol (EE2).

Methods.—Patients ranged in age from 16 to 29 years; 11 had idiopathic hirsutism, and 29 had polycystic ovary syndrome. None had hypertension, clinical signs of virilization, drug-induced hyperandrogenism, or evidence of an androgen-producing neoplasm. Randomization was to finasteride (5 mg/d) or CPA (25 mg/d on days 5-14) plus EE2 (20 µg/d on days 5-25). Oligomenorrhea was present in 65% of the finasteride group and in 70% of the CPA plus EE2 group. Hirsutism scores and hormone levels were measured at baseline and at 9 months.

Results.—The 2 groups were similar in age, body mass index, initial Ferriman-Gallwey score for hirsutism, and other measured baseline variables. Both treatment groups showed significant decreases in the mean Ferriman-Gallwey score (from 23.7 to 11.3 in the finasteride group and from 22.3 to 11.4 in the CPA plus EE2 group). Serum levels of total testosterone increased and dihydrotestosterone decreased significantly with finasteride. Treatment with CPA plus EE2 significantly decreased serum and total free testosterone, androstenedione, dehydroepiandrosterone sulfate, and dihydrotestosterone but increased sex hormone–binding globulin levels. All patients completed the trial with no signs of adverse effects or changes in hematochemical variables.

Conclusion.—Patients treated for hirsutism with either finasteride or CPA plus EE2 achieved significant and similar reductions in the Ferriman-Gallwey score, despite different mechanisms of action in the 2 therapies and different changes in androgen levels. In part because of its contraceptive effect, the combined therapy of CPA plus EE2 may be the treatment of choice for hyperandrogenic hirsutism in sexually active women; moreover, CPA is less expensive than finasteride.

▶ Although both treatments yielded similar results, finasteride and the combined CPA–EE2 regimen had significantly different effects on serum hormone levels.

B. H. Thiers, MD

8 Pigmentary Disorders

Topical Tacrolimus Therapy for Vitiligo: Therapeutic Responses and Skin Messenger RNA Expression of Proinflammatory Cytokines
Grimes PE, Morris R, Avaniss-Aghajani E, et al (Univ of California, Los Angeles)
J Am Acad Dermatol 51:52-61, 2004   8–1

Introduction.—The reported increase in tumor necrosis factor–α (TNF-α) levels in lesional and perilesional skin of patients with vitiligo suggests that immunomodulatory drugs may have a role in its treatment. Topical tacrolimus, which is believed to inhibit T-cell activation, was evaluated for its benefits and its effects on cytokine expression in affected patients.

Methods.—Twenty-three patients enrolled in the study and 19 (11 women and 8 men) completed therapy. All had mild to moderate generalized vitiligo of less than 10 years' duration. Tacrolimus 0.1% ointment was applied twice daily for 24 weeks in addition to a daily morning application of a broad-spectrum sunscreen. Each patient had a baseline severity assessment and follow-up examinations at weeks 4, 8, 12, 16, 20, and 24. Laboratory studies were performed at baseline and at 12 and 24 weeks.

Results.—Overall disease severity showed a statistically significant decrease by week 24 compared with baseline and a similar decrease for face and neck sites at weeks 12 and 24. Only minimal repigmentation occurred on hands, feet, ankles, and wrists. Six patients (31%) achieved greater than 50% repigmentation and 13 experienced greater than 75% repigmentation of head and neck lesions (Fig 4; see color plate XVI). Reported side effects were generally mild and no patient discontinued treatment because of adverse events. Both laboratory parameters and T-cell profiles (the latter significantly decreased at baseline) were unchanged at 12 and 24 weeks, but TNF-α expression in treated skin showed a statistically significant decrease at 24 weeks.

Conclusion.—Tacrolimus 0.1% ointment demonstrated efficacy and safety for repigmentation in vitiligo. At least some repigmentation occurred in 17 of 19 patients in this series. The suppression of TNF-α by topical tacrolimus may be associated with repigmentation.

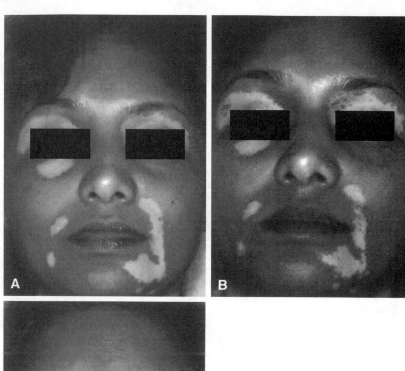

FIGURE 4.—A 36-year-old Asian-Indian women, with 6-year duration of vitiligo, at baseline (A), 8 weeks (B; follicular repigmentation), and 24 weeks (C; 51% to 75% repigmentation). (Reprinted by permission of the publisher from Grimes PE, Morris R, Avaniss-Aghajani E, et al: Topical tacrolimus therapy for vitiligo: Therapeutic responses and skin messenger RNA expression of proinflammatory cytokines. *J Am Acad Dermatol* 51:52-61, 2004. Copyright 2004 by Elsevier.)

▶ The authors allude to the "hit-or-miss" nature of vitiligo treatment. I have found this to be no less true with tacrolimus/pimecrolimus than with other popular therapies. In general, patients with limited vitiligo or vitiligo of fairly recent onset tend to respond better than those with extensive pigmentary loss of long duration.

B. H. Thiers, MD

Calcipotriene and Corticosteroid Combination Therapy for Vitiligo

Travis LB, Silverberg NB (St Luke's-Roosevelt Hosp Ctr, New York)
Pediatr Dermatol 21:495-498, 2004   8–2

Introduction.—The most widely prescribed therapies for vitiligo, cortico-steroids and photochemotherapy, are not beneficial in all patients. Psoralen and ultraviolet A (PUVA) is not recommended for children, and topical ste-roids also have adverse effects with prolonged use. Calcipotriene, recently reported to be effective for vitiligo in adult patients, was administered in combination with corticosteroids to young patients with vitiligo.

Methods.—Study participants were 12 otherwise healthy patients (6 males and 6 females) with an average age of 13.1 years (range, 3-28 years). The 2 adult patients in the group were included because of a recent relapse of pediatric-onset vitiligo. The treatment consisted of topical steroid oint-ments: a thin coat was applied to affected areas in the morning. Class 5 cor-ticosteroids were prescribed for the eyelids, and class 2 or 3 corticosteroids were prescribed for the body. Calcipotriene ointment (maximum, 100 g/wk) was applied to all affected areas in the evening. Skin examinations took place every 6 weeks, and therapy continued until repigmentation occurred or for at least 3 months if no repigmentation was seen.

Results.—The vitiligo type was vulgaris in 7 patients, acro-orofacial in 7, and segmental in 2. Patients' ethnicities were African American in 4 patients, Hispanic in 4, Arab in 2, Asian in 1, and white in 1. Ten patients (83%) re-sponded to treatment, and the average time was 4.5 weeks to the first re-sponse. After an average of 4.5 months of calcipotriene–corticosteroid treat-ment, responders showed a mean pigmentation rate of 95%, and none had new lesions develop during the protocol. Treatment failure occurred in 2 young Arab boys.

Conclusion.—The development of hyperpigmentation in patients with psoriasis who were treated with calcipotriene and phototherapy suggested that the drug might be useful for vitiligo. In this small series of patients, the high percentage of responders indicates that a combination of calcipotriene and corticosteroid ointments is more effective than monotherapy with either agent. Four of 10 responders previously had poor results with topical corti-costeroids alone.

▶ In a small group of children with vitiligo, the authors noted good repigmen-tation using a combination of calcipotriene and medium- to high-strength topi-cal corticosteroids. An enhanced response might be obtained from the addi-tion of either natural sunlight or narrowband UVB to this topical regimen.

S. Raimer, MD

Parametric Modeling of Narrowband UV-B Phototherapy for Vitiligo Using a Novel Quantitative Tool: The Vitiligo Area Scoring Index

Hamzavi I, Jain H, McLean D, et al (Univ of British Columbia, Vancouver, Canada)

Arch Dermatol 140:677-683, 2004   8–3

Background.—Currently, no quantitative tool exists for assessing the response of vitiligo to treatment. In the current research, the Vitiligo Area Scoring Index (VASI) was developed and used to model the response of vitiligo to narrowband UV-B (NB-UV-B) phototherapy with the use of parametric tests.

Methods.—Twenty-two patients were enrolled in the prospective, bilateral left–right, randomized controlled comparison study. All participants were older than 18 years and had stable vitiligo involving at least 5% of their total body surface in a symmetric distribution. Treatment consisted of NB-UV-B 3 times a week to 1 side of the body for a total of 60 treatments or 6 months. The contralateral side of each patient served as the control. The VASI was used to assess repigmentation. This instrument is based on a composite estimate of the overall area of vitiligo patches at baseline and the degree of macular repigmentation within these patches over time. The VASI was validated against physician and patient global evaluations. Overall decreases in the VASI for NB-UV-B and control groups were modeled by multilevel regression with random effects and compared parametrically.

Findings.—The VASI scores showed good correlation with patient and physician global evaluations. The extent of repigmentation after 6 months was 42.9% on the treated side and 3.3% on the untreated side. Significant differences between the treated and untreated sides became apparent within the first 2 months of therapy. Repigmentation was much more likely to occur on the legs, trunk, and arms than on the feet and hands.

Conclusions.—The VASI is a simple, quantitative clinical tool useful for assessing vitiligo parametrically. The application of this tool demonstrated that patients undergoing NB-UV-B can achieve about 42.9% repigmentation after 6 months of treatment, and the greatest responses occur over the trunk and nonacral parts of the extremities.

▶ Hamzavi et al have developed a clinical tool to objectively assess the response to vitiligo treatment. Using this tool, they report that patients with vitiligo treated with NB-UVB achieve approximately 42% repigmentation after 6 months of treatment. The identification of prognostic factors for a response or a lack of response to treatment was not an objective of the current study.

B. H. Thiers, MD

The Use of the 308-nm Excimer Laser for the Treatment of Vitiligo

Hadi SM, Spencer JM, Lebwohl M (Mount Sinai School of Medicine, New York)
Dermatol Surg 30:983-986, 2004   8–4

Introduction.—Many treatment approaches are available for patients with vitiligo, yet most are either only slightly effective or have significant side effects. The 308-nm excimer laser has recently been reported to be an effective and safe method for treating vitiligo. The effectiveness of the new 308-nm excimer laser for the treatment of vitiligo was evaluated.

Methods.—A retrospective medical record review was performed in 32 patients with 55 spots of vitiligo. A population-based sample was evaluated that included males and females, adults and children, with diverse ethnic backgrounds. Treatment was initiated with the lowest dose, which is 100 mJ/cm^2 (comparable to 1 minimal erythema dose value and 1 multiplier). Depending on Fitzpatrick skin type, the dose was gradually increased in a stepwise fashion. In patients with skin types I to II, the same dose was repeated twice before increasing it to help prevent burns. Patients underwent 30 sessions or until 75% repigmentation, whichever came first.

Results.—Of 55 spots treated, 29 (52.8%) had 75% pigmentation or better and 35 (63.7%) had 50% pigmentation or better. Best results were attained on the face (Figs 1 and 2; see color plate XVII): of 21 spots treated, 15 (71.5%) had 75% pigmentation and 16 (76.2%) had 50% pigmentation or better. Other areas (neck, extremities, trunk, and genitals) experienced moderate response compared with the face. Least responsive were the hands and feet; of 5 spots treated, only 20% had 50% pigmentation or better.

Conclusion.—Slightly more than half of the cohort experienced 75% or more pigmentation of their vitiligo lesions after 30 treatments or less; the

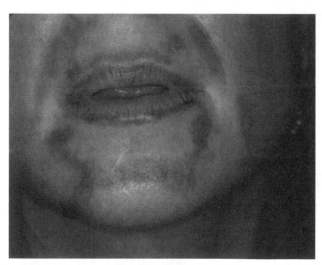

FIGURE 1.—Prelaser photo of a patient with vitiligo (before). (Courtesy of Hadi SM, Spencer JM, Lebwohl M: The use of 308-nm excimer laser for the treatment of vitiligo. *Dermatol Surg* 30:983-986, 2004. Reprinted by permission of Blackwell Publishing.)

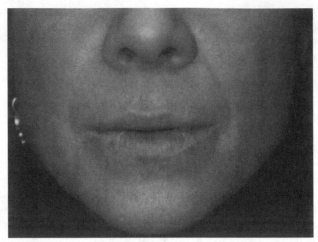

FIGURE 2.—Pigmentation after 25 sessions of treatment with the 308-nm excimer laser (after). (Courtesy of Hadi SM, Spencer JM, Lebwohl M: The use of 308-nm excimer laser for the treatment of vitiligo. *Dermatol Surg* 30:983-986, 2004. Reprinted by permission of Blackwell Publishing.)

majority of responders had Fitzpatrick skin type III and above. All control patches remained unchanged. The 308-nm excimer laser is effective in the treatment of vitiligo.

▶ The use of the excimer laser offers hope for repigmenting vitiligo lesions. Typically, multiple treatments are required and the efficacy is somewhat dependent on the anatomic location. Very few of the patients in this study were followed for an extended period. Thus, the durability of the repigmentation achieved with the excimer laser is uncertain, and further clinical trials are indicated, especially to address the long-term retention of the restored pigment.

J. Cook, MD

9 Collagen Vascular and Related Disorders

Pimecrolimus 1% Cream for Cutaneous Lupus Erythematosus
Kreuter A, Gambichler T, Breuckmann F, et al (Ruhr-Univ Bochum, Germany; Old-church Hosp, Greater London)
J Am Acad Dermatol 51:407-410, 2004   9–1

Introduction.—Glucocorticosteroids are used topically in the treatment of cutaneous lupus erythematosus (LE), despite the side effects associated with prolonged application. Newer anti-inflammatory substances such as tacrolimus and pimecrolimus have the potential to replace corticosteroids as a safer treatment option for cutaneous LE. In the current study, 11 patients were treated with pimecrolimus 1% cream.

Methods.—Patients ranged in age from 11 to 76 years and had a duration of LE ranging from 1 month to 23 years. Diagnoses included subacute cutaneous LE (2 cases), discoid LE (4 cases), systemic LE (3 cases), and LE tumidus (2 cases). No other topical therapy was applied for at least 8 weeks before initiation of pimecrolimus, and additional therapy during the study was limited to sunscreens and emollients. Pimecrolimus was applied twice daily on affected areas for 3 consecutive weeks. Skin involvement before and after therapy was scored for erythema, infiltration, and squamation.

Results.—All patients experienced significant regression of skin lesions (Fig 1) after therapy (Fig 2). The overall clinical score decreased from a mean of 6.45 to a mean of 2.73 after 3 weeks of topical pimecrolimus treatment. Two patients had new lesions after the end of therapy, but 9 exhibited sustained clinical improvement during 8 weeks of follow-up.

Discussion.—Topical pimecrolimus showed significant efficacy and safety for the treatment of the cutaneous lesions of LE. The agent acts by preventing the cascade of immune and inflammatory signals in a variety of skin diseases. Early erythematous lesions of subacute cutaneous LE and LE tumidus showed a better response than long-standing discoid LE, perhaps because the latter lesions have substantially more hyperkeratosis.

▶ Similar studies have suggested the usefulness of topical tacrolimus ointment for cutaneous LE.[1,2]

B. H. Thiers, MD

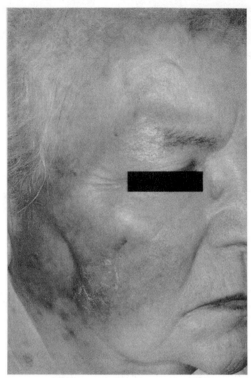

FIGURE 1.—Facial lesions of subacute cutaneous lupus erythematosus (patient No. 1) before treatment. (Reprinted by permission of the publisher from Kreuter A, Gambichler T, Breuckmann F, et al: Pimecrolimus 1% cream for cutaneous lupus erythematosus. *J Am Acad Dermatol* 51:407-410, 2004. Copyright 2004 by Elsevier.)

References

1. Lampropoulos CE, Sangle S, Harrison P, et al: Topical tacrolimus therapy of resistant cutaneous lesions in lupus erythematosus: A possible alternative. *Rheumatology (Oxford)* 43:1383-1385, 2004.
2. Walker SL, Kirby B, Chalmers RJ: The effect of topical tacrolimus on severe recalcitrant chronic discoid lupus erythematosus. *Br J Dermatol* 147:405-406, 2002.

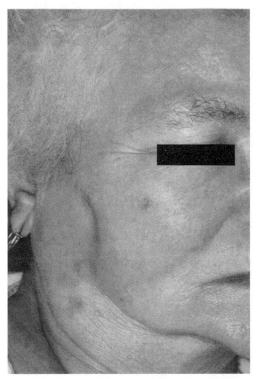

FIGURE 2.—Almost complete clearance after 3 weeks of pimecrolimus 1% cream. (Reprinted by permission of the publisher from Kreuter A, Gambichler T, Breuckmann F, et al: Pimecrolimus 1% cream for cutaneous lupus erythematosus. *J Am Acad Dermatol* 51:407-410, 2004. Copyright 2004 by Elsevier.)

Neonatal Lupus and a Seronegative Mother

Gattorno M, Di Rocco M, Buoncompagni A, et al (Univ of Genoa, Italy; Univ of Milan, Italy)
Lancet 363:1038, 2004   9–2

Background.—Lysinuric protein intolerance (LPI) is an autosomal recessive disease caused by defects in the membrane transport of lysine, arginine, and ornithine. Clinical and serologic features of patients with LPI are suggestive of neonatal systemic lupus erythematosus (SLE). A newborn with LPI initially suspected to have neonatal SLE is described.

>   *Case Report.*—Girl was born with a diffuse vasculitic rash and mild hepatosplenomegaly with elevated transaminase levels. At age 3 months, she was seen with a persistent rash, stunted growth, and loss of appetite. Physical examination revealed massive hepatosplenomegaly and hypotonia. Laboratory tests revealed thrombocytopenia, anemia, and markedly increased levels of lactate dehydrogenase and ferritin.

The antinuclear antibody (ANA) titer was 1:320 with a speckled pattern, and anti-Ro/SSA antibodies were present. Coomb's test results were negative, and she was thought to have neonatal SLE. However, subsequent electrocardiographic findings were normal, and the mother was negative for ANA and anti-Ro/SSA and anti-La/SSB antibodies. Bone marrow aspiration revealed hemophagocytic lymphohistiocytosis.

The working diagnosis was changed to LPI, and plasma and urine concentrations of lysine, arginine, and ornithine were measured. Levels of each of these amino acids were below normal in plasma and above normal in urine. Molecular analysis of the SLC7A7 gene indicated that the child was homozygous for the 967G→A mutation, which confirmed the diagnosis of LPI. The patient began treatment with steroids and citrulline, which rapidly resolved the rash, anemia, and thrombocytopenia. At her last follow-up visit 3.6 years later, the patient still tested positive for ANA and anti-Ro/SSA antibodies, and she had intermittent episodes of cytopenia requiring steroids and immunosuppressive therapy.

Conclusion.—These findings underscore the need to include LPI in the differential diagnosis of neonatal SLE.

▶ The diagnosis of neonatal lupus still remains a possibility. A skin biopsy specimen would have been helpful. Although the child appeared to have LPI, the lupus-like rash and the detectable ANA and anti-Ro/SSA antibodies still require explanation.

B. H. Thiers, MD

Antihistone and Anti–Double-Stranded Deoxyribonucleic Acid Antibodies Are Associated With Renal Disease in Systemic Lupus Erythematosus
Cortés-Hernández J, Ordi-Ros J, Labrador M, et al (Vall d'Hebron Hosps, Barcelona)
Am J Med 116:165-173, 2004   9–3

Purpose.—We sought to assess the nephritogenic antibody profile of patients with systemic lupus erythematosus (SLE), and to determine which antibodies were most useful in identifying patients at risk of nephritis.

Methods.—We studied 199 patients with SLE, 78 of whom had lupus nephritis. We assayed serum samples for antibodies against chromatin components (double-stranded deoxyribonucleic acid [dsDNA], nucleosome, and histone), C1q, basement membrane components (laminin, fibronectin, and type IV collagen), ribonucleoprotein, and phospholipids. Correlations of these antibodies with disease activity (SLE Disease Activity Index) and nephropathy were assessed. Patients with no initial evidence of nephropathy were followed prospectively for 6 years.

Results.—Antibodies against dsDNA, nucleosomes, histone, C1q, and basement membrane components were associated with disease activity ($P <$ 0.05). In a multivariate analysis, anti-dsDNA antibodies (odds ratio [OR] = 6; 95% confidence interval [CI]: 2 to 24) and antihistone antibodies (OR = 9.4; 95% CI: 4 to 26) were associated with the presence of proliferative glomerulonephritis. In the prospective study, 7 (6%) of the 121 patients developed proliferative lupus glomerulonephritis after a mean of 6 years of follow-up. Patients with initial antihistone (26% [5/19] vs. 2% [2/95], $P =$ 0.0004) and anti-dsDNA reactivity (6% [2/33] vs. 0% [0/67], $P = 0.048$) had a greater risk of developing proliferative glomerulonephritis than patients without these autoantibodies.

Conclusion.—In addition to routine anti-dsDNA antibody assay, antihistone antibody measurement may be useful for identifying patients at increased risk of proliferative glomerulonephritis.

▶ The authors present data to suggest that antihistone antibody measurement may, like anti-dsDNA antibody detection, help identify patients with SLE at risk for developing proliferative glomerulonephritis.

B. H. Thiers, MD

Sequential Therapies for Proliferative Lupus Nephritis
Contreras G, Pardo V, Leclercq B, et al (Univ of Miami)
N Engl J Med 350:971-980, 2004   9–4

Background.—Long-term cyclophosphamide treatment has been shown to improve renal survival rates in patients with proliferative lupus nephritis. However, the benefits of this therapy must be weighed against its considerable toxicity. Research has demonstrated that mycophenolate mofetil inhibits purine synthesis, exerts antiproliferative effects on lymphocytes, and profoundly attenuates the production of autoantibodies by B cells. The safety and efficacy of IV cyclophosphamide followed by oral mycophenolate mofetil or azathioprine were compared with those of long-term IV cyclophosphamide.

Methods.—Fifty-nine patients with lupus nephritis were included in the study. Twelve had World Health Organization class III disease, 46 had class IV disease, and 1 had class Vb disease. Induction therapy in all patients consisted of up to 7 monthly boluses of IV cyclophosphamide, 0.5 to 1 g per square meter of body surface area, plus corticosteroids. Thereafter, patients were assigned randomly to 1 of 3 maintenance groups: quarterly IV injections of cyclophosphamide, oral azathioprine (1-3 mg/kg/body weight per day), or oral mycophenolate mofetil (500-3000 mg/d). Maintenance treatment lasted for 1 to 3 years.

Findings.—Five patients died during maintenance therapy, including 4 in the cyclophosphamide group and 1 in the mycophenolate mofetil group. Chronic renal failure developed in 3 patients in the cyclophosphamide group, in 1 in the azathioprine group, and in 1 in the mycophenolate mofetil group. The event-free survival rate at 72 months was higher in the myco-phenolate mofetil and azathioprine groups than in the cyclophosphamide group. The relapse-free survival rate was also superior in the mycophenolate mofetil group than in the cyclophosphamide group. Patients receiving my-cophenolate mofetil or azathioprine maintenance therapy had a significantly lower incidence of hospitalization, amenorrhea, infections, nausea, and vomiting than did patients receiving long-term cyclophosphamide.

Conclusions.—Following short-term IV cyclophosphamide administra-tion with mycophenolate mofetil or azathioprine maintenance therapy ap-pears to be more effective than long-term IV cyclophosphamide in patients with proliferative lupus nephritis. This new approach to maintenance ther-apy also appears to be safer.

▶ Although long-term therapy with cyclophosphamide enhances renal surviv-al in patients with proliferative lupus nephritis, considerable adverse effects, including amenorrhea, infections, leukopenia, nausea/vomiting, and diarrhea, may occur. The data offered by Contreras et al demonstrate the utility of my-cophenolate mofetil or azathioprine as viable alternatives to cyclophospha-mide for long-term maintenance.[1]

B. H. Thiers, MD

Reference

1. Balow JE, Austin HA III: Maintenance therapy for lupus nephritis-Something old, something new. *N Engl J Med* 350:1044-1046, 2004.

Mannose-Binding Lectin Variant Alleles and the Risk of Arterial Throm-bosis in Systemic Lupus Erythematosus
Øhlenschlaeger T, Garred P, Madsen HO, et al (Bispebjerg Hosp, Copenhagen; Hvidovre Hosp, Copenhagen; Univ of Copenhagen)
N Engl J Med 351:260-267, 2004   9–5

Background.—An important complication of systemic lupus erythemato-sus (SLE) is cardiovascular disease. Variant alleles of the mannose-binding lectin (MBL) gene correlate with both SLE and severe atherosclerosis. Whether MBL variant alleles are associated with an increase in the risk of arterial thrombosis in patients with SLE was investigated.

Methods.—Ninety-one Danish patients with SLE were included in the prospective study. MBL alleles were genotyped by polymerase chain reac-tion assay. Arterial and venous thromboses after SLE diagnoses were con-firmed with the use of appropriate diagnostic tools. The median follow-up period was 9.1 years.

Findings.—Thirty patients were heterozygous for MBL variant alleles, with the A/O genotype, and 7 were homozygous, with the O/O genotype. Fifty-four patients had no MBL variant alleles, with a genotype of A/A. Dur-ing follow-up, arterial thromboses developed in 6 of 7 patients with the O/O genotype, compared with 18 of the 84 patients in the other 2 genotype groups. The O/O genotype carried a hazard ratio of 5.8, which increased to 7.0 after adjustment for other known risk factors. Venous thromboses occurred in 14 patients and were unassociated statistically with the MBL genotype.

Conclusion.—Homozygosity for MBL variant alleles correlates with an increased risk of arterial thrombosis in patients with SLE. The risk of venous thrombosis was not increased in the patients studied. Thus, MBL appears to play a specific role in protecting against arterial thrombosis.

▶ A specific role for MBL in providing protection against arterial thrombosis is suggested by the lack of an increased risk of venous thrombosis in patients with SLE homozygous for MBL variant alleles. This suggests a specific role for MBL in protecting against atherosclerosis. Future studies may explore the utility of MBL genotyping to identify patients (both with and without SLE) at high risk for cardiovascular disease.

B. H. Thiers, MD

Antiphospholipid Antibodies and Subsequent Thrombo-occlusive Events in Patients With Ischemic Stroke
Levine SR, for the APASS Investigators (Mount Sinai School of Medicine, New York; et al)
JAMA 291:576-584, 2004   9–6

Introduction.—Several potential hematologic markers of hypercoagulability, including antiphospholipid antibody (aPL), have been linked with vascular thrombo-occlusive events in most case-control investigations. In prospective trials, aPL positivity has been correlated with initial thrombotic events, including strokes, but the correlation has been inconsistent. The role of aPL in predicting ischemic events, especially recurrent ischemic strokes, is controversial. The effect of baseline aPL positivity on subsequent thrombo-occlusive events, including recurrent strokes, was examined in the Antiphospholipid Antibodies and Stroke Study (APASS), a prospective cohort investigation within the Warfarin vs Aspirin Recurrent Stroke Study (WARSS), a randomized double-blind trial of 2206 participants performed at multiple United States clinical sites between June 1993 through 2000.

Methods.—In WARSS, adjusted dose warfarin (target international normalized ratio, 1.4-2.8) and aspirin (325 mg/d) were compared for prevention of recurrent strokes or death. The APASS participants were 1770 WARSS participants (80%) who had usable baseline blood samples obtained before randomization to the WARSS and were evaluated for aPL status within 90 days of the index stroke. The primary outcome measures were as follows: 2-year rate of the composite end point of death from any cause, ischemic stroke, transient ischemic attack, myocardial infarction, deep vein thrombosis, pulmonary embolism, and other systemic thrombo-occlusive events.

Results.—Seven hundred twenty APASS participants (41%) had aPL-positive status. No increased risk of thrombo-occlusive events associated with baseline aPL status was observed in patients treated with either warfarin (relative risk [RR], 0.99; 95% CI, 0.75-1.31; $P = .94$) or aspirin (RR, 0.94; 95% CI, 0.70-1.28; $P = .71$). The overall event rate was 22.2% and 21.8% among participants with aPL-positive or aPL-negative status, respectively. No treatment $\times$ aPL interaction was seen ($P = .91$). Patients with baseline positivity for both lupus anticoagulant antibodies (LA) and anticardiolipin antibodies (aCL) tended to experience a higher event rate (31.7%) than did those who had negative results for both antibodies (24.0%) (unadjusted RR, 1.36; 95% CI, 0.97-1.92; $P = .07$). No specific LA test or aCL isotope or titer was linked with an increased risk of thrombo-occlusive events.

Conclusion.—The presence of aPL (either LA or aCL) among patients with ischemic strokes is not predictive of an increased risk for subsequent vascular occlusive events over 2 years or a differential response to aspirin or warfarin therapy. It seems that routine screening for aPL in patients with ischemic strokes is not necessary.

▶ The APASS protocol sought to evaluate the effect of baseline aPL positivity on subsequent thrombo-occlusive events, including recurrent strokes. No such correlation was found. Thus, routine screening for aPL in patients with ischemic stroke is not recommended. The challenges in reducing stroke risk and directions for future research were discussed in an accompanying editorial.[1]

B. H. Thiers, MD

Reference

1. Hanley DF: The challenge of stroke prevention. *JAMA* 291:621-622, 2004.

Increased Prevalence of Human Parvovirus B19 DNA in Systemic Sclerosis Skin

Ohtsuka T, Yamazaki S (Dokkyo Koshigaya Hosp, Saitoma, Japan)
Br J Dermatol 150:1091-1095, 2004   9–7

Background.—Some evidence suggests human parvovirus B19 infection is involved in systemic sclerosis (SSc). Because most abnormalities in SSc occur in the skin, the presence of human parvovirus B19 DNA in the skin of patients with SSc was investigated.

Methods.—In all, 48 patients with SSc, 16 with systemic lupus erythematosus, 8 with dermatomyositis, 6 with morphea, 8 with graft-versus-host disease, and 97 healthy research subjects were studied. Skin specimens from the dorsal aspect of the forearm were obtained from each study participant, including lesional skin in each patient. Genomic DNA was extracted from the specimens and was examined via nested polymerase chain reaction that used 2 different parvovirus B19 primers.

Results.—With the first 284-base pair (bp) primer, human parvovirus B19 DNA was significantly more common in patients with SSc (75%) than in those with other conditions or in control subjects (52%). Similarly, with the second 103-bp primer, human parvovirus B19 DNA was also significantly more common in patients with SSc (75%) than in those with other conditions or in control subjects (55%).

Conclusion.—Persistent human parvovirus B19 infection may be involved in the etiology of the skin abnormalities seen in SSc.

▶ Further study will be needed to assess the pathogenetic importance of these findings. An association of parvovirus B19 with SSc as well as with rheumatoid arthritis has previously been postulated.[1,2]

B. H. Thiers, MD

References

1. Ferri C, Longombardo G, Azzi A, et al: Parvovirus B19 and systemic sclerosis. *Clin Exp Rheumatol* 17:267-268, 1999.
2. Altschuler EL: The historical record is consistent with the recent finding of parvovirus B19 infection of bone marrow in systemic sclerosis patients. *Clin Exp Rheumatol* 19:228, 2001.

Patient Initiated Outpatient Follow Up in Rheumatoid Arthritis: Six Year Randomised Controlled Trial

Hewlett S, Kirwan J, Pollock J, et al (Univ of Bristol, England)
BMJ 330:171-175, 2005   9–8

Background.—In the United Kingdom, patients with rheumatoid arthritis (RA) undergo physician-initiated hospital reviews every 3 to 6 months. Many patients are healthy at the time of the review, and thus the scheduled review can be a burden. Conversely, many patients with disease exacerbation cannot receive a hospital appointment in a timely manner because of the number of routine reviews scheduled. A new system, in which patients with RA initiate these hospital reviews according to their disease status, has been shown to be safe and cost-effective through 4 years of follow-up. This study extends follow-up to 6 years, to ensure that skipping routine physician-initiated hospital reviews does not result in long-term physical consequences.

Methods.—The subjects were 209 patients with RA for 2 years or more. Half were randomly assigned to traditional hospital review directed by their physician every 3 to 6 months, whereas the other half initiated their own hospital reviews and were seen within 10 days of their request for an appointment. The 2 groups were compared in terms of clinical outcomes (pain, disease activity, early morning stiffness, inflammatory indices, disability, grip strength, range of motion in joints, bone erosion), psychologic status (anxiety, depression, helplessness, self-efficacy, satisfaction, confidence in the health care delivery system), and the number of visits to hospital physicians or general practitioners for RA.

Results.—After 6 years of follow-up, the only clinical parameter that differed significantly between the 2 groups was that patients who made their own appointments had less deterioration in range of motion at the elbow than did the patients in the traditional care group. The only psychologic parameters that differed significantly between the 2 groups were that patients in the direct access group were more satisfied with their care and more confident in the system at 2, 4, and 6 years. Also, patients in the direct access group made 38% fewer hospital appointments (median, 8 vs 13) during follow-up.

Conclusion.—Over 6 years of follow-up, clinical and psychologic outcomes in patients with RA who initiated their own hospital reviews were at least as good as those in patients who attended regular physician-scheduled hospital reviews. Furthermore, patients who initiated their own reviews made 38% fewer hospital medical appointments to achieve this level of care. If initiated on a large scale, this approach to managing RA could improve costs, hospital and other health care utilization, and patient satisfaction.

▶ The traditional UK system of routine hospital follow-up in patients with chronic disease is a drain on NHS resources and a burden for patients if they are well. Ironically, the patient is often well at the assigned review time but unable to rapidly access support when it is required. Hewlett et al show that in patients with RA, replacing traditional reviews with access initiated by the patient could be advantageous. Such a system is preferred by patients and general practitioners and significantly decreases the number of hospital medical appointments. The advantage of rapid specialist access is a concept to be appreciated by American health insurers as well.

B. H. Thiers, MD

Effect of a Treatment Strategy of Tight Control for Rheumatoid Arthritis (the TICORA Study): A Single-blind Randomised Controlled Trial

Grigor C, Capell H, Stirling A, et al (Gartnavel Gen Hosp, Glasgow, Scotland; Glasgow Royal Infirmary, Scotland; Univ of Glasgow, Scotland; et al)
Lancet 364:263-269, 2004   9–9

Background.—Current strategies for treating rheumatoid arthritis include the use of disease-modifying antirheumatic agents. Unfortunately, only a minority of patients obtain a good response. Whether a strategy of intensive outpatient management for sustained, tight control of disease activity would yield better outcomes than routine outpatient care was investigated.

Methods and Findings.—One hundred eleven patients were enrolled in the single-blind, randomized controlled study at 2 centers. One patient withdrew after randomization, and 7 quit during the study. The mean decline in disease activity score was greater among patients assigned to intensive care than among those assigned to routine care; the decreases in disease activity score were 3.5 and 1.9, respectively. Patients in the intensive treatment group were more likely to have a good response or to be in remission than were those receiving routine care. Four patients died during the study, including 3 assigned to routine care. None of the deaths could be attributed to the type of treatment.

Conclusion.—Intensive outpatient management of rheumatoid arthritis markedly improves outcomes in disease activity, radiographic disease progression, physical functioning, and quality of life.

▶ Surprisingly, costs were not different between patients undergoing intensive management and those receiving routine treatment. Unfortunately, it is still uncertain whether the improvement in patient outcomes will translate into long-term savings, such as a reduced need for joint replacement and a reduction in work disability.

B. H. Thiers, MD

Therapeutic Effect of the Combination of Etanercept and Methotrexate Compared With Each Treatment Alone in Patients With Rheumatoid Arthritis: Double-blind Randomised Controlled Trial

Klareskog L, for the TEMPO (Trial of Etanercept and Methotrexate With Radiographic Patient Outcome) Study Investigators (Karolinska Inst/Karolinska Hosp, Stockholm; Univ Hosp, Maastricht, The Netherlands; Gold Coast Rheumatology, Southport, Queensland, Australia; et al)
Lancet 363:675-681, 2004   9–10

Background.—Etanercept and methotrexate are each effective for treating rheumatoid arthritis (RA). Whether their combination might be more effective than either drug alone in patients with refractory RA was investigated.

Methods.—The research subjects were 682 patients (77% women; mean age, 52 years) with adult-onset, active RA whose treatment with at least 1 disease-modifying antirheumatic drug other than methotrexate had failed. Patients were randomly assigned to receive 52 weeks of therapy with either etanercept alone (25 mg subcutaneously twice a week), oral methotrexate alone (up to 20 mg every week), or their combination. The primary end point was the numeric index of the American College of Rheumatology response (ACR-N) area under the curve (AUC) during the first 24 weeks of treatment. In addition, radiographs were taken at week 52 and compared with baseline images to determine changes in total joint damage, joint space narrowing, and erosion.

Results.—The ACR-N AUC at 24 weeks was significantly higher in the combination group (18.3%-years [95% CI, 17.1-19.6%-years]) than in the etanercept alone (14.7%-years [95% CI, 13.5-16.0-years] $P < .0001$) or the methotrexate alone (12.2%-years [95% CI, 11.0-13.4-years] $P < .0001$, respectively) groups. The ACR-N AUC was also significantly greater with etanercept monotherapy than with methotrexate monotherapy. The mean total Sharp score at 52 weeks decreased by –0.54 (95% CI, –1.00 to –0.07) in the combination group, but increased by 0.52 (95% CI, 0.10-1.15; P = .0006) in the etanercept group and by 2.80 (95% CI, 1.08-4.51; P < .0001) in the methotrexate group. The between-group difference with etanercept and methotrexate monotherapies was also significant. Joint space narrowing scores and erosion scores followed a similar pattern. Infection and other adverse events occurred with similar frequency in the 3 groups.

Conclusion.—Etanercept and methotrexate in combination was significantly more effective than either drug alone in reducing disease activity, improving functional disability, and slowing the radiographic progression of RA.

▶ Klareskog et al show that, in patients with RA, the combination of etanercept and methotrexate is significantly better than either drug alone for reducing disease activity, improving functional disability, and retarding radiographic progression. Nevertheless, a sizeable number of patients have continued active inflammation even with combination therapy.[1,2] Quite likely, similar studies in patients with psoriasis would demonstrate a synergistic effect between the 2 drugs. These findings underscore the difficulty in effectively and safely suppressing the aberrant immune response in immunologically mediated diseases and show that, even with the new innovative biologic therapies, the goal of a single magic bullet for immune-mediated diseases has still not been attained.[3]

B. H. Thiers, MD

References

1. Schnabel A: Disease-modifying antirheumatic drugs: Enhancing efficacy by combination. *Lancet* 363:670-671, 2004.
2. Schottelius AJG: Biology of tumor necrosis factor-α—Implications for psoriasis. *Exp Dermatol* 13:193-222, 2004.
3. Olsen NJ, Stein CM: New drugs for rheumatoid arthritis. *N Engl J Med* 350:2167-2179, 2004.

Newer Disease-Modifying Antirheumatic Drugs and the Risk of Serious Hepatic Adverse Events in Patients With Rheumatoid Arthritis
Suissa S, Ernst P, Hudson M, et al (McGill Univ, Montreal)
Am J Med 117:87-92, 2004   9–11

Background.—Spontaneous cases of hepatic adverse events have been reported in patients with rheumatoid arthritis who were being treated with leflunomide, one of the newer disease-modifying antirheumatic drugs (DMARDs). We assessed the risk of hepatic events associated with the use of leflunomide and other DMARDs.

Methods.—Two cohorts comprising 41,885 patients with rheumatoid arthritis who had been dispensed a DMARD between September 1, 1998, and December 31, 2001, were formed using claims databases. Follow-up was from the first dispensing date to the occurrence of a serious or nonserious hepatic event. A nested case-control approach was used to estimate adjusted rate ratios of hepatic events associated with DMARDs dispensed during the prior year, as compared with methotrexate monotherapy.

Results.—There were 25 cases of serious hepatic events (rate, 4.9 per 10,000 per year) and 411 nonserious hepatic events (rate, 80.0 per 10,000 per year). There was no increase in the rate of serious hepatic events with either leflunomide (rate ratio [RR] = 0.9; 95% confidence interval [CI]: 0.2 to 4.9) or traditional DMARDs (RR = 2.3; 95% CI: 0.8 to 6.5). However, the rate was increased with biologic DMARDs (RR = 5.5; 95% CI: 1.2 to 24.6). The rate of nonserious hepatic events was also increased with biologic DMARDs (RR = 1.5; 95% CI: 1.0 to 2.3), but not with leflunomide (RR = 0.9; 95% CI: 0.7 to 1.3) and traditional DMARDs (RR = 1.1; 95% CI: 0.8 to 1.4).

Conclusions.—We found no evidence of an excess risk of serious or nonserious hepatic events with the use of leflunomide as compared with methotrexate. Still, the increased risk observed with the new biologic DMARDs should be investigated further.

▶ The authors sought to confirm or refute previous reports suggesting an association between leflunomide and serious hepatic adverse events. Although no excess risk of hepatotoxicity was noted with leflunomide compared with methotrexate, the authors did find an unexpected increase in the risk of serious hepatic events associated with the use of biologic DMARDs, namely infliximab and etanercept. It is currently uncertain whether this risk is real or whether these newer drugs have been given to patients with more severe disease or to patients who are at greater risk of liver damage.

B. H. Thiers, MD

Heart Failure in Rheumatoid Arthritis: Rates, Predictors, and the Effect of Anti-Tumor Necrosis Factor Therapy
Wolfe F, Michaud K (Univ of Kansas, Wichita)
Am J Med 116:305-311, 2004   9–12

Introduction.—Patients with rheumatoid arthritis are at increased risk for cardiovascular morbidity and mortality. Anti-tumor necrosis factor (TNF) therapy, increasingly used to treat rheumatoid arthritis, theoretically could reduce the risk of heart failure because the failing heart, in contrast to the normal heart, produces TNF. However, clinical trials of TNF blockade in patients with advanced heart failure have shown either some harm or little benefit. Participants in the National Data Bank for Rheumatic Diseases study of the outcomes of arthritis were studied during a 2-year period for prevalence of heart failure, factors associated with heart failure, and the effects of anti-TNF therapy.

Methods.—The study included 13,171 patients with rheumatoid arthritis and 2568 with osteoarthritis. Information on demographic and clinical variables was obtained during 6-month assessment periods. Self-reports or reviews of medical records provided data on heart failure diagnoses. Incident cases were those occurring in individuals without a history of cardiovascular disease, including the use of cardiovascular medications.

Results.—After adjusting for differences in demographic characteristics, heart failure was more common among patients with rheumatoid arthritis (3.9%) than among those with osteoarthritis (2.3%). Men made up only 23% of the rheumatoid arthritis group, but the frequency of heart failure was greater in men (5.2%) than in women (3.0%). An association was noted between increased age and a greater frequency of heart failure. Anti-TNF-treated patients had a lower rate of heart failure (3.1%) than those not receiving the therapy (3.8%), even after adjusting for baseline differences. Patients with rheumatoid arthritis and no pre-existing cardiovascular disease had a very low risk of heart failure (0.4%).

Conclusion.—Patients with rheumatoid arthritis have a greater risk of heart failure than patients with osteoarthritis. This increased risk occurs in those with pre-existing cardiovascular disease and may be related to increased inflammatory activity, a fact that could explain the decreased rate of heart failure in patients treated for rheumatoid arthritis with anti-TNF agents.

▶ Data from heart failure models in mice suggests that blockade of circulating TNF may limit ventricular dysfunction. In contrast, clinical trials of TNF blockade in humans with advanced heart failure have shown little benefit or even harm.[1] The risk of myocardial infarction appears to be increased in patients with rheumatoid arthritis, although little is known about heart failure in that condition. The effect of anti-TNF therapy on heart failure is of special interest because the failing heart produces that cytokine, although the normal heart does not.[2] The data presented by Wolfe and Michaud indicate that while the risk of heart failure may indeed be increased in patients with rheumatoid arthritis, this risk may be ameliorated to some degree by anti-TNF therapy.

B. H. Thiers, MD

References

1. Kwon HJ, Cote TR, Cuffe MS, et al: Case reports of heart failure after therapy with a tumor necrosis factor antagonist. *Ann Intern Med* 138:807-811, 2003.
2. Feldman AM, Combes A, Wagner D, et al: The role of tumor necrosis factor in the pathophysiology of heart failure. *J Am Coll Cardiol* 35:537-544, 2000.

Fatal Exacerbation of Rheumatoid Arthritis Associated Fibrosing Alveolitis in Patients Given Infliximab

Ostor AJK, Crisp AJ, Somerville MF, et al (Addenbrooke's Hosp, Cambridge, England; Norfolk and Norwich Univ, England)
BMJ 329:1266, 2004   9–13

Background.—Tumor necrosis factor α (TNF α) antibodies are being used increasingly to treat autoimmune conditions, yet the long-term safety of these antibodies is unclear. Three patients in whom rapid fatal exacerbations of rheumatoid arthritis (RA)-related fibrosing alveolitis developed after they took infliximab are reported.

Patients and Outcomes.—The patients were 2 women and 1 man, aged 60 to 75 years. All had long-standing RA, were taking azathioprine, and had a previous diagnosis of asymptomatic fibrosing alveolitis. After 2 doses of infliximab, 3 mg/kg, in 2 patients and 3 doses in 1, sudden onset of breathlessness occurred. Lung function deteriorated in all 3 patients, 2 of whom died 1 month after infliximab therapy. The third patient died 9 months after treatment. Extensive examinations revealed no infection or other cause for respiratory decline.

Conclusions.—The authors caution against the use of infliximab in patients with underlying lung disease. All patients on immune-modulating drugs must be carefully monitored.

▶ The cause of the pulmonary deterioration in these patients is unknown. It is possible that infection may have played a role despite the lack of isolation of an organism. Pulmonary disease has been associated with all 3 biologic agents licensed for the treatment of RA, ie, infliximab, etanercept, and adalimumab.

B. H. Thiers, MD

Efficacy of B-Cell–Targeted Therapy With Rituximab in Patients With Rheumatoid Arthritis

Edwards JCW, Szcepański L, Szechiński J, et al (Univ College London; Med Univ School of Lubin, Poland; Univ School of Wroclaw, Poland; et al)
N Engl J Med 350:2572-2581, 2004   9–14

Background.—Approximately 1% of the adult population is affected by rheumatoid arthritis, which is characterized by chronic inflammation in the synovial membrane of affected joints. The progression of this systemic autoimmune disease results in loss of daily function due to chronic pain and fatigue. Most patients also suffer deterioration of cartilage and bone in the affected joints, which may lead to permanent disability. An open-label study reported that selective depletion of B cells with the use of rituximab provided sustained clinical improvements for patients with rheumatoid arthritis. These observations were investigated in a randomized controlled study.

Methods.—A total of 161 patients with active rheumatoid arthritis despite treatment with methotrexate were randomly assigned to receive 1 of 4 treatments: oral methotrexate (control); rituximab; rituximab plus cyclophosphamide; or rituximab plus methotrexate. Responses defined according to the criteria of the American College of Rheumatology (ACR) and the European League against Rheumatism (EULAR) were assessed at week 24 (primary analyses) and week 48 (exploratory analyses).

Results.—At week 24, the proportion of patients with 50% improvement in disease symptoms was significantly greater, according to the ACR criteria, with the rituximab-methotrexate (43%) and the rituximab-cyclophosphamide combination (41%) than with methotrexate alone (13%). In all of the groups treated with rituximab, a significantly higher portion of patients had a 20% improvement in disease symptoms according to the ACR criteria (65% to 76% vs 38%) or had EULAR responses (83% to 85% vs 50%). All of the ACR responses were maintained at week 48 in the rituximab-methotrexate group. Most of the adverse events occurred with the first rituximab infusion. At 24 weeks, serious infections occurred in 1 patient (2.5%) in the control group and in 4 patients (3.3%) in the rituximab groups. Peripheral blood immunoglobulin concentrations remained within normal ranges.

Conclusions.—Patients with active rheumatoid arthritis despite methotrexate treatment were effectively treated with a single course of 2 infusions of rituximab either alone or in combination with cyclophosphamide or continued methotrexate. This therapy provided significant improvement in disease symptoms at weeks 24 and 48.

▶ The response of rheumatoid arthritis to rituximab suggests the importance of the CD20+ B-cell subpopulation in the pathophysiology of rheumatoid arthritis. This surface antigen is expressed only on pre-B and mature-B cells but not on stem cells. It is lost before differentiation of B-cells into plasma cells. The observation that rituximab reduced disease activity without changing serum immunoglobulin levels supports the proposition that B-cells have an antibody-independent role in the pathogenesis of rheumatoid arthritis and systemic autoimmunity in general.[1] A more complete review of drug therapy for rheumatoid arthritis has recently been published.[2]

B. H. Thiers, MD

References

1. Tsokos GC: B cells, be gone—B-cell depletion in the treatment of rheumatoid arthritis. *N Engl J Med* 350:2546-2548, 2004.
2. O'Dell JR: Therapeutic strategies for rheumatoid arthritis. *N Engl J Med* 350:2591-2602, 2004.

Trial of Atorvastatin in Rheumatoid Arthritis (TARA): Double-blind, Randomised Placebo-controlled Trial

McCarey DW, McInnes IB, Madhok R, et al (Univ of Glasgow, Scotland)
Lancet 363:2015-2021, 2004   9–15

Background.—Rheumatoid arthritis is associated with a rapid onset of clinically significant functional impairment and accelerated vascular risk with attendant early mortality. HMG-CoA reductase inhibitors (statins) have been shown to modify clinically significant vascular risk in patients without inflammatory disease and may have an immunomodulatory function. However, no data have clearly shown that statins modulate autoimmune disease activity or modify vascular risk factors in the context of high-grade inflammation. Whether statins reduce inflammatory factors in rheumatoid arthritis and modify surrogates for vascular risk was determined.

Methods.—A total of 116 patients with rheumatoid arthritis were included in the double-blind placebo-controlled trial. The patients were randomly assigned to receive 40 mg atorvastatin or placebo as an adjunct to existing disease-modifying antirheumatic drug therapy. The patients were monitored over 6 months, and disease activity variables and circulating vascular risk factors were assessed. The main outcome measures were change in disease activity score (DAS28) and proportion meeting European League Against Rheumatism (EULAR) response criteria. Analysis was by intention to treat.

Results.—DAS28 improved significantly at 6 months after patients started atorvastatin compared with placebo. A DAS28 EULAR response was achieved in 18 of 58 patients (31%) in the atorvastatin group compared with 6 of 58 patients (10%) taking placebo. C-reactive protein levels and the erythrocyte sedimentation rate declined by 50% and 28%, respectively, relative to placebo. The swollen joint count also fell. The frequency of adverse events was similar for the atorvastatin and placebo groups.

Conclusion.—Statins can produce modest but clinically evident anti-inflammatory effects and can modify vascular risk factors in the setting of high-grade autoimmune inflammation.

▶ This study demonstrates that the lipid-lowering statin class of drugs may provide modest benefit in the treatment of rheumatoid arthritis. The mechanism presumably involves some immunomodulatory function,[1] as beneficial effects were noted on inflammatory markers such as the erythrocyte sedimentation rate, fibrinogen, C-reactive protein, and interleukin-6 levels. These statistically significant changes were of a magnitude that might affect the risk of future cardiovascular disease, above and beyond the obvious benefits of the cholesterol-lowering effects of the drugs.[2] Because rheumatoid arthritis is associated with accelerated vascular risk and early mortality, future studies of the salutory effects of the statins in this disorder are warranted.

B. H. Thiers, MD

References

1. Namazi MR: Statins: Novel additions to the dermatologic arsenal? *Exp Dermatol* 13:337-339, 2004.
2. Klareskog L, Hamsten A: Statins in rheumatoid arthritis: Two birds with one stone? *Lancet* 363:2011-2012, 2004.

Pulmonary Artery Aneurysms in Behçet Syndrome

Hamuryudan V, Er T, Seyahi E, et al (Univ of Istanbul, Turkey; Abant Izzet Baysal Univ, Duzce, Turkey)
Am J Med 117:867-870, 2004   9–16

Background.—Patients with Behçet syndrome have pulmonary artery aneurysms develop that can be seen on chest radiography as nodular opacities (Fig 1, A). Almost all these patients present with hemoptysis, and a study published in 1994 showed about 50% of patients with Behçet syndrome and pulmonary artery aneurysms die within 1 year after the onset of hemoptysis. Prognosis of these patients has improved since then. This study reassesses the prognosis of patients with Behçet syndrome and pulmonary artery aneurysms diagnosed since 1992.

Methods.—The medical records of 26 patients with Behçet syndrome (25 men and 1 woman, mean age 32.6 years) who received a diagnosis of pulmonary artery aneurysm since January 1, 1992, were reviewed. Outcomes in these patients were compared with those in a previous report of 24 patients

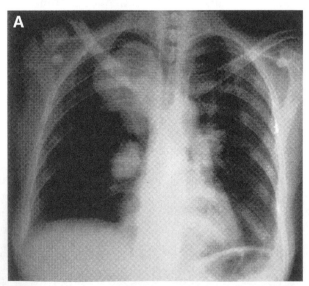

FIGURE 1.—**A,** Posteroanterior chest radiograph showing multiple pulmonary artery aneurysms. (Reprinted from Hamuryudan V, Er T, Seyahi E, et al: Pulmonary artery aneurysms in Behçet's syndrome. *Am J Med* 117:867-870, 2004. Copyright 2004, with permission from Excerpta Medica, Inc.)

who received the diagnosis before 1992. Treatment in both cohorts consisted of 3 methylprednisolone pulses, followed by prednisolone and cyclophosphamide therapy for 2 years, after which the drugs could be continued, stopped, or replaced with azathioprine.

Results.—Each of the 26 patients had received a diagnosis of Behçet syndrome before the development of pulmonary artery aneurysms. Twenty-six patients (88%) presented with hemoptysis, 21 (81%) also had deep vein thrombosis of the lower extremities, and other venous abnormalities (vena cava thrombosis, intracardiac thrombus, arterial aneurysms at other sites) were present as well. The time from diagnosis with Behçet syndrome to the first symptom of a pulmonary artery aneurysm was similar in the current cohort and the 1992 cohort (64.8 vs 63.1 months, respectively). However, patients in the current cohort had a significantly shorter time from the first symptom until diagnosis of an aneurysm (2.6 vs 6.4 months). Three patients were treated with embolization of the aneurysm sac with n-butyl cyanoacrylate; 1 patient is alive 4 years later, whereas the other 2 patients died 1 and 15 months after embolization. As of June 2003, 16 patients in the current cohort (61%) were alive, 6 (23%) were dead, and 4 (15%) were lost to follow-up. Of the 6 patients who died, 4 did so within 1 year after the onset of hemoptysis. Kaplan-Meier analysis showed survival of the present cohort was significantly better (5-year survival rate, 62%) than that of patients diagnosed before 1992.

Conclusion.—Survival in patients with Behçet syndrome and pulmonary artery aneurysm has improved during the past decade. This improvement is likely because of earlier recognition and treatment, and because of the use of endovascular embolization in select patients with treatment-resistant hemoptysis. Misdiagnosis of hemoptysis as being caused by pulmonary tuberculosis or pulmonary thromboembolism can delay the diagnosis and the initiation of treatment in these patients.

▶ The authors suggest that the improvement in outcomes results from early recognition and treatment rather than any specific change in treatment. Because the study was retrospective and uncontrolled, no conclusions can be made about the optimal duration of treatment. For patients in whom hemoptysis persists despite treatment, endovascular embolization may have value.[1]

B. H. Thiers, MD

Reference

1. Cantasdemir M, Kantarci F, Mihmanli I, et al: Emergency endovascular management of pulmonary artery aneurysms in Behçet's disease: Report of two cases and a review of the literature. *Cardiovasc Intervent Radiol* 25:533-537, 2002.

Necrotizing Vasculitis Associated With Familial Mediterranean Fever

Hatemi G, Masatlioglu S, Gogus F, et al (Istanbul Univ, Turkey)
Am J Med 117:516-519, 2004   9–17

Introduction.—Vasculitis may be linked with familial Mediterranean fever. Henoch-Schönlein purpura occurs in 5% to 8% of these patients compared with 0.8% of the general population. Necrotizing vasculitis that resembles polyarteritis nodosa occurs in about 1% of patients with Mediterranean fever; this is about 100-fold times higher than expected. Patients with necrotizing vasculitis associated with familial Mediterranean fever were evaluated.

Methods.—Of 30 patients with polyarteritis nodosa, 8 had familial Mediterranean fever. Their records were reviewed to identify clinical and laboratory characteristics, histologic findings where appropriate, the type and duration of treatment, and outcomes.

Results.—The mean age of onset of familial Mediterranean fever in the 6 males and 2 females evaluated was 7 years; the mean age of onset of vasculitis was 25 years. The most frequent presenting symptoms for vasculitis were fever, weight loss, myalgias, arthralgias, and arthritis. One patient had eye involvement that resulted in loss of vision in the right eye. One patient had peripheral neuropathy; electromyography revealed mononeuritis multiplex. A splenic subcapsular hematoma was detected in 1 patient. Of 6 patients tested for hepatitis B surface antigen, 1 had positive findings. All 5 patients tested for antineutrophil cytoplasmic antibodies had negative findings. All patients were treated with corticosteroids in addition to colchicine. There was 1 death, and 1 patient was lost to follow-up; the remaining 6 continued treatment with corticosteroids and other immunosuppressive agents for a mean duration of 48 months.

Conclusion.—A link between polyarteritis nodosa and familial Mediterranean fever is well established. The vasculitis observed in some patients with familial Mediterranean fever involves both medium and small vessels and has characteristics of classic polyarteritis nodosa, along with microscopic polyangiitis. Referring to this disorder as *necrotizing vasculitis associated with familial Mediterranean fever* may best reflect the spectrum of vascular pathologic features.

▶ Although the necrotizing vasculitis associated with familial Mediterranean fever may represent polyarteritis nodosa, some differences can be detected. Thus, the authors prefer to use the term *necrotizing vasculitis* to describe the associated vasculopathy rather than the more specific term *polyarteritis nodosa*.

B. H. Thiers, MD

10 Blistering Disorders

A New Model for Dermatitis Herpetiformis That Uses HLA-DQ8 Transgenic NOD Mice

Marietta E, Black K, Camilleri M, et al (Mayo Clinic, Rochester, Minn; Sir Paul Boffa Hosp, Floriana, Malta)

J Clin Invest 114:1090-1097, 2004   10–1

Background.—Dermatitis herpetiformis (DH) is an autoimmune skin disorder presenting as a severely pruritic papulovesicular rash on the elbows, forearms, buttocks, knees, and scalp. DH is also often associated with enteropathy. Both the rash and the enteropathy resolve when the patient begins a gluten-free diet. DH and celiac disease are tightly associated with DQ2 and DQ8, and HLA-DQ8+ transgenic mice are often used as a model for studying DH. A new mouse model of DH that incorporates the HLA-DQ8 transgene (which sensitizes to gliadin) and the NOD background (which contributes to autoimmunity) is described.

Methods.—Transgenic DQ8+ mice lacking endogenous mouse MHC II (Ab° DQ8+ mice) were backcrossed with NOD mice for 10 generations, and intercrossed to produce congenic NOD Ab° DQ8+ mice. At 7 to 16 weeks of age, 90 of these mice were injected with pertussis toxin (50 ng in 100 µL phosphate-buffered saline solution). Three days later, they began receiving crude gluten intraperitoneally or by gavage twice a week. Animals were ini-

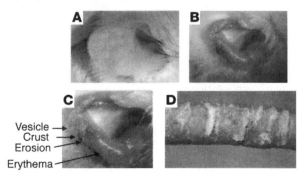

FIGURE 1.—Progression of cutaneous blistering. **A**, Normal unaffected ear. **B**, Blistered ear of an NOD Ab° DQ8+ mouse sensitized to gluten. **C**, Magnified view of the ear in B. **D**, Tail of an affected mouse. (Republished with permission of the Journal of Clinical Investigation from Marietta E, Black K, Camilleri M, et al: A new model for dermatitis herpetiformis that uses HLA-DQ8 transgenic NOD mice. *J Clin Invest* 114:1090-1097, 2004. Reproduced by permission of the publisher via Copyright Clearance Center, Inc.)

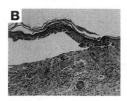

FIGURE 2.—Histopathology of a blistered ear. Hematoxylin and eosin–stained sections from the lesional areas of blistered ears from gluten-sensitized NOD Ab° DQ8⁺ mice. **B**, Full-thickness epidermal separation from the dermis of a gluten-sensitized NOD Ab° DQ8⁺ mouse. Original magnification ×20. (Republished with permission of the Journal of Clinical Investigation from Marietta E, Black K, Camilleri M, et al: A new model for dermatitis herpetiformis that uses HLA-DQ8 transgenic NOD mice. *J Clin Invest* 114:1090-1097, 2004. Reproduced by permission of the publisher via Copyright Clearance Center, Inc.)

tially fed chow containing gluten and were monitored twice a week for blistering and weight loss. Some of the animals that had overt gluten sensitivity develop were subsequently fed a gluten-free chow; some animals were also given dapsone (1 mg/kg/d) for 4 to 6 weeks. Histologic evidence of enteropathy was also assessed in 3 mice with blistering.

Results.—Fifteen of these 90 gluten-sensitized mice (16.7%) had blistering develop on both ears after 2 to 5 months of ingesting a diet containing gluten (Fig 1; see color plate XVII). Histopathologic examining of lesional skin specimens from the ears showed neutrophil infiltration of the dermis and deposition of IgA at the dermal-epidermal junction, similar to that seen in DH (Fig 2B; see color plate XVII). Nine of these 15 mice began ingesting a gluten-free chow, with (n = 3) or without (n = 6) dapsone. Blisters began to resolve within 2 to 3 weeks, regardless of dapsone treatment, and the time to complete resolution was associated with the extent of the blistering while receiving the gluten-containing chow. Rechallenge with gluten in 3 of these 9 animals resulted in the reappearance of blistering. The intestines of 3 other animals with blistering were examined histopathologically, and none showed small bowel pathology.

Conclusion.—These Ab° DQ8⁺ mice manifested the 3 main features of DH in humans: gluten-dependent blistering, local deposits of granular IgA beneath the basement membrane zone, and subepidermal blisters with high levels of neutrophils and monocytes within the dermis. This model will be useful for determining the specificity of the IgA deposition in DH and for examining the pathologic effects of gluten ingestion on the skin in this disorder.

▶ Although the mouse model for DH described by the authors develops skin lesions similar to the human disease, there is no apparent association with small bowel disease. Despite these differences, the model may prove useful for studying the pathogenic mechanisms underlying the cutaneous manifestations of this fascinating disease.

B. H. Thiers, MD

Pemphigus Vulgaris Acantholysis Ameliorated by Cholinergic Agonists

Nguyen VT, Arredondo J, Chernyavsky AI, et al (Univ of California, Davis; Mayo Clinic, Rochester, Minn; Gifu Univ, Japan)

Arch Dermatol 140:327-334, 2004   10–2

Introduction.—Patients with pemphigus vulgaris (PV), an autoimmune, IgG antibody-mediated disease of skin and mucosa, are usually treated with long-term systemic glucocorticosteroids. Autoantibodies to adhesion molecules mediating intercellular adhesion and to keratinocyte cholinergic receptors regulating cell adhesion develop. Activation of these receptors mimics anti-acantholytic effects of glucocorticosteroids in vitro. Experiments in mice sought to determine whether a cholinergic agonist could abolish PV IgG-induced acantholysis.

Methods.—Neonatal athymic nude mice were injected with PV IgG (experiment) or normal human IgG (control). One subgroup received PV IgG alone and the other received PV IgG together with a test drug (carbachol 0.04 µg/g body weight). Skin specimens were obtained after the animals were killed and prepared for direct and indirect immunofluorescence assays, immunoblotting, and phosphorylation assays.

Results.—Gross skin lesions were seen within 24 to 40 hours of the first injection of PV IgG. None of the mice injected with normal human IgG exhibited gross or microscopic signs of pemphigus or any deposition of human IgGs in their skin during 40 hours of observation. No skin lesions developed in carbachol-treated mice, and their skin samples showed only limited areas of epidermal acantholysis. Carbachol caused an elevation of the relative amount of E-cadherin in keratinocytes without changing that of plakoglobin. The phosphorylation level of E-cadherin and plakoglobin was increased by PV IgG, but this effect was diminished in the presence of carbachol. Treatment with pyridostigmine bromide (360 mg/d), an acetylcholinesterase inhibitor, allowed a patient with active PV to control the disease with a reduced dose of prednisone.

Conclusion.—Activation of the keratinocyte acetylcholine axis can ameliorate pemphigus acantholysis and upregulate the expression of adhesion molecules, protecting them from PV IgG-induced phosphorylation.

▶ The anti-acantholytic activity of cholinergic drugs deserves further exploration, and suggests a possible new avenue of treatment for patients with acantholytic disorders. Pyridostigmine bromide as a treatment for PV has been studied recently in a clinical trial.[1]

B. H. Thiers, MD

Reference

1. Grando SA: New approaches to the treatment of pemphigus. *J Invest Dermatol Symp Proc* 9:84-91, 2004.

Treatment of Refractory Pemphigus Vulgaris With Rituximab (Anti-CD20 Monoclonal Antibody)

Dupuy A, Viguier M, Bédane C, et al (Hôpital Saint-Louis Assistance Publique–Hôpitaux de Paris; Hôpital Dupuytren. Limoges, France)
Arch Dermatol 140:91-96, 2004   10–3

Introduction.—Systemic corticosteroid treatment has significantly improved the prognosis of patients with pemphigus vulgaris (PV), but the therapy has adverse effects and must be administered on a long-term basis to those patients who never achieve complete remission. Rituximab, a monoclonal anti-CD20 antibody, may prove more effective and safer than high-dose corticosteroids and immunosuppressive adjuvant treatments. The responses of the 3 patients reported here suggest that rituximab could be of value in treating refractory PV.

Methods.—Patients were a man, 20, and 2 women, aged 34 and 42 years. All had an unambiguous diagnosis of refractory PV according to clinical, histologic, and immunofluorescence criteria. Rituximab was given IV once weekly, over a 4- to 6-hour period, at a dosage of 375 mg per square of height in meters. Each treatment course consisted of 4 infusions.

Results.—All 3 patients achieved a clinical response, and 2 were judged to have a complete response. The improvement in disease activity was paralleled by a decline in titers of circulating anti-epidermal autoantibodies, and circulating B cells remained undetectable for 6 to 10 months. Bacterial infections occurred in 2 patients in the weeks after rituximab infusions. Two patients experienced a clinical relapse, 1 at 6 months and the other at 10 months. PV was controlled in 1 of these patients by a second course of rituximab.

Conclusion.—Systemic corticosteroids remain the standard of treatment for PV, but rituximab, which induces depletion of B cells, may offer benefits to patients with corticoresistant and corticodependent disease. The adverse effect profile of rituximab is favorable, and life-threatening events have been rare.

▶ The autoantibodies in patients with PV have been shown to be pathogenic, and antibody levels appear to correlate with disease activity. Thus, the effectiveness of rituximab, a monoclonal anti-CD20 antibody that induces depletion of B-cells, is not surprising and should be confirmed in prospective controlled studies involving larger numbers of patients.

B. H. Thiers, MD

Therapy of Refractory Pemphigus Vulgaris With Monoclonal Anti-CD20 Antibody (Rituximab)

Morrison LH (Oregon Health Sciences Univ, Portland)
J Am Acad Dermatol 51:817-819, 2004   10–4

Introduction.—High-dose corticosteroids and immunosuppressive agents are often used to treat pemphigus vulgaris (PV), but their adverse effects and lack of benefit in some patients have prompted a search for new therapies. Rituximab, an anti-CD20 monoclonal antibody directed against B cells, was examined for its therapeutic value in patients with PV.

Methods.—The patients, 2 men and 1 woman, had PV confirmed by histologic examination and immunofluorescence. Treatment consisted of IV rituximab (375 mg/m^2) once weekly for 4 consecutive weeks. All patients tolerated the infusions with no adverse effects, and the results of blood chemistry and complete blood cell count studies showed no abnormalities.

> *Case 1.*—Man, 51, had PV involving 75% of the scalp and oral cavity. Skin lesions had failed to improve with various therapies administered over a 4-year period, including prednisone, methotrexate, dapsone, IV immunoglobulin, and cyclophosphamide (2.5 mg/kg). Four weeks after rituximab was added to the regimen, erosions were 95% epithelialized. Prednisone was tapered at this time, and cyclophosphamide was continued at the same dose. Prednisone was then discontinued at 9 months, and cyclophosphamide was discontinued at 10 months. After 18 months, the patient remained in complete remission.

Discussion.—Patients with PV whose disease was unresponsive to a variety of immunosuppressive therapies improved shortly after rituximab was added to their regimens. Two went into remission, and a third continued to show steady improvement. Autoantibody titers fell sharply, which suggests that pathogenic antibodies were reduced by the drug. Future studies of rituximab in larger patient series should assess the risk of the development of infectious complications.

▶ It should be remembered that patients with autoimmune diseases who are treated with rituximab and immunosuppressant agents may be at a higher risk for infections.

B. H. Thiers, MD

Castleman's Tumours and Production of Autoantibody in Paraneoplastic Pemphigus

Wang L, Bu D, Yang Y, et al (Peking Univ, Beijing, China)
Lancet 363:525-531, 2004

10–5

Introduction.—The role of neoplasms in the pathogenesis of paraneoplastic pemphigus is controversial. Detailed data are not available, perhaps because of the limited number of affected individuals. Clinically, an IgG autoantibody against epidermal proteins is frequently used as a diagnostic marker for the disease. It may also be involved in autoimmune injuries. The mechanism by which the autoantibody is produced, along with the role of Castleman's tumors in the production of the autoantibody and in the pathogenesis of paraneoplastic pemphigus, was examined.

Methods.—Seven patients with paraneoplastic pemphigus associated with Castleman's disease were evaluated. The effect of removal of the tumors on the mucocutaneous lesions was monitored in 6 patients; the autoantibody titer was assessed with indirect immunofluorescence in 4 patients. Tumor cells from 1 patient were cultured, and the secreted autoantibody was assayed. The gene sequence and expression of the variable region of the immunoglobulin heavy chain were characterized in tumor B cells from all patients with the use of reverse transcriptase-polymerase chain reaction, DNA sequencing, and in situ hybridization.

Results.—Cutaneous lesions disappeared within 6 to 11 weeks after tumor resection. Mucosal lesions also gradually improved during this time but persisted for 5 to 10 months overall. Autoantibody titers diminished and became undetectable within 5 to 9 weeks in 3 of the 4 patients evaluated. Secreted autoantibodies were observed in cultured tumor cells; these were similar to those seen in patients' serum. The tumor B cells of all 7 patients shared and expressed 2 rearrangement patterns of complementary determining region 3 of IgV_H.

Conclusion.—Castleman's tumors seem to be involved in the production of autoantibodies and have a significant role in the pathogenesis of paraneoplastic pemphigus. Clonal rearrangement, resulting in similar variable regions of IgV_H, was observed in tumor B cells isolated from all 7 patients.

▶ When paraneoplastic pemphigus is associated with Castleman's disease and other benign tumors, a remarkable improvement in symptoms is often noted after resection of the neoplasm. The role of the neoplasm in the pathogenesis of paraneoplastic pemphigus is uncertain. Wang et al suggest that B-cell clones within the tumor produce autoantibodies against desmosomal and hemidesmosomal proteins, such as envoplakin and periplakin, and that these autoantibodies are an essential factor in the pathogenesis of the skin disease. They recommend that patients with refractory pemphigus be evaluated for the presence of Castleman's tumors and that, if found, complete resection of the tumor may be the most effective treatment available for the associated blistering disease.

B. H. Thiers, MD

11 Genodermatoses

Gene Therapy of X-Linked Severe Combined Immunodeficiency by Use of a Pseudotyped Gammaretroviral Vector
Gaspar HB, Parsley KL, Howe S, et al (Univ College London)
Lancet 364:2181-2187, 2004   11–1

Introduction.—Severe combined immunodeficiencies (SCID) are a heterogeneous group of inherited disorders characterized by the abnormal development or function of T, B, and natural killer cells. Defects in the gene encoding the common cytokine-receptor γ chain (γc) result in the X-linked form (SCID-X1), which is responsible for about 50% of all cases of SCID. γc is an important component of the high-affinity cytokine-receptor complexes for interleukins 2, 4, 7, 9, 15, and 21. Abnormal signaling through these receptors results in several immunologic defects, particularly severe disruption of the development of T cells and natural killer cells, and the intrinsic dysfunction of B cells. The outcomes of 4 children undergoing gene therapy for cellular and humoral immune recovery were evaluated, as was the safety of the procedure.

Methods.—All 4 children underwent molecular confirmation of SCID-X1 by identification of a mutation in γc; all 4 lacked an HLA-identical sibling donor. Autologous CD34-positive hemopoietic bone marrow stem cells were transduced ex vivo and were returned to patients without preceding cytoreductive chemotherapy. Patients were monitored for integration and expression of the γc vector and for functional immunologic recovery.

Results.—All patients demonstrated marked improvements in clinical and immunological characteristics. In 2 patients, it was possible to withdraw prophylactic medication. No serious adverse events were documented. The T cells responded normally to mitogenic and antigenic stimuli; the T-cell-receptor (TCR) repertoire was vastly diverse. When assessable, humoral immunity, as judged by antibody production, was also restored and was linked with increasing rates of somatic mutation in immunoglobulin genes.

Conclusion.—Gene therapy for SCID-X1 is highly effective in the restoration of functional cellular and humoral immunity.

▶ This important article describes the successful application of gene therapy in 4 patients with SCID-X1. This rare disease results from mutations in the gene encoding the γc chain of the common cytokine receptor (γc), which, as the name implies, is a component of several interleukin receptors essential for normal immune function. These patients present early in life with recurrent infections and failure to thrive; laboratory studies reveal the virtual absence of T lymphocytes and natural killer cells, and severely dysfunctional B cells. Here, the authors describe the use of a gammaretroviral vector carrying the human γc gene to transduce autologous bone-marrow–derived CD34+ cells in vitro during a culture period of 96 hours. At the time of reinfusion of the cells, a high transduction efficiency was observed (27%-58%). Following gene therapy, increases in T cell and natural killer cell numbers and function were observed in all patients within weeks. At the time of the latest follow-up described by the investigators, which ranged from 12 to 29 months, all patients were healthy and enjoying normal development. Immunoglobulin replacement therapy was discontinued in 2 patients. It is important to note that no serious adverse events occurred as a result of this therapy.

Currently, the only alternative treatment for SCID-X1 is bone marrow transplantation, which is successful when there is a high degree of histocompatibility between donor and patient. Gene therapy offers several advantages and has now been shown to have a high success rate. In an accompanying editorial, Cavazzana-Calvo and Fischer note that 18 patients with SCID have now been treated with gene therapy, with clear success in 17 subjects.[1] These results offer strong encouragement to the application of gene therapy in a variety of genetic diseases.

G. M. P. Galbraith, MD

Reference

1. Cavazzana-Calvo M, Fischer A: Efficacy of gene therapy for SCID is being confirmed. *Lancet* 364:2155-2156, 2004.

Immunodeficiency and Infections in Ataxia-Telangiectasia
Nowak-Wergzyn A, Crawford TO, Winkelstein JA, et al (Johns Hopkins Univ, Baltimore, Md; Mount Sinai School of Medicine, New York)
J Pediatr 144:505-511, 2004   11–2

Introduction.—Patients with the autosomal recessive multisystem disorder ataxia-telangiectasia (A-T) may experience progressive neurodegeneration, ocular and cutaneous telangiectasia, immunodeficiency, and premature aging. However, their immune functioning is quite variable, and few cases of progressive immunodeficiency have been reported. The records of 100 consecutive patients with A-T were reviewed so that the immunodeficiency associated with the disorder could be better characterized.

Methods.—Patients underwent multidisciplinary assessments at the Johns Hopkins Ataxia-Telangiectasia Clinical Center (ATCC). All displayed characteristic neurologic features, and 96% had oculocutaneous telangiectasia. The median patient age at the initial ATCC visit was 11.3 years, 85% of patients were white, and 53% were male. Elevated serum alpha-fetoprotein levels were present in all but 1 of 80 patients who had alpha-fetoprotein concentrations recorded. Patient records were reviewed for a history of infections and the results of laboratory assessments of the immune system.

Results.—The most common humoral immune abnormalities were serum IgG4 deficiency (in 65% of patients) and IgA deficiency (63%); IgG2 deficiency was present in 48%, IgE deficiency was present in 23%, and IgG deficiency was present in 18%. No patient had IgM deficiency. Lymphopenia affected 71% of patients: 75% had reduced CD19B lymphocytes, 69% had reduced CD4 T lymphocytes, and 51% had reduced CD8 T lymphocytes. Sixty-six percent of 52 tested patients had elevated percentages of natural killer cells. The frequency or severity of immune abnormalities did not appear to increase with age. Recurrent upper and lower respiratory tract infections were common, particularly otitis media (46% of patients) and sinusitis (27%); 15% had a history of pneumonia. Uncomplicated varicella infections had occurred in 44%, and 17% were affected with warts. Most patients had received all routine childhood immunizations, and none had a recognized complication of a live viral vaccine. At their first ATCC visit, 13% of patients were receiving IV immune globulin replacement therapy.

Discussion.—Laboratory evidence of immune dysfunction is common in patients with A-T, but systemic bacterial and opportunistic infections are uncommon. No association was found between a predisposition to recurrent upper respiratory tract infections and the presence of an IgG, IgA, or IgG subclass deficiency. In addition, immunodeficiency in A-T is only rarely progressive.

▶ Despite laboratory evidence of a high prevalence of impaired cell-mediated immunity, very few individuals in this large series of patients with A-T developed severe infections, and none had complications after receiving live virus vaccines. The incidence of common warts was increased. Progressive immunodeficiency occurred only rarely. The authors found no age-dependent risk of chronic or recurrent upper respiratory infections or nonrespiratory infections. They postulated that the increased incidence of lower respiratory infections with increasing age could be explained by progressive abnormalities of chewing and swallowing leading to pulmonary aspiration.

S. Raimer, MD

A Combined Syndrome of Juvenile Polyposis and Hereditary Haemorrhagic Telangiectasia Associated With Mutations in *MADH4 (SMAD4)*
Gallione CJ, Repetto GM, Legius E, at al (Duke Univ, Durham, NC; Universidad del Desarrollo, Santiago, Chile; Univ Hosp Gasthuisberg, Leuven, Belgium; et al)
Lancet 363:852-859, 2004   11–3

Background.—Juvenile polyposis is an autosomal dominant condition associated with a predisposition to malignancy that affects the gastrointestinal epithelium. Hereditary hemorrhagic telangiectasia, also known as

Osler–Weber–Rendu disease, is an autosomal dominant disorder of vascular dysplasia that affects many organs. Both of these conditions are uncommon, but there are many reports of patients and families with both disorders or of patients with juvenile polyposis who demonstrate selected symptoms of hereditary hemorrhagic telangiectasia. Some genetic as well as clinical overlap exists between these 2 disorders. Juvenile polyposis is caused by mutations in *MADH4* (encoding SMAD4) or *BMPR1A*, and hereditary hemorrhagic telangiectasia is caused by mutations in *ENG* (endoglin) or *ACVRL1 (ALK1)*; however, all 4 genes encode proteins involved in the transforming growth-factor-β signaling pathway. The genetic basis of the syndrome of combined juvenile polyposis and hereditary hemorrhagic telangiectasia was investigated.

Methods.—Blood samples were obtained from 7 unrelated families segregating both phenotypes. DNA from the proband of each family was sequenced for the *ACVRL1, ENG,* and *MADH4* genes. Mutations were examined for familial cosegregation with phenotype and their presence or absence in population controls.

Results.—None of the patients had mutations in the *ENG* or *ACVRL1* genes, but all patients had *MADH4* mutations. Three patients had new *MADH4* mutations. In 1 patient, the mutation was passed on to a similarly affected child. Each mutation cosegregated with the syndromic phenotype in other affected family members.

Conclusions.—Mutations in *MADH4* seem to cause a syndrome that consists of both juvenile polyposis and hereditary hemorrhagic telangiectasia phenotypes. Genetic testing is recommended for patients with either phenotype to identify those at risk for this combined syndrome because patients may present to different medical specialties. Patients with juvenile polyposis who have *MDAH4* mutations should be screened for the vascular lesions associated with hereditary hemorrhagic telangiectasia, particularly occult arteriovenous malformations in visceral organs that might otherwise manifest suddenly and have serious medical consequences.

▶ Gallione et al studied 7 families whose members had features of 2 seemingly unrelated disorders: juvenile polyposis and hereditary hemorrhagic telangiectasia. Although these conditions were believed to be caused by different genes, all families with both phenotypes had mutations in a single gene, *MADH4* (also known as *SMAD4*). This gene was previously thought to be associated only with juvenile polyposis. The results emphasize the need for patients with features of either of these disorders to have genetic screening. Individuals with *MADH4* mutations should be carefully examined to determine whether they have clinical features of more than one disorder. The existence of this overlap syndrome demonstrates that mutations in 1 gene can produce a number of complex phenotypes.

B. H. Thiers, MD

Cutaneous Manifestations of Proteus Syndrome: Correlations With General Clinical Severity

Nguyen D, Turner JT, Olsen C, et al (Uniformed Services Univ of the Health Sciences, Bethesda, Md; NIH, Bethesda, Md)

Arch Dermatol 140:947-953, 2004   11–4

Introduction.—The rare disorder known as Proteus syndrome is characterized by progressive asymmetric overgrowth of multiple tissues and an increased risk of the development of certain neoplasms. Because skin abnormalities such as epidermal nevi, vascular malformations, and lipomas are seen in other syndromes, misdiagnosis may occur. The range of cutaneous findings in Proteus syndrome was determined in a prospective cohort study, and these findings were then correlated with disease severity.

Methods.—A total of 24 consecutive patients (14 male and 10 female; age range, 10 months-40 years; median age, 12 years) were evaluated at the National Institutes of Health between November 1996 and February 2001. Patient medical records were reviewed, and cutaneous lesions were diagnosed on the basis of their clinical appearance; in some cases, a diagnosis was confirmed by histologic examination.

Results.—All patients exhibited progressive disproportionate overgrowth; some required a wheelchair because of severe leg deformities, and a few had mental retardation. Skin abnormalities, seen in all cases, included cerebriform connective tissue nevi, epidermal nevi, cutaneous vascular malformations, and lipomas (each present in at least 16 of 24 patients). The size of the skin abnormalities ranged from 3-mm macules and papules to massive lesions. In 20 patients, the cerebriform connective tissue nevi were on the soles of the feet (5 also had palm involvement). Epidermal nevi appeared in linear streaks along the lines of Blaschko. Some patients had localized alterations in skin pigmentation and hair or nail growth. Extracutaneous manifestations were classified as skeletal overgrowth, visceral overgrowth, other overgrowth, tumors, cysts, vascular abnormalities, deformity, or hypoplasia–maldevelopment. All patients exhibited overgrowth of the hands or feet, and 23 had overgrowth of the arms or legs. The skull was enlarged in 14 cases, and the spleen was enlarged in 8. Scoliosis was seen in 17 patients, and chest asymmetry was seen in 13. Four patients died during the study at ages ranging from 1 year 9 months to 17 years; pulmonary emboli were the cause of death in 3.

Discussion.—Patients with Proteus syndrome who have a greater number of skin abnormalities tend to have a greater number of extracutaneous abnormalities. A trend was seen for the number of abnormalities to increase up to the age of 8 years. The wide array of abnormalities in this disorder requires a multidisciplinary approach.

▶ This study documents the cutaneous and extracutaneous findings in 24 patients with Proteus syndrome. A greater number of skin abnormalities in these patients correlated with an increased incidence of extracutaneous abnormalities, which suggests that patients with numerous skin findings need a thorough evaluation for internal problems. The correlation between a variety of skin lesions and the number of internal abnormalities is consistent with the theory that Proteus syndrome results from mosaicism. An early postzygotic mutation would be expected to be associated with more skin and internal abnormalities than a later postzygotic mutation.

S. Raimer, MD

Mutation of Perinatal Myosin Heavy Chain Associated With a Carney Complex Variant

Veugelers M, Bressan M, McDermott DA, et al (Cornell Univ, New York; Brigham and Women's Hosp, Boston; Univ of Kentucky, Lexington; et al)
N Engl J Med 351:460-469, 2004   11–5

Introduction.—Approximately 7% of cardiac myxomas, the most common primary cardiac tumor in adults, are components of Carney complex, a familial autosomal dominant multiple neoplasia syndrome. *PRKAR1A* mutations can cause this complex, but the disorder is genetically heterogeneous. Clinical and genetic studies were performed to identify the cause of a Carney

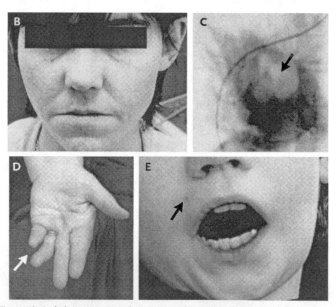

FIGURE 1.—Clinical phenotypes (Panels B, C, D, and E) in Family 1. Panel B shows the typical spotty pigmentation of the periorbital region and of the vermilion borders of the lips in family member III-19, who had previously received a diagnosis of a cardiac myxoma. In Panel C, ventriculography in family member II-7 revealed mitral regurgitation and a left atrial mass (*arrow*), that was resected and was shown to be a cardiac myxoma. Panel D shows a flexion deformity of the fourth and fifth digits (*arrow*), typical of pseudocamptodactyly, in family member II-3. Panel E shows trismus in family member IV-20 as well as typical spotty facial pigmentation (*arrow*). (Reprinted by permission of *The New England Journal of Medicine* from Veugelers M, Bressan M, McDermott DA, et al: Mutation of perinatal myosin heavy chain associated with a Carney complex variant. *N Engl J Med* 351:460-469, 2004. Copyright 2004, Massachusetts Medical Society. All rights reserved.)

complex variant associated with distal arthrogryposis (the trismus-pseudocamptodactyly syndrome).

Methods.—A large family (Fig 1) with familial cardiac myxoma and the trismus-pseudocampodactyly syndrome (Family 1) was identified and examined along with 2 families with trismus and pseudocamptodactyly (Families 2 and 3). Studies included clinical evaluations and genetic and mutational analyses. Positional cloning and mutational analyses of candidate genes were performed to identify the genetic cause of disease in the 3 families.

Results.—Clinical evaluations indicated that the Carney complex co-segregated with the trismus-pseudocamptodactyly syndrome in Family 1, and genetic analyses showed linkage of the disease to chromosome 17p12-p13.1. Sequence analysis revealed a missense mutation (Arg674Gln) in the perinatal myosin heavy-chain gene (*MYH8*) in Family 1, and the same mutation was also found in Families 2 and 3. Arg674 is highly conserved evolutionarily, localizes to the actin-binding domain of the perinatal myosin head, and is close to the ATP-binding site. Patients with cardiac myxoma syndromes but without arthrogryposis were found to have nonsynonymous *MYH8* polymorphisms.

Conclusion.—The R674Q mutation of the *MYH8* gene encoding perinatal myosin heavy chain causes a variant form of the Carney complex associated with distal arthrogryposis. Arthrogryposis manifests as typical trismus-pseudocamptodactyly syndrome, with congenital contractures. The findings demonstrate a novel role for perinatal myosin in both the development of skeletal muscle and cardiac tumorigenesis.

▶ The Carney complex describes the association of spotty cutaneous pigmentation with familial cardiac myxomas and neoplasms involving other organs. Veugelers and colleagues demonstrate the genetic basis for a novel heart-hand syndrome representing a variant of this disorder, and speculate on the importance of perinatal myosin in the pathogenesis of its salient clinical features.

B. H. Thiers, MD

Long-term Safety and Efficacy of Enzyme Replacement Therapy for Fabry Disease

Wilcox WR, Banikazemi M, Guffon N, et al (Univ of California, Los Angeles; Mount Sinai School of Medicine, New York; Hôpital Edouard Herriot, Lyon, France; et al)
Am J Hum Genet 75:65-74, 2004   11–6

Background.—Fabry disease, an X-linked lysosomal storage disease, is caused by deficient α-galactosidase A activity and the resulting accumulation of globotriaosylceramide (GL-3) and related glycosphingolipids in the plasma and tissue lysosomes throughout the body. Classically affected males show vascular endothelial GL-3 accumulation in the kidney, brain, and heart. Early death results from renal failure, strokes, and cardiovascular disease. The efficacy and safety of recombinant human α-galactosidase A (rh-αGalA) replacement in patients with Fabry disease have been demonstrated in a multicenter phase 3 trial. The continued safety and efficacy of this treatment was examined after 30 months of an ongoing open-label extension study.

Methods and Findings.—All 58 patients enrolled originally in the phase 3 trial subsequently received 1 mg/kg of rh-αGalA biweekly in the ongoing extension study. During the 30-month extension study, mean plasma GL-3 levels were continuously normal, even in patients in whom IgG antibodies against rh-αGalA developed. Sustained capillary endothelial GL-3 clearance was observed in 98% of patients undergoing skin biopsies after treatment for 30 or 36 months. In addition, mean serum creatinine levels and the estimated glomerular filtration rate remained stable after 30 to 36 months. Infusion-related reactions and anti-rh-αGalA IgG antibody titers declined over time. Seven patients with seroconversion had no detectable IgG antibodies after 30 to 36 months. Fifty-nine percent had 4-fold or greater reductions in antibody titers. Three patients had to be withdrawn from the study by 30 months because of positive serum IgE or skin test results. However, all 3 were later successfully rechallenged.

Conclusions.—In this study, enzyme replacement therapy with rh-αGalA for 30 to 36 months resulted in continuously reduced plasma GL-3 levels, sustained endothelial GL-3 clearance, and stable kidney function in patients with Fabry disease. The safety profile of rh-αGalA was favorable.

▶ This article, an open-label extension of a trial previously abstracted in the 2002 YEAR BOOK OF DERMATOLOGY AND DERMATOLOGIC SURGERY,[1] confirms that long-term enzyme replacement with α-galactosidase A exhibits a favorable benefit:risk ratio. Periodic skin biopsies can be used to monitor the efficacy of enzyme replacement therapy in Fabry disease.[2]

B. H. Thiers, MD

Reference

1. Eng CM, Guffon N, Wilcox WR, et al: Safety and efficacy of recombinant human α-galactosidase A replacement therapy in Fabry's disease. *N Engl J Med* 345:9-16, 2001.
2. Thurberg BL, Randolph Byers H, Granter SR, et al: Monitoring the 3-year efficacy of enzyme replacement therapy in Fabry disease by repeated skin biopsies. *J Invest Dermatol* 122:900-908, 2004.

Cord-Blood Transplants From Unrelated Donors in Patients With Hurler's Syndrome

Staba SL, Escolar ML, Poe M, et al (Duke Univ, Durham, NC; Univ of North Carolina, Chapel Hill; Emmes Corp, Rockville, Md; et al)
N Engl J Med 350:1960-1969, 2004   11–7

Background.—Hurler's syndrome is an autosomal recessive metabolic storage disease that is caused by a deficiency of α-L-iduronidase; this results in the accumulation of heparan and dermatan sulfate substrates (glycosaminoglycans) in various tissues. In severe phenotypes, Hurler's syndrome is characterized by severe, progressive deterioration of the CNS, cardiac disease, skeletal abnormalities, corneal clouding, hepatomegaly, and death in childhood, with symptoms beginning by 2 years of age. Allogeneic bone marrow transplantation can be effective in preventing the progression of selected heritable enzyme deficiencies and provides maximal benefit when performed early in life. However, many children who might benefit from transplantation do not have an appropriately matched donor. The purpose of this study was to investigate the feasibility of using cord blood transplants from unrelated donors and a myeloablative preparative regimen that does not involve total-body irradiation in young children with Hurler's syndrome.

Methods.—A group of 20 consecutive children with Hurler's syndrome received busulfan, cyclophosphamide, and antithymocyte globulin before undergoing cord blood transplants from unrelated donors. The main outcome measures were engraftment, adverse effects, and effects on disease symptoms.

Results.—The cord blood donors had normal α-L-iduronidase activity and were discordant for up to 3 of 6 HLA markers. Neutrophil engraftment occurred at a median of 24 days after transplantation. Grade II or III acute graft-versus-host disease developed in 5 patients, but none of the patients had extensive graft-versus-host disease. Of the 20 children in the study group, 17 were alive at a median of 905 days after transplantation, with complete donor chimerism and normal peripheral blood α-L-iduronidase activity. The event-free survival rate was 85%. Transplantation was found to improve the patients' neurocognitive performance and ameliorate the somatic features of Hurler's syndrome.

Conclusions.—Cord blood from unrelated donors may be an excellent source of stem cells for transplantation in patients with Hurler's syndrome. This approach can provide for sustained engraftment without total-body irradiation and can effect beneficial changes in the natural history of the disease.

▶ The lysosomal storage diseases that comprise the mucopolysaccharidoses are caused by a deficiency of enzymes that degrade glycosaminoglycans. Mucopolysaccharidosis type I is caused by a deficiency of the enzyme α-L-iduronidase; it is an autosomal recessive disorder that is associated with a wide range of clinical presentations. Its most severe form, Hurler's syndrome, is characterized by a progressive deterioration of the CNS and death in childhood. The clinical spectrum includes mental retardation, macrocephaly, corneal clouding, coarse facies, hearing loss, joint stiffness, hepatosplenomegaly, valvular heart disease, airway obstruction and short stature. Since the first report of successful bone marrow transplantation for Hurler's syndrome in 1981, more than 300 such procedures, initially of bone marrow and more recently of umbilical cord blood, have been performed worldwide in patients with this disorder. Staba and colleagues report that cord blood transplantation may be as effective as bone marrow transplantation in alleviating some, although perhaps not all, of the protean manifestations of this disease.[1]

B. H. Thiers, MD

Reference

1. Muenzer J, Fisher A: Advances in the treatment of mucopolysaccharidosis type I. *N Engl J Med* 350:1932-1934, 2004.

▶ The authors report that hematopoietic stem cell transplantation with cord blood from partially HLA-matched, unrelated donors favorably altered the natural history of Hurler's syndrome in a group of young children. Bone marrow transplants have been reported to be of benefit in this condition; however, the limited availability of donors is a major obstacle. Suitable donors are difficult to identify in a timely fashion, and rapid intervention is critical to prevent significant tissue damage. Umbilical cord blood is prospectively HLA-typed, screened for infection, and readily available for transplantation. One additional advantage of this technique is that engraftment and full donor chimerism can be achieved without the use of irradiation. Cord blood transplantation appears to be a good therapeutic option for young patients with Hurler's syndrome who lack an HLA-matched related bone marrow donor who is not a carrier of the disease.

S. Raimer, MD

Gastrointestinal Involvement in Chronic Granulomatous Disease
Marciano BE, Rosenzweig SD, Kleiner DE, et al (NIH, Bethesda, Md)
Pediatrics 114:462-468, 2004   11–8

Background.—Chronic granulomatous disease (CGD) is a rare disorder of phagocyte oxidative metabolism. The abnormal inflammatory responses in CGD result in exuberant and persistent tissue granuloma formation, which can affect diverse organs; however, involvement of the gut is the most common symptom and may be present either at CGD diagnosis or later. However, the extent of gastrointestinal (GI) tract involvement in patients with CGD is unknown. The clinical presentation, prevalence, and consequences of GI involvement in patients with CGD were assessed.

Methods.—A review was conducted of the medical records of 140 patients with CGD (of whom 67% were cases of X-linked inheritance) followed at the National Institutes of Health. GI manifestations in these patients were abstracted, and all available GI pathology was reviewed.

Results.—GI involvement was recorded in 46 (32.8%) of 140 patients, 89% of whom had X-linked inheritance. The age at initial GI manifestations ranged from 0.8 to 30 years (median age, 5 years), and 70% of affected patients were seen with GI involvement in the first decade of life. Abdominal pain was the most frequent symptom (100%), and hypoalbuminemia was the most frequent sign (70%). Prednisone controlled the signs and symptoms in most of the affected patients, but relapse occurred in 71% of patients. GI involvement had no effect on mortality rate and was not associated with interferon-γ use.

Conclusions.—GI involvement is a common and recurring problem in patients with CGD, particularly in patients with X-linked inheritance. At this time there is no clear evidence for an infectious cause. Interferon-γ use does not affect the frequency of GI involvement, and mortality is not affected by GI involvement. GI involvement should be investigated in patients with CGD who manifest abdominal pain, delay in growth, or hypoalbuminemia.

▶ Although dermatologists are not the primary caretakers of patients with CGD, they often do see these patients because of its cutaneous manifestations. This population is continuously at risk for the development of life-threatening infections because of the inability of their phagocytes to kill bacteria and fungi. To further complicate the situation, approximately one third of these patients have debilitating GI involvement requiring long-term or intermittent corticosteroid therapy for management.

S. Raimer, MD

Nutritional Status and Gastrointestinal Structure and Function in Children With Ichthyosis and Growth Failure

Fowler AJ, Moskowitz DG, Wong A, et al (Univ of California San Francisco)
J Pediatr Gastroenterol Nutr 38:164-169, 2004   11–9

Introduction.—Growth failure may occur in patients with ichthyosis, a heterogeneous group of inherited disorders characterized by thickened, scaly skin. Previous studies have implicated a hypermetabolic state induced by epidermal inflammation and hyperproliferation or malabsorption and nutritional deficiencies caused by enteropathy. Children with severe ichthyosis and growth failure were evaluated for the extent to which enteropathies and nutritional deficiencies contributed to their conditions.

Methods.—The 10 children (7 boys, 3 girls) included in the study ranged in age from 2.83 to 13.6 years. All had weight decreasing across centiles for more than 6 months, weight or height below the fifth percentile, or weight for height below the fifth percentile. Laboratory tests and a nutritional assessment were performed, and 7 of 10 patients underwent upper and lower endoscopic analysis under general anesthesia.

Results.—Three patients had Netherton's syndrome and 2 had ichthyosis en confetti; additional diagnoses were harlequin ichthyosis, psoriasis, lamellar ichthyosis, congenital ichthyosiform erythroderma, and trichothiodystrophy. Three of 10 patients had mild deficiencies in 1 or more nutrient levels. Ferritin levels were low but normal in all studied patients, and no patient was anemic or deficient in essential fatty acids. Levels of IgE were elevated in 6 patients, especially in the 3 with Netherton's syndrome. Mild steatorrhea, present in 2 patients, was the most significant abnormality noted in gastrointestinal functional studies. Constipation was a common finding, as were elevated hematocrit levels and mildly elevated serum calcium and magnesium levels.

Conclusion.—In all 10 patients with severe ichthyosis and growth failure, the total caloric intake exceeded established requirements for age, height, and weight. Nutritional deficiencies and gastrointestinal abnormalities were uncommon and appear to be unlikely causes of growth failure. An impaired skin barrier, however, may increase caloric needs and contribute to chronic dehydration. Nutritional supplementation and fluid replacement may be appropriate and effective treatments.

▶ After an evaluation of the nutritional status and gastrointestinal structure and functioning of 10 children with various forms of ichthyosis and growth failure, the authors conclude that gastrointestinal dysfunction and nutritional deficiencies are unlikely causes of growth failure in these children. Rather, they postulate that growth failure results from the impaired skin barrier and associated increased caloric needs and chronic dehydration. Early caloric supplementation that can maximize growth potential may be desirable for these children.

S. Raimer, MD

The Importance of Screening for Sight-Threatening Retinopathy in Incontinentia Pigmenti
Wong GAE, Willoughby CE, Parslew R, et al (Royal Liverpool Children's Hosp, England)
Pediatr Dermatol 21:242-245, 2004   11–10

Background.—Incontinentia pigmenti (IP) is a rare, X-linked dominant disorder caused by mutations in the NF-kB essential modulator (NEMO) gene. Female infants with IP will have characteristic abnormalities of the skin, teeth, and hair. However, the ocular and neurologic sequelae are responsible for the major morbidity in IP. Two cases were presented to highlight the severe ocular manifestations of this condition and underscore the need for close ophthalmologic surveillance.

> *Case 1.*—Girl, 4 years, initially was seen by a general pediatrician shortly after birth with a bullous eruption on the arms and trunk. A diagnosis of IP was confirmed by skin biopsy specimen findings. When she was 8 weeks old, the girl's parents noticed abnormal visual behavior, with poor fixing and following. A formal ophthalmologic

assessment at the age of 6 months detected bilateral total retinal detachment.

Case 2.—Girl, 6 years, with no family history of IP was born with a pustular eruption on the trunk, limbs, and scalp typical of stage I cutaneous lesions of IP. The child had no neurologic or developmental abnormalities. Initial ocular examination at the age of 10 months was normal, as were examinations at 14 months, 18 months, 2 years, 3 years, and 4 years. At routine indirect ophthalmoscopy at the age of 5 years, the child was found to have a left peripheral retinal hemorrhage with some overlying vitreous hemorrhage. A decision against active treatment was made. At follow-up at the age of 6 years, the child had normal vision with no recurrent retinal or vitreous hemorrhage.

Conclusions.—Many eye abnormalities have been reported in patients with incontinentia pigmenti. Most of these features are secondary, nonspecific events related to the retinal pathology of IP, including strabismus, nystagmus, myopia, uveitis, corneal changes, cataract, microphthalmos, optic nerve atrophy, and iris hypoplasia. Retinal vascular abnormalities, which can lead to retinal detachment, are the primary cause of severe visual defects in patients with incontinentia pigmenti.

▶ This report emphasizes the need for early ophthalmologic examinations in children with incontinentia pigmenti to look for retinal vascular abnormalities that can lead to retinal detachment. Eye examinations should be repeated frequently throughout early childhood.

S. Raimer, MD

Liver Transplantation as a Cure for Acute Intermittent Porphyria
Soonawalla ZF, Orug T, Badminton MN, et al (Queen Elizabeth Hosp, Birmingham, England; Univ of Wales, Cardiff, England; Univ of Liverpool, England)
Lancet 363:705-706, 2004   11–11

Background.—Acute intermittent porphyria can cause frequent, crippling acute neurovisceral attacks associated with increased hepatic production of porphyrin precursors. This results in long-term damage, a poor quality of life, and a shortened life expectancy. No cure has been found, but replacing the deficient hepatic enzymes may restore excretion of porphyrin precursors to normal levels and prevent severe attacks. Liver transplantation is one way to replace hepatic enzymes. The medium-term outcome of liver transplantation in a young patient severely affected by recurrent attacks of acute intermittent porphyria was reported.

Case Report.—Woman, 19, had acute intermittent porphyria. For a 2.5-year period, she had regular, severe attacks characterized by intense abdominal pain, leg pain, foot drop, hyponatremia, and hypotension and associated with dark red urine. After detailed consulting and counseling with the patient and her family, a liver transplantation was planned. She underwent orthotopic liver transplantation from an identical blood group A Rh+ cadaveric donor. At surgery, the patient's native liver had a normal macroscopic appearance. Her postoperative course was uncomplicated. For the first 3 months she received prednisolone, azathioprine, and tacrolimus for immunosuppression. Thereafter, she received azathioprine and tacrolimus. Levels of urinary haem precursor rapidly returned to normal. No further porphyria attacks occurred. At 1.5 years after liver transplantation, the patient has normal nerve conduction and maintains a good quality of life.

Conclusions.—Acute intermittent porphyria can be treated effectively by liver transplantation. Replacing hepatic enzymes can restore normal excretion of 5-aminolevulinic acid and porphobilinogen and prevent severe attacks.

▶ Acute intermittent porphyria results from a deficiency of porphobilinogen deaminase, an early enzyme in the heme biosynthetic pathway. It is a devastating disease associated with severe abdominal pain, a poor quality of life, and shortened life expectancy. This article demonstrates that liver transplantation can serve to replace the deficient hepatic enzyme, restore excretion of porphyrin precursors to normal, and prevent severe attacks. An excellent review of the diagnosis and treatment of the acute porphyrias has recently been published.[1]

B. H. Thiers, MD

Reference

1. Anderson KE, Bloomer JR, Bonkovsky HL, et al: Recommendations for the diagnosis and treatment of the acute porphyrias. *Ann Intern Med* 142:439-450, 2005.

Skeletal Effects and Functional Outcome With Olpadronate in Children With Osteogenesis Imperfecta: A 2-Year Randomised Placebo-Controlled Study
Sakkers R, Kok D, Engelbert R, et al (Wilhemina Children's Hosp-Univ Med Centre Utrecht, The Netherlands; Reinier de Graaf Group Hosp, Delft-Voorburg, The Netherlands)
Lancet 363:1427-1431, 2004   11–12

Introduction.—Bisphosphonates, which suppress osteoclast-mediated bone resorption and decrease bone turnover in patients with osteoporosis, are now being used in many children with osteogenesis imperfecta. The effects of daily olpadronate on incident fractures, dual X-ray absorptiometry outcomes, and functional outcomes were assessed in children with osteogenesis imperfecta in a randomized double-blind trial at one center in The Netherlands.

Methods.—The 34 children recruited for the study received either olpadronate (10 mg/m² daily) or placebo for 2 years. Calcium and vitamin D supplements were given to all participants to avoid nutritional deficiencies, and routine care continued as usual. Measures of functional outcomes included the degree of ambulation and muscle strength. Gastrointestinal side effects were also recorded.

Results.—The 2 groups were similar in mean age (approximately 10 years) and body height and weight at baseline. No patient in either group reported signs or symptoms of an acute phase reaction, and the only gastrointestinal complaint occurred in a child taking placebo. In both unadjusted analyses and analyses adjusted for baseline differences, the olpadronate group showed a greater rise in spinal dual X-ray absorptiometry values at follow-up. The relative fracture risk was reduced by 31% with olpadronate therapy, but functional and anthropomorphic variables did not differ between groups. In addition, neither group had changes in urinary markers of bone resorption at follow-up.

Conclusion.—Two years of treatment with oral olpadronate reduced the fracture risk in the long bones of children with osteogenesis imperfecta. The treatment appeared to be safe but did not result in catch-up growth. The duration of olpadronate therapy was too short to determine whether the course of the disease might be altered, and more studies are needed before the age at which treatment should start and its necessary duration can be recommended.

▶ In this randomized placebo-controlled study, the number of fractures was decreased in children with osteogenesis imperfecta who were treated with the oral bisphosphonate olpadronate (10 mg/m²/d) for 2 years, when compared with control children. Unfortunately, no functional improvement was seen in these children. However, there is hope that functional improvement might occur with early initiation of treatment and/or a longer treatment duration, although this remains to be proven.

S. Raimer, MD

Activating Gsα Mutations: Analysis of 113 Patients With Signs of McCune-Albright Syndrome—A European Collaborative Study
Lumbroso S, Paris F, Sultan C (Centre Hospitalier Universitaire (CHU) de Montpellier, France)
J Clin Endocrinol Metab 89:2107-2113, 2004   11–13

Introduction.—The McCune-Albright syndrome (MAS) is a sporadic disorder associated with a triad of physical signs: cafè-au-lait pigmented skin lesions, polyostotic fibrous dysplasia, and endocrine dysfunction. The disorder is caused by postzygotic activating mutations of arginine 201 in the guanine-nucleotide–binding protein (G protein) α-subunit (Gsα), leading to a mosaic distribution of cells bearing constitutively active adenylate cyclase. Various atypical or partial presentations have been reported. Presented were findings of a systematic search for Gsα mutations in patients with at least 1 of the signs of MAS.

Methods.—Of 113 patients with MAS (98 women, 15 men), 24% were seen with the classic triad, 33% with 2 signs, and 40% with only 1 classic sign of MAS. A polymerase chain reaction–sensitive method identified the mutation in 43% of the cohort. When an affected tissue was available, the mutation was seen in over 90% of patients, regardless of the number of signs. Skin was a noteworthy exception since only 3 of the 11 skin samples tested positive. The mutation was seen in 46% of blood samples among patients with the classic triad, 21% of those with 2 signs, and 8% of those with 1 sign.

Discussion/Conclusion.—These findings highlight the frequency of partial forms of MAS and the usefulness of sensitive techniques to verify the diagnosis at the molecular level. The mutation was seen in 33% of 39 cases of isolated peripheral precocious puberty. These findings widen the definition of MAS. It appears that monostotic fibrous dysplasia, isolated peripheral precocious puberty, neonatal liver cholestasis, and the classic triad of MAS are all components of a wide spectrum of diseases based on the same molecular defect.

▶ MAS is an uncommon disorder with a variable clinical presentation. A proportion of patients display the triad of cafè-au-lait skin pigmentation, endocrine dysfunction frequently manifesting as precocious puberty, and polyostotic fibrous dysplasia. However, many patients exhibit only 1 or 2 of the classic signs. Previous studies have identified the presence of postzygotic mutations in the α subunit of G proteins (usually a substitution mutation of arginine at position 201), leading to activation of adenylate cyclase in certain cells.

In this study, the investigators used a polymerase chain reaction–based method to examine a heterogeneous population of patients for the presence of Gα subunit mutations. The data obtained showed that, overall, the mutations were more likely to be found in patients with the classic triad of presentation (59%) but were also identified in at least 33% of patients with isolated clinical signs of disease. When available affected tissues were examined, the mutations were detected in all of the testicular, thyroid, muscle and endometrial tissues, but relatively rarely in the affected skin (27%). This study highlights the importance of genetic mutation studies in the diagnosis of this syndrome, particularly in patients with atypical presentations.

G. M. P. Galbraith, MD

Klippel-Trénaunay Syndrome: The Importance of "Geographic Stains" in Identifying Lymphatic Disease and Risk of Complications

Maari C, Frieden IJ (Univ of Montreal; Univ of California, San Francisco)
J Am Acad Dermatol 51:391-398, 2004   11–14

Background.—Klippel-Trénaunay syndrome (KTS) is a relatively rare congenital vascular anomaly that is classically defined as the triad of vascular stain, soft tissue and/or bony hypertrophy, and venous varicosities. Many (though not all) cases of KTS are a result of mixed malformations with capillary, lymphatic, and venous elements (so-called CLVM). Whether the morphologic characteristics of the associated vascular stains in KTS are predictive of the presence of lymphatic involvement and/or complications was determined.

Methods.—A retrospective review was conducted of all cases of KTS seen between January 1989 and September 2001 at an outpatient dermatology practice and a tertiary care medical center. The review identified 40 patients who were then classified by type of cutaneous vascular stain, either "geographic" or "blotchy/segmental" (Table 1). Patients were further classified as having definite, probable, possible, or no evidence of lymphatic disease. A chart review was also conducted for other associated manifestations and complications of KTS.

Results.—Of the 22 patients with sharply demarcated geographic stains, 21 had definite or probable evidence of lymphatic disease. Of the 17 patients with blotchy port-wine stains, 16 had possible or no evidence of lymphatic disease. Determination of the type of stain had 95% sensitivity and 94% specificity in differentiation of definite or probable presence of definite or probable lymphatic disease from possible or no evidence of lymphatic disease (Table 4). Complications occurred in 19 (86%) of 22 patients with a geographic stain versus 7 (41%) of 17 with a blotchy/segmental stain.

Conclusions.—The presence of a geographic vascular stain is a predictor of the risk of both associated lymphatic malformation and complications in patients with KTS. These stains are present at birth, so this clinical observa-

---

TABLE 1.—Comparative Features of Geographic vs
Non-geographic Stains

Geographic:
- Extremely sharply demarcated
- Irregular shape, resembling a country or continent
- Dark red/purple color (most cases)

Blotchy/Segmental:
- Blotchy or indistinct demarcation from normal skin in at least some areas (Often have sharp demarcation from normal skin at midline)
- Often large, typically with a segmental distribution
- Light pink or red-pink color

TABLE 4.—Type of Stain per Category

Category	Geographic Stain	Blotchy Stain
Definite	13 patients	0 patient
Probable	8 patients	1 patient
Possible	0 patient	1 patient
No LM	1 patient	15 patients

Abbreviation: LM, Lymphatic malformation.
(Reprinted by permission of the publisher from Maari C, Frieden IJ: Klippel-Trénaunay syndrome: The importance of "geographic stains" in identifying lymphatic disease and risk of complications, *J Am Acad Dermatol* 51:391-398, 2004. Copyright 2004 by Elsevier.)

tion can aid in the identification of persons with KTS at greatest risk for complications and thus, those that require closer observation.

▶ The authors correlate the presence and morphology of vascular stains in patients with KTS with associated lymphatic malformations and the frequency of complications. Thus, the clinical features of vascular anomalies help guide the management of affected patients.

S. Raimer, MD

PHACES Syndrome: A Review of Eight Previously Unreported Cases With Late Arterial Occlusions
Bhattacharya JJ, Luo CB, Álvarez H, et al (Southern Gen Hosp, Glasgow, Scotland; Hôpital de Bicêtre, France; Ramathibodi Hosp, Bangkok, Thailand)
Neuroradiology 46:227-233, 2004   11–15

Introduction.—The neural crest has been implicated in the pathogenesis of the PHACES syndrome. This syndrome is characterized by posterior fossa malformations, facial hemangiomas, arterial anomalies, aortic coarctation and other cardiac disorders, ocular abnormalities, and stenotic arterial disease. Six children with various components of PHACES syndrome and 2 additional children with possible PHACES were reviewed for clinical and imaging features.

Methods.—Patients were 5 girls and 3 boys ranging in age from 1 month to 14 years at the time of the assessment. All were referred for evaluation of complex hemangiomas. The diagnosis was considered definite in 6 cases because of the presence of a cervicofacial hemangioma. The diagnosis was considered possible in 2 children without a hemangioma. Two radiologists reviewed case notes and imaging studies (Table 1). Six children underwent angiography, and cross-sectional imaging was available in 7; 6 underwent MRI, and 1 had a CT scan available for review.

Results.—In the 6 definite cases, hemangiomas were apparent soon after birth, usually on the left and involving the maxillofacial region. Parotid or oral involvement was present in 2 cases. Five patients had eyelid or intraorbital extension of the hemangioma. Arterial anomalies of the head and neck

TABLE 1.—Clinical and Imaging Features of 6 Patients With Definite PHACES Syndrome and 2 (7 and 8) With Possible Partial Expression

Patient, Age (Months)/Sex	Clinical Features	Posterior Cranial Fossa	Haemangiomas	Anomalous Arteries	Aortic Coarctation	Eyes	Stenoses
1 4 years/f	Headache; progressive neurological deficit	Normal	Maxilla	Vertebrobasilar; internal and external carotid	Yes	Haemangioma	Yes
2 3/m	Left facial mass; seizures	Dandy-Walker; left cerebellar hypoplasia	Face, lip, orbit	Internal and external carotid, spinal	No	Haemangioma	No
3 6/f	Headache; progressive neurological deficit; chorea	Normal	Eyelid	Internal carotid, trigeminal	No	Haemangioma	Yes
4 1/f	Left facial mass	Normal	Face, orbit, parotid	No	Yes	Haemangioma	No
5 3/m	Left orbital and back masses	Dandy-Walker; haemangioma	Orbit, parotid, back	Right subclavian	Yes	Haemangioma	No
6 9/f	Left facial mass	Dandy-Walker	Maxilla, eyelid	No	No	Haemangioma	No
7 14 years/f	Headache	Normal	No	Vertebral; posterior inferior cerebellar; internal carotid	No	Normal	Yes
8 14 years/m	Aphasia; progressive neurological deficit; hemiplegia	Normal	No	Internal carotid, middle cerebral aneurysms	No	Normal	Yes

Abbreviation: PHACES, Posterior cranial fossa malformations, hemangiomas, arterial anomalies, coarctation of the aorta and cardiac defects, abnormalities of the eye, and stenotic arterial disease.
(Courtesy of Bhattacharya JJ, Luo CB, Alvarez H, et al: PHACES syndrome: A review of eight previously unreported cases with late arterial occlusions. *Neuroradiology* 46:227-233, 2004. Copyright 2004 Springer-Verlag.)

were present in 4 patients, and 4 had cardiac and associated abnormalities. Progressive intracranial arterial occlusions appeared in 4 patients between the ages of 4 and 14 years.

Discussion.—The cases described in this study illustrate the spectrum of abnormalities in the PHACES syndrome. Abnormalities varied considerably among patients, but large cervicofacial hemangiomas were considered the identifying feature, and posterior cranial fossa abnormalities were the most common intracranial finding. The embryonic insult responsible for the syndrome may occur before or during the phases of vasculogenesis but must occur before migration of the neural crest and mesodermal cells to account for the widespread lesions. Many elements of the PHACES syndrome could reflect an abnormality of cell proliferation and apoptosis. A familial tendency does not seem to be evident.

▶ The authors observed a relatively high percentage of arterial stenosis in their patients with PHACES syndrome. They suggest that the *S* in PHACES should stand for stenosis of arteries rather than for sternal abnormalities because stenosis appears to be more commonly associated with the other characteristic findings of this syndrome. In their series, the symptoms of arterial stenosis developed later than in previously reported cases.

S. Raimer, MD

12 Drug Actions, Reactions, and Interactions

Adverse Drug Reactions as Cause of Admission to Hospital: Prospective Analysis of 18 820 Patients
Pirmohamed M, James S, Meakin S, et al (Univ of Liverpool, England)
BMJ 329:15-19, 2004   12–1

Introduction.—Most studies on the epidemiology of adverse drug reactions (ADRs) in the United Kingdom (UK) were performed more than a decade ago and were limited in scope. To provide more recent estimates of the burden of ADRs on hospitals, admissions to 2 large hospitals in the UK were prospectively analyzed.

Methods.—The study was conducted from November 2001 to April 2002 at a teaching hospital and a district general hospital. All patients older than 16 years were assessed to determine whether admission was caused by an ADR. Excluded were patients with accidental or deliberate overdose and those who relapsed because of noncompliance. Outcomes of interest included type of ADR, length of stay, ability to avoid the ADR, costs of admission, and mortality rates.

Results.—Of the total of 18,820 admissions over the 6-month period, 1225 (6.5%) were determined to have resulted from an ADR. The ADR directly led to admission in 80% of cases. Compared with patients without ADRs, those with ADRs were significantly older and more likely to be female. The median bed stay for patients with ADRs was 8 days, and the projected annual cost (in US dollars) of such admissions in the UK was $847 million. The overall fatality rate was 0.15%. Gastrointestinal bleeding was the most common ADR; drugs frequently involved were low-dose aspirin, diuretics, warfarin, and nonsteroidal anti-inflammatory drugs other than aspirin. Most reactions to drugs were judged to be definitely or possibly avoidable.

Conclusion.—ADRs cause considerable morbidity and substantially increase costs for the National Health Service in the UK. The fatality rate observed in this study suggests that more than 10,000 ADR-related deaths may occur annually in the UK. Many hospital admissions for ADRs may be prevented by simple improvements in prescribing, with emphasis on identifying potential drug interactions.

▶ An estimate based on small studies, many of which were done before 1990, suggests that ADRs account for 5% of hospital admissions; the incidence of fatal reactions in all patients admitted to the hospital has been estimated at 0.13%. Pirmohamed et al performed a large prospective analysis of ADRs as the cause of hospital admission in the United Kingdom. They found that ADRs accounted for 1 of 16 hospital admissions and 4% of hospital bed capacity. Most of these ADRs were predictable from the known pharmacology of the drugs, and many were deemed preventable in that they represented known drug interactions. More than 2% of patients admitted with an ADR died, suggesting that ADRs were responsible for the death of 0.15% of all admitted patients. ADRs to older drugs were more likely to cause admission than reactions to newer drugs.

B. H. Thiers, MD

Effects of Geriatric Evaluation and Management on Adverse Drug Reactions and Suboptimal Prescribing in the Frail Elderly
Schmader KE, Hanlon JT, Pieper CF, et al (Veterans Affairs Med Ctr, Durham, NC; Duke Univ, Durham, NC; Univ of Minnesota, Minneapolis; et al)
Am J Med 116:394-401, 2004   12–2

Introduction.—Frail elderly patients are at increased risk for suboptimal prescribing and for serious adverse drug reactions. Homeostatic reserve and functional status are often impaired in such patients, who are likely to be taking multiple medications for a variety of comorbid conditions. A program of inpatient or outpatient geriatric evaluation and management was compared with a program of usual care for the ability to reduce adverse drug reactions and suboptimal prescribing.

Methods.—The study included patients in 11 Veterans Affairs hospitals who were 65 years or older and met criteria for frailty. Excluded were patients admitted from a nursing home and those with a severe disabling disease, terminal condition, or severe dementia. The study intervention had a core team that included a geriatrician, social worker, and nurse. In addition, pharmacists performed regular reviews of medications. Research assistants at each site created study charts to identify potential drug-related adverse events within the 12-month study period. Blinded physician-pharmacist pairs determined adverse drug reaction causality.

Results.—Diarrhea and renal insufficiency were the most common adverse drug reactions during the inpatient and outpatient periods; the most common serious adverse drug reactions were renal failure and hypoglycemia. For the serious reactions, no inpatient geriatric unit effects were noted during the inpatient or outpatient follow-up examinations. Compared with usual care, outpatient geriatric clinic care led to a 35% reduction in the risk of a serious adverse drug reaction and significantly reduced the number of conditions with omitted drugs. During the inpatient period, inpatient geriatric unit care significantly reduced underuse and unnecessary and inappropriate drug use.

Conclusion.—A program of outpatient evaluation and management can reduce, relative to usual care, the incidence of serious adverse drug reactions in frail, elderly populations. Inpatient and outpatient geriatric evaluation and management was also found to reduce suboptimal prescribing.

▶ The authors demonstrate that inpatient and outpatient geriatric evaluation and management may improve suboptimal prescribing, and outpatient geriatric evaluation and management may reduce the risk of serious adverse drug reactions in the frail elderly. Nevertheless, the risk of serious adverse drug reactions in frail, hospitalized elderly patients remains high even in specialized inpatient units, a finding that those of us who do hospital consultations would readily acknowledge.

B. H. Thiers, MD

Drug Provocation Tests in Patients With a History Suggesting an Immediate Drug Hypersensitivity Reaction
Messaad D, Sahla H, Benahmed S, et al (Hôpital Arnaud de Villeneuve, Montpellier, France)
Ann Intern Med 140:1001-1006, 2004   12–3

Background.—Drug hypersensitivity reactions may be life-threatening; thus, patients with drug hypersensitivity must avoid the medication to which they are allergic. However, how many patients with a suspected allergy to a certain drug are truly allergic to that drug? This question was examined by performing provocation testing in a hospitalized setting.

Methods.—The medical records of 898 patients were reviewed; these patients were referred for provocation testing because they had a history of immediate (within 24 hours) hypersensitivity to a certain drug but now required the drug in question. Patients with severe skin reactions or positive results on skin testing for β-lactams were not eligible for provocation testing. After a thorough clinical history was obtained, patients were admitted to the hospital, where they were given increasing doses of the suspected drug up to the usual daily dose.

Results.—In all, 1372 drug provocation tests were performed, most commonly with β-lactams (30.3%), aspirin (14.5%), other nonsteroidal anti-inflammatory drugs (11.7%), paracetamol (8.9%), macrolides (7.4%), and quinolones (2.4%). In 241 tests (17.6%), drug provocation prompted the same symptom (although milder and of shorter duration) as the initial episode, including anaphylactic shock (5.4% of positive tests), anaphylaxis without shock (7.0%), laryngeal edema (4.1%), bronchospasm (7.9%), urticaria (66.4%), and maculopapular eruption (9.1%). In every case, adverse reactions were completely and promptly controlled by treatment with prednisolone, epinephrine, or H_1-antihistamines.

Conclusion.—Fewer than 1 in 5 of these patients with suspected drug hypersensitivity were confirmed to be allergic to the suspected drug by provocation testing.

► Often a physician must decide whether a patient who claims hypersensitivity to a specific drug is truly allergic to it. Messaad et al gave the implicated drug or drugs to 898 patients referred for evaluation of suspected drug hypersensitivity. Of 1372 tests performed, only 17.6% confirmed the report of hypersensitivity. Of the 241 positive tests, none involved a reaction that could not be readily controlled with steroids, epinephrine, or antihistamines. The data suggest that drug provocation tests, when administered by experienced clinicians in a carefully monitored setting, are a safe method for confirming immediate hypersensitivity. The authors do advise that drug provocation tests not be performed on patients with severe comorbid illnesses.

B. H. Thiers, MD

Cross-Reactivity and Tolerability of Cephalosporins in Patients With Immediate Hypersensitivity to Penicillins

Romano A, Guéant-Rodriguez R-M, Viola M, et al (Università Cattolica del Sacro Cuore, Rome; Istituto di Ricovero e Cura A Carattere Scientifico, Troina, Italy; Institut Natl de la Santé et de la Recherche Médicale, Vandoeuvre, France; et al)
Ann Intern Med 141:16-22, 2004   12–4

Introduction.—Data concerning sensitization to cephalosporins vary in patients who have documented IgE-mediated hypersensitivity to penicillins. The administration of cephalosporins in these patients is commonly deferred because of the risk of cross-reactivity. Cross-reactivity with cephalosporins and its potential determinants was prospectively examined in a large group of well-characterized penicillin-allergic patients.

Methods.—A total of 128 consecutive patients with anaphylactic shock or urticaria (81 and 47 patients, respectively) were evaluated; each had positive results on skin tests for at least 1 of the penicillin reagents. All patients underwent skin testing with cephalothin, cefamandole, cefuroxime, ceftazidime, ceftriaxone, and cefotaxime. Patients with negative results for the final 4 cephalosporins underwent challenge with cefuroxime axetil and ceftriaxone.

Results.—Positive skin test results for cephalosporins occurred in 14 patients (10.9%; 95% CI, 6.1%-17.7%); positive tests were mostly for cephalothin or cefamandole. Skin test results using the minor determinant penicillin mixture were positive in 10 of 14 patients (71.4%) who had cross-reactivity and in 44 of 114 patients (38.6%) without cross-reactivity (odds ratio, 3.90; 95% CI, 1.17-13.40; P = .0189). All 101 patients who had negative skin test results for cefuroxime, ceftazidime, ceftriaxone, and cefotaxime tolerated cefuroxime axetil and ceftriaxone (tolerability rate, 100%; 95% CI, 96.4%-100%).

Conclusion.—These data verify the advisability of avoiding cephalosporin treatment in patients who have positive skin test results for penicillin. For patients who particularly need cephalosporin treatment, skin tests with cephalosporins with a graded challenge are recommended.

▶ Estimates of cephalosporin sensitivity in patients with IgE-mediated hypersensitivity to penicillins vary; the most recent review[1] estimates a 4.4% positivity rate. The usefulness of cephalosporin skin tests is not well documented in penicillin-allergic patients. In this study, about 11% of the 128 patients with a history of documented penicillin allergies had a positive result on cephalosporin skin testing. Importantly, patients with negative skin test results tolerated a subsequent cephalosporin challenge without an allergic reaction. The results suggest that physicians should avoid using cephalosporins in patients with documented penicillin allergy unless they have a negative cephalosporin skin test result. The subject of adverse drug events has recently been reviewed in detail.[2]

B. H. Thiers, MD

References

1. Kelkar PS, Li JT: Cephalosporin allergy. *N Engl J Med* 345:804-809, 2001.
2. Nebeker JR, Barach P, Samore MH: Clarifying adverse drug events: A clinician's guide to terminology, documentation, and reporting. *Ann Intern Med* 140:795-801, 2004.

Characterization of Human T Cells That Regulate Neutrophilic Skin Inflammation

Schaerli P, Britschgi M, Keller M, et al (Inselspital, Bern, Switzerland; Univ of Bern, Switzerland; Univ Hosp Zürich, Switzerland)
J Immunol 173:2151-2158, 2004   12–5

Introduction.—Drug hypersensitivity reactions can act as imitators of many T-cell–mediated diseases. Understanding their pathomechanism may contribute markedly to enhancing knowledge of basic immunologic processes. The severe pustular drug eruption acute generalized exanthematous pustulosis (AGEP) was used as a model to better understand the interplay between T cells and neutrophils. About 90% of AGEP cases are associated with the intake of drugs, especially antibacterials such as aminopenicillins.

There are 3 special features of AGEP as follows: (1) an acute generalized formation of numerous, mostly nonfollicular intraepidermal or subcorneal sterile pustules (less than 5 mm); (2) neutrophils that appear after T-cell infiltration; and (3) the possibility of inducing the reaction by patch testing with the corresponding drug, whereby a massive release of CXCL8/IL-8 by both keratinocytes and isolated drug-specific T cells can be seen upon stimulation. Phenotypic and functional features of CXCL-8 producing (CXCL8+)

CD4+ T cells obtained from patients with AGEP and healthy controls were described.

Findings.—Supernatants from CXCL8+ T cells were strongly chemotactic for neutrophils, CXCR1, and CXCR2 transfectants. This was not observed for tranfectants that expressed CXCR4, CX3CR1, human chemokine receptor, and RDC1. Neutralizing experiments showed that chemotaxis was primarily mediated by CXCL8 and not by granulocyte chemotactic protein-2/CXCL6, epithelial cell-derived neutrophil attractant-78/CXCL5, or growth-related oncogene-α,β, γ/CXCL1,2,3.

About 2.5% of CD4+ T cells in normal peripheral blood also produced CXCL8. In addition to CXCL8, AGEP T cells produced large amounts of the monocyte/neutrophil–activating cytokine GM-CSF. Most released IFN-γ and the proinflammatory cytokine tumor necrosis factor–α. Apoptosis in neutrophils treated with conditioned medium from CXCL8+ T cells was decreased by 40%. In lesional skin, CXCL8+ T cells consistently expressed the chemokine receptor CCR6, indicating there may be a prominent role for CCR6 in early inflammatory T cell recruitment.

Conclusion.—CXCL8-producing T cells facilitate skin inflammation by organizing neutrophilic infiltration and ensuring neutrophil survival, which produces sterile eruptions like those seen in patients with AGEP. This mechanism may be relevant for other T cell–mediated diseases with neutrophilic inflammation.

▶ Whereas acute inflammation in response to a bacterial or viral insult relies upon a primary neutrophil response, other inflammatory conditions appear to depend on T-lymphocyte–mediated recruitment of neutrophils. These investigators studied the involvement of regulatory T cells in a human model of sterile inflammation: acute generalized exanthematous pustulosis, a severe reaction to drugs—particularly antimicrobials—resulting in widespread intraepidermal pustules and erythema.

Previous studies have shown that in such patients, drug-specific T cells were a significant source of interleukin-8 (also termed CXCL8 in description of its recognition by chemokine receptors) which is a prototype neutrophil chemoattractant. In this study, T cells were isolated from the blood of 3 patients with AGEP and the affected skin of 2. Control cells were derived from healthy donors. The investigators determined that drug-specific T cells derived from the affected patients displayed a Th1 cytokine profile, with release of substantial quantities of GM-CSF and interferon-γ.

T-cell supernatants were strongly chemotactic for neutrophils. This activity was only partially abrogated by antibodies to CXCL8, suggesting that the T cells produced another, as yet unidentified, neutrophil chemoattractant. These supernatants also enhanced neutrophil survival by suppressing apoptosis. The authors postulate that this may have been due to the release of GM-CSF by the T cells. Interestingly, a small percentage of peripheral T cells from healthy individuals were also found to produce CXCL8 in response to mitogen stimulation. The significance of this finding is not clear and warrants further study.

G. M. P. Galbraith, MD

Oral Erythromycin and the Risk of Sudden Death From Cardiac Causes

Ray WA, Murray KT, Meredith S, et al (Vanderbilt Univ, Nashville, Tenn; Nashville Veterans Affairs Med Ctr, Tenn)

N Engl J Med 351:1089-1096, 2004   12–6

Background.—Erythromycin is a commonly used macrolide antimicrobial agent that has been considered to be largely without serious toxicity. However, erythromycin has been associated with case reports of torsades de pointes in patients receiving the drug in both oral and IV forms. Erythromycin is extensively metabolized by cytochrome P-450 3A (CYP3A) isozymes, so commonly used medications that inhibit the effects of CYP3A may increase plasma erythromycin concentration and increase the risk of ventricular arrhythmias and sudden death. The association between erythromycin use and the risk of sudden death from cardiac causes and whether this risk is increased with the concurrent use of strong inhibitors of CYP3A were investigated.

Methods.—The group for this study was a previously identified Tennessee Medicaid cohort that included 1,249,943 person-years of follow-up and 1476 cases of confirmed sudden death from cardiac causes. The CYP3A inhibitors identified in the study were nitromidazole antifungal agents, diltiazem, verapamil, and troleandomycin. Amoxicillin, an antimicrobial agent with similar indications that does not prolong cardiac repolarization, was studied along with former use of erythromycin to evaluate possible confounding by indication.

Results.—The multivariate adjusted rate of sudden death from cardiac causes among patients currently using erythromycin was twice as high as the rate among patients who had not used any of the study antibiotic medications. There was no significant increase in the risk of sudden death among patients who were former users of erythromycin or among patients who were currently using amoxicillin. The adjusted rate of sudden death from cardiac causes was 5 times greater among patients with concurrent use of erythromycin and CYP3A inhibitors compared with patients who had used neither CYP3A inhibitors nor any of the study antibiotic medications. However, there was no increase in the risk of sudden death among patients who concurrently used amoxicillin and CYP3A inhibitors or patients who concurrently used any of the study antibiotic medications and who had formerly used CYP3A inhibitors.

Conclusion.—Erythromycin should not be used concurrently with strong inhibitors of CYP3A, including nitromidazole antifungal agents, some calcium-channel blockers, and some antidepressant drugs.

▶ Interacting drugs that are metabolized by CYP3A, such as erythromycin and -azole antifungal agents, are commonly used in dermatology. When used together, prolongation of the QT interval and devastating cardiac arrhythmias may occur.[1] Such toxicity led to withdrawal from the market of the first generation of non-sedating antihistamines, including terfenadine and astemizole. The report by Ray and colleagues stresses that not only these antihistamines (whose concentrations can be increased by concomitant use of erythromycin) but erythromycin itself in sufficiently high concentrations can cause torsades de pointes. This demonstrates the importance of taking a complete drug history from all patients.[2]

B. H. Thiers, MD

References

1. Roden DM: Drug-induced prolongation of the QT interval. *N Engl J Med* 350:1013-1022, 2004.
2. Liu BA, Juurlink DN: Drugs and the QT interval—Caveat Doctor. *N Engl J Med* 351:1053-1056, 2004.

Clopidogrel Versus Aspirin for Secondary Prophylaxis of Vascular Events: A Cost-Effectiveness Analysis
Schleinitz MD, Weiss JP, Owen DK (Brown Univ, Providence, RI; Rhode Island Hosp, Providence; Stanford Univ, Palo Alto, Calif; et al)
Am J Med 116:797-806, 2004   12–7

Purpose.—Clopidogrel is more effective than aspirin in preventing recurrent vascular events, but concerns about its cost-effectiveness have limited its use. We evaluated the cost-effectiveness of clopidogrel and aspirin as secondary prevention in patients with a prior myocardial infarction, a prior stroke, or peripheral arterial disease.

Methods.—We constructed Markov models assuming a societal perspective, and based analyses on the lifetime treatment of a 63-year-old patient facing event probabilities derived from the Clopidogrel versus Aspirin in Patients at Risk of Ischemic Events (CAPRIE) trial as the base case. Outcome measures included costs, life expectancy in quality-adjusted life-years (QALYs), incremental cost-effectiveness ratios, and events averted.

Results.—In patients with peripheral arterial disease, clopidogrel increased life expectancy by 0.55 QALYs at an incremental cost-effectiveness ratio of $25,100 per QALY, as compared with aspirin. In poststroke patients, clopidogrel increased life expectancy by 0.17 QALYs at a cost of $31,200 per QALY. Aspirin was both less expensive and more effective than clopidogrel in post-myocardial infarction patients. In probabilistic sensitivity analyses, our evaluation for patients with peripheral vascular disease was robust. Evaluations of stroke and myocardial infarction patients were sensitive predominantly to the cost and efficacy of clopidogrel, with aspirin therapy more effective and less expensive in 153 of 1000 simulations (15.3%) in poststroke patients and clopidogrel more effective in 119 of 1000 simulations (11.9%) in the myocardial infarction sample.

Conclusion.—Clopidogrel provides a substantial increase in quality-adjusted life expectancy at a cost that is within traditional societal limits for patients with either peripheral arterial disease or a recent stroke. Current evidence does not support increased efficacy with clopidogrel relative to aspirin in patients following myocardial infarction.

▶ Can clopidogrel be the much sought-after "super-aspirin"? In their study, Schleinitz et al found very different cost-effectiveness ratios among the 3 groups of cardiovascular diseases that were studied. Clopidogrel is currently too expensive to be prescribed to everyone with cardiovascular disease world-wide and may be ineffective in some patients. The decision to use clopidogrel or aspirin must be tailored to the individual patient, with consideration of the magnitude of risk of recurrent cardiovascular events, concurrent treatment with drugs that can potentially interact with antiplatelet agents, and the patient's resistance profile to these drugs.[1]

B. H. Thiers, MD

Reference

1. Gaspoz J-M, de Moerloose P: Aspirin or clopidogrel for secondary prevention of cardiovascular events: Is there a winner? *Am J Med* 116:850-852, 2004.

Taking Glucocorticoids by Prescription Is Associated With Subsequent Cardiovascular Disease
Wei L, MacDonald TM, Walker BR (Ninewells Hosp and Med School, Dundee, Scotland; Univ of Edinburgh, Scotland; Western Gen Hosp, Edinburgh, Scotland)
Ann Intern Med 141:764-770, 2004   12–8

Introduction.—The use of glucocorticoids is linked with adverse systemic effects (eg, obesity, hypertension, and hyperglycemia) that may predispose to cardiovascular disease. The effect of glucocorticoid use on cardiovascular disease has yet to be quantified and was therefore evaluated to ascertain whether the use of exogenous glucocorticoids increases the risk of cardiovascular disease.

Methods.—A cohort investigation was performed with the use of a record linkage database that identified 68,781 glucocorticoid users and 82,202 nonusers without previous hospitalization for cardiovascular disease who were evaluated between 1993 and 1996. The average daily dose of glucocorticoid exposure during follow-up was classified as low (ie, inhaled, nasal, and topical only), medium (ie, oral, rectal, or parental; <7.5 mg of prednisolone equivalent), or high (≥7.5 mg of prednisolone equivalent). The association between glucocorticoid exposure and cardiovascular outcomes was investigated.

Results.—A total of 4383 cardiovascular events occurred in 257,487 person-years of follow-up for a rate of 17.0 (95% CI, 16.5%-17.5%) per 1000 person-years in the comparator group; 5068 events occurred in 212,287 person-years for a rate of 23.9 (95% CI, 23.2%-24.5%) per 1000 person-years in the group exposed to glucocorticoids (22.1, 27.2, and 76.5 in the low, medium, and high groups, respectively). The absolute difference in risk was 6.9 (95% CI, 6.0-7.7) per 1000 person-years (5.1, 10.1, and 59.4, for those in the low, medium, and high groups, respectively). After adjustment was made for known covariates, the relative risk for a cardiovascular event in patients receiving high-dose glucocorticoids was 2.56 (95% CI, 2.18-2.99).

Conclusion.—Treatment with high-dose glucocorticoids seems to be linked with an increased risk of cardiovascular disease.

▶ The authors sought to document whether individuals who take glucocorticoids have an increased risk of cardiovascular disease. They found a clear dose–response relationship, with the use of glucocorticoids associated with an increased risk of cardiovascular events. Individuals who received high doses of the drugs were more than 2.5 times as likely to experience a cardiovascular event as patients who did not use glucocorticoids. One key question is whether the association of glucocorticoid use with cardiovascular disease reflects a true effect of glucocorticoids or an association with the underlying disease for which they were prescribed. However, the authors argue that their study design appropriately adjusted for known covariates.

B. H. Thiers, MD

Skin Cancers and Non-Hodgkin Lymphoma Among Users of Systemic Glucocorticoids: A Population-Based Cohort Study

Sørensen HT, Mellemkjaer L, Nielsen GL, et al (Aarhus Univ Hosp, Denmark; Danish Cancer Society, Copenhagen; Dartmouth Med School, Hanover, NH)
J Natl Cancer Inst 96:709-711, 2004   12–9

Background.—The risk of skin cancer may be increased in patients treated with glucocorticoids. This possibility was further investigated with the use of data from a population-based database and national registry.

Methods.—Information was obtained from the North Jutland Prescription Database and the Danish Cancer Registry. Observed and expected numbers of cases of skin cancer and non-Hodgkin lymphoma were compared among 59,043 individuals receiving prescriptions for glucocorticoids between 1989 and 1996.

Findings.—The overall risks for squamous cell carcinomas and basal cell carcinomas of the skin were increased among the glucocorticoid users, especially among those with 15 or more prescriptions. Among such individuals, the standardized incidence ratios were 2.45 for squamous cell carcinomas and 1.52 for basal cell carcinomas. The risk for non-Hodgkin lymphoma was also increased among patients with 10 to 14 prescriptions; the standardized incidence ratio was 2.68.

Conclusions.—The incidences of skin cancers and non-Hodgkin lymphoma have increased worldwide, which suggests a possible common etiology. The current cohort study indicates that immunosuppression by glucocorticoids may be a shared risk factor for certain skin cancers and lymphomas.

▶ The findings, indicating a modestly increased risk for nonmelanoma skin cancer and non-Hodgkin lymphoma in patients receiving multiple prescriptions for systemic steroids are not particularly surprising, given the known risk of these disorders in patients receiving other forms of immunosuppressive therapy. Although this was a large population-based study, clinical details regarding comorbid diseases, the intensity of sun exposure, and compliance with the prescriptions was lacking. Moreover, no data were presented regarding the reason for the prescriptions, and it is possible that some of the diseases for which steroids were prescribed (eg, autoimmune disorders) may themselves be associated with an increased lymphoma risk.

B. H. Thiers, MD

Skin Manifestations of Inhaled Corticosteroids in COPD Patients: Results From Lung Health Study II
Tashkin DP, for the Lung Health Study Research Group (Case Western Reserve Univ, Cleveland, Ohio)
Chest 126:1123-1133, 2004   12–10

Background.—Inhaled corticosteroids (ICSs) are often used to treat stable chronic obstructive pulmonary disease (COPD). ICS therapy, however, is associated with easy skin bruising, other cutaneous manifestations (eg, acne, rash, impaired skin healing), and other systemic effects (eg, adrenal suppression, lost of bone mineral density [BMD]). The cutaneous and systemic effects of ICS therapy in patients with COPD were examined.

Methods.—The subjects were 1116 patients (37.2% women; mean age, 56.3 years) with mild to moderate COPD; all were smokers or recent ex-smokers. Patients were randomly assigned to receive either triamcinolone acetonide, 6 puffs twice a day (1200 µg/d), or placebo. Compliance with ICS use was assessed by weighing the canisters; good compliance was defined as 6 or more puffs per day. Every 6 months over the 4.5-year study, patients completed a questionnaire to identify skin changes and to assess their severity. Also, subsets of these patients had their hypothalamic-pituitary-adrenal (HPA) axis function (n = 221) or their BMD of the femoral neck and lumbar spine (n = 412) evaluated at baseline and at years 1 and 3.

Results.—Among the patients with poor compliance, the incidence of skin changes did not differ significantly between the ICS and placebo groups. Among those with good compliance, however, patients in the ICS group were significantly more likely to report easy bruising (11.2% vs 3.4%) and slow skin healing (2.4% vs 0.5%), whereas patients in the placebo group were significantly more likely to report rash (6.4% vs 4.9%). The greatest risk of bruising was seen in men 56 years old or older with good compliance to ICS therapy. Skin bruising did not correlate significantly with either suppression of adrenal function or loss of BMD.

Conclusion.—ICS therapy at moderate to high doses increases the incidence of easy bruising and impairs skin healing in patients with COPD. Skin bruising in ICS users, however, is not associated with systemic toxicity.

▶ The findings are hardly surprising, as systemic absorption of inhaled drugs has been previously demonstrated. It should be noted that there was no association between skin bruising and other markers of systemic corticosteroid toxicity, such as loss of BMD or suppression of adrenal function.

B. H. Thiers, MD

Inhaled Corticosteroids and the Risk of Fractures in Children and Adolescents
Schlienger RG, Jick SS, Meier CR (Univ of Basel, Switzerland; Boston Univ)
Pediatrics 114:469-473, 2004   12–11

Background.—Inhaled corticosteroids are recommended for children and adolescents with mild persistent or more severe asthma. However, few studies have assessed the risks of this treatment. Some research has suggested that long-term or moderate to high-dose inhaled steroid therapy suppresses bone formation or negatively affects bone mineral density in young persons. Whether children and adolescents exposed to inhaled corticosteroids have an increased risk of bone fractures was investigated.

Methods.—This population-based, nested case-control analysis included 3744 patients, 5 to 17 years old, with a diagnosis of fracture and 21,757 matched control subjects. The use of inhaled steroids by the patients before the index date was compared with that of the control subjects.

Findings.—Current exposure to inhaled steroids did not markedly alter fracture risk compared with nonuse, even in persons with longer-term exposure. Compared with nonusers, users of inhaled steroids with 20 or more prescriptions, adjusted for use of other antiasthmatic drugs and oral steroid use, had a risk estimate of 1.21.

Conclusions.—Inhaled steroid treatment does not appear to materially affect the risk of bone fracture in children and adolescents. However, longer-term exposure to inhaled steroids in children and adolescents with concomitant or past oral steroid use may slightly increase the risk of fracture.

▶ Exogenous corticosteroid therapy has been associated with effects on adrenal function and growth as well as on bone metabolism and bone mineral density. Dermatologists have voiced similar concerns over excessive use of topical steroids, especially in children. Although the findings of Schlienger et al are reassuring, they relate only to inhaled steroids and cannot be extrapolated to topical steroids.

B. H. Thiers, MD

Long-term, High-Dose Glucocorticoids and Bone Mineral Content in Childhood Glucocorticoid-Sensitive Nephrotic Syndrome

Leonard MB, Feldman HI, Shults J, et al (Children's Hosp, Philadelphia; Univ of Pennsylvania, Philadelphia)

N Engl J Med 351:868-875, 2004   12–12

Background.—Declines in bone mineral density (BMD) have been described in a variety of pediatric disorders that require glucocorticoid therapy. However, some of the detrimental effects on bone attributed to glucocorticoids may result from the underlying inflammatory disease. Unlike other pediatric conditions that require long-term glucocorticoid therapy in childhood, glucocorticoid-sensitive nephrotic syndrome, a condition without substantial systemic inflammatory involvement, remits completely and quickly with glucocorticoid therapy. Unfortunately, there is a relapse of nephrotic syndrome in most children after reduction or discontinuation of glucocorticoids, resulting in protracted, repeated courses of glucocorticoids. The effects of long-term glucocorticoid treatment on bone mineral content (BMC) in children with glucocorticoid-sensitive nephrotic syndrome were determined.

Methods.—Dual x-ray absorptiometry of the whole body and spine was performed in 60 children and adolescents with nephrotic syndrome and in 195 control subjects. Linear regression analysis of log-transformed values was used to compare the BMC in patients with that in control subjects.

Results.—The patients had received an average of 23,000 mg of glucocorticoids and were shorter and had a greater body mass index (BMI) than the control subjects. The BMC of the spine, adjusted for bone area, age, sex, degree of maturation, and race, did not differ significantly between patients and control subjects. The BMC of the spine was significantly less in patients than in the control subjects, after adjustment for the z score for BMI. Whole-body BMC, after adjustment for height, age, sex, degree of maturation, and race, was significantly higher in patients than control subjects. However, the association with the nephrotic syndrome was eliminated by the addition of the z score for BMI to the model.

Conclusions.—Intermittent treatment with high-dose glucocorticoids during childhood did not appear to be associated with deficits in BMC of the spine or whole body in relation to age, bone size, sex, and degree of maturation. Glucocorticoid-induced increases in BMI in this study were associated with increased whole-body mineral content and maintenance of spinal BMC.

▶ It is reassuring that children with nephrotic syndrome, having received an average of 23,000 mg of prednisone over a mean of 4.4 years, had similar BMC of the lumbar spine and whole body as that of a control population after adjustment for age, sex, bone area, maturity and race. Unfortunately, bone mass, as determined by dual-energy x-ray absorptiometry, was the only measure of skeletal health considered; bone geometry and quality, which can also influence bone strength, were not evaluated. Although it would appear from the study that demineralization of bones from intermittent high-dose systemic glucocorticosteroid treatment is much less of a problem in growing children than it is in adults, treated children will need long-term follow-up to ensure that their bone strength as adults is not diminished.

S. Raimer, MD

Risk of Cardiovascular Events and Rofecoxib: Cumulative Meta-analysis
Jüni P, Nartey L, Reichenbach S, et al (Univ of Berne, Switzerland; Univ of Bristol, England)
Lancet 364:2021-2029, 2004   12–13

Introduction.—Rofecoxib (Vioxx), the cyclo-oxygenase 2 (COX2) inhibitor marketed by Merck, was withdrawn from the market on September 30, 2004, after a placebo-controlled trial found increased cardiovascular risk in patients taking the drug for more than 18 months. The 2000 Vioxx Gastrointestinal Outcomes Research study had attributed the apparent increase in cardiovascular adverse effects associated with the drug to the cardioprotective effects of naproxen, the nonsteroidal anti-inflammatory drug (NSAID) with which it was compared. But findings of a cumulative meta-analysis indicate that there was evidence of a real increase in adverse effects associated with rofecoxib before September 2004.

Methods.—Randomized trials comparing rofecoxib (12.5-50 mg daily) with another NSAID or placebo were identified by a search of databases such as MEDLINE and relevant files of the Food and Drug Administration. Also included were cohort and case-control studies that examined the association between naproxen use and cardiovascular risk. Trial quality was assessed according to 2 components: concealment of allocation of patients to treatment groups and external review of serious cardiovascular events.

Results.—Eighteen randomized trials and 11 observational studies met inclusion criteria. The analysis of primary end point, myocardial infarction, was based on 64 events from 16 comparisons between rofecoxib and control, with 52 events in rofecoxib groups and 12 in control groups. An increased risk of myocardial infarction was apparent in 2000, when 14,247 patients had been randomly assigned and 44 events had occurred. The cardioprotective effect of naproxen, examined in 8 case-control and 3 retrospective cohort studies, was too small (combined estimate 0.86) to have explained the relative increase in cardiovascular events with rofecoxib. Neither type of control group (placebo, non-naproxen NSAID, or naproxen) nor duration of trial appeared to influence the relative risk (2.30 by the end of 2000) associated with rofecoxib therapy.

Conclusion.—The withdrawal of Vioxx by its manufacturer in 2004 was based on findings of a fairly small trial designed for a different purpose. This cumulative meta-analysis, however, indicates that the increased risk of myocardial infarction was quite evident by the end of 2000. In addition, patients were at risk even when rofecoxib was taken for a few months, and cardiovascular toxicity was not dose dependent.

▶ The withdrawal of rofecoxib (Vioxx) from the market was one of the land-mark medical events of 2004. The authors argue that data existed several years earlier to justify its removal.

B. H. Thiers, MD

The Effectiveness of Five Strategies for the Prevention of Gastrointestinal Toxicity Induced by Non-Steroidal Anti-Inflammatory Drugs: Systematic Review
Hooper L, Brown TJ, Elliott RA, et al (Univ of Manchester, England; North West Genetics Knowledge Park, Manchester, England)
BMJ 329:948-952, 2004   12–14

Background.—Different strategies are available to protect patients from nonsteroidal anti-inflammatory drug (NSAID)-induced gastrointestinal toxicity. The efficacy of 5 such strategies was investigated: H_2 receptor antagonists plus nonselective NSAIDs, proton pump inhibitors plus nonselective NSAIDs, misoprostol plus nonselective NSAIDs, cyclooxygenase 2 (COX-2) selective NSAIDs, and COX-2 specific NSAIDs.

Methods.—In a search of the literature, 112 randomized controlled trials were identified. Inclusion criteria were assessment of a gastroprotective strategy compared with placebo, duration of more than 21 days, and measurement of review outcomes. Studies exclusively of children or healthy volunteers were excluded.

Findings.—A total of 74,666 participants were included in the 112 trials. Five studies were judged to be at low risk of bias. Overall, 138 deaths and 248 serious gastrointestinal events were reported. Comparing protective strategies with placebo, the authors found no evidence for the efficacy of H_2 receptor antagonists for any primary outcomes. Proton pump inhibitors may have decreased the risk of symptomatic ulcers.

Misoprostol reduced the risk of serious gastrointestinal complications and symptomatic ulcers. In addition, COX-2 selective agents decreased the risk of symptomatic ulcers, and COX-2–specific agents reduced the risk of symptomatic ulcers and possibly serious gastrointestinal complications. All but COX-2 selective agents lowered the risk of endoscopic ulcers.

Conclusion.—Misoprostol, COX-2 selective and specific NSAIDs, and probably proton pump inhibitors significantly decrease the risk of symptomatic ulcers. Misoprostol and probably COX-2 specific agents may significantly decrease the risk of serious gastrointestinal complications. More research is needed on H_2 receptor antagonists and proton pump inhibitors.

▶ The known gastrointestinal side effects of NSAIDs range from mild dyspepsia to death from gastric hemorrhage and perforation. Agents to mitigate against such adverse events are commonly co-prescribed with these drugs. This study confirms that misoprostol, COX-2 specific and selective NSAIDs, and probably proton pump inhibitors significantly reduce the risk of symptomatic ulcers. Additionally, misoprostol and probably COX-2 specific NSAIDs reduce the risk of serious gastrointestinal complications, but the quality of data is low.

B. H. Thiers, MD

Interaction of St John's Wort With Conventional Drugs: Systematic Review of Clinical Trials
Mills E, Montori VM, Wu P, et al (McMaster Univ, Hamilton, Ont, Canada; Mayo Clinic College of Medicine, Rochester, Minn; London School of Hygiene and Tropical Medicine, London; et al)
BMJ 329:27-30, 2004   12–15

Introduction.—Findings of both case reports and clinical trials indicate that interactions occur between the herbal medicine St John's wort and prescribed drugs. A systematic review of clinical trials was conducted to evaluate the pharmacokinetic effect of St John's wort on the metabolism of conventional drugs.

Methods.—Nine electronic databases were searched for relevant articles, and the bibliographies of retrieved studies were reviewed for further materials; experts in the field were also contacted. Two reviewers who selected studies for inclusion independently extracted data. Each study was assessed for the quality of its methods.

Results.—The review included 22 trials published between 1999 and April 2004. The average number of participants in the trials was 12; 17 trials enrolled healthy volunteers, and 5 studied patients who needed the drugs for health reasons. Steady state pharmacokinetics was examined in 18 trials, and 15 assayed the St John's wort preparation for accuracy of the stated dosage. Seventeen of 19 trials with available plasma data found a decrease in systemic bioavailability of the conventional drug when coadministered with the herbal preparation.

Discussion.—St John's wort may reduce the bioavailability of many conventional drugs. Studies of the issue, however, varied widely in methods, enrolled small numbers of patients, and contained few safeguards against bias. Clinicians and patients should be aware of the potential effects of St John's wort on prescribed drugs. Better research is needed to provide more reliable information.

▶ Previous studies have suggested decreased systemic bioavailability of certain prescription drugs with concomitant administration of St John's wort. Mills et al emphasize the need for higher quality research to convincingly determine whether such drug interactions do, in fact, occur.

B. H. Thiers, MD

Brief Communication: American Ginseng Reduces Warfarin's Effect in Healthy Patients: A Randomized, Controlled Trial
Yuan C-S, Wei G, Dey L, et al (Univ of Chicago)
Ann Intern Med 141:23-27, 2004   12–16

Introduction.—Individuals who use prescription medications frequently concurrently take herbal supplements. A reduced anticoagulant effect of warfarin was observed after consumption of ginseng in a widely cited case report. The interaction between American ginseng and warfarin was examined in a randomized, double-blind, placebo-controlled trial.

Methods.—During a 4-week investigation, 20 young, healthy volunteers received warfarin for 3 days during week 1 and 4. Beginning in week 2, participants were assigned to receive either American ginseng or placebo. Measurements of the international normalized ratio (INR) and plasma warfarin levels were obtained at appropriate intervals.

Results.—The peak INR significantly diminished after 2 weeks of ginseng administration compared with placebo (difference between ginseng and placebo, -0.19 [95% CI, -0.36 to -0.07; $P = .0012$). The INR area under the curve, peak plasma warfarin level, and warfarin area under the curve were also statistically significantly decreased in the ginseng group compared with the placebo group. A positive association was observed between peak INR and peak plasma warfarin level.

Conclusion.—American ginseng decreases the anticoagulant effect of warfarin. Physicians need to warn patients about ginseng use when taking warfarin.

▶ Yuan et al demonstrate that ginseng consumption decreases plasma warfarin levels and lowers the INR. The results emphasize that nonprescription drugs or other substances can have a significant effect on prescription drug metabolism.[1-3]

B. H. Thiers, MD

References

1. Ernst E: The risk-benefit profile of commonly used herbal therapies: Ginkgo, St John's wort, ginseng, echinacea, saw palmetto, and kava. *Ann Intern Med* 136:42-53, 2002.
2. Kaufman DW, Kelly JP, Rosenberg L, et al: Recent patterns of medication use in the ambulatory adult population of the United States: The Slone survey. *JAMA* 287:337-344, 2002.
3. Zhou S, Chan E, Pan SQ, et al: Interaction of drugs with St. John's wort. *J Psychopharmacol* 18:262-276, 2004.

Activation of Autoimmunity Following Use of Immunostimulatory Herbal Supplements

Lee AN, Werth VP (Univ of Chicago; Univ of Pennsylvania, Philadelphia)
Arch Dermatol 140:723-727, 2004   12–17

Background.—In vitro and in vivo experiments have supported the notion that many herbal supplements have immunostimulatory properties, which explains the beneficial effects of such supplements in preventing or ameliorating disease. However, there appear to be no reports of immunostimulatory herbal supplements exacerbating disorders of immune system overactivity. In the current article, 3 patients had onset or flares of autoimmune disease after ingesting herbal supplements with proven immunostimulatory effects.

Patients and Findings.—The patients were 2 men and 1 woman, aged 55, 57, and 45 years, respectively. Patient 1 was a white man given a diagnosis of pemphigus vulgaris in 1995. He also had chronic uveitis, necessitating long-term systemic steroid treatment, and secondary osteoporosis. At the current presentation, he had not taken corticosteroids for 4 months. Subsequently, his disease was controlled with prednisone, dapsone, and azathioprine. After complete lesion clearance, prednisone and azathioprine were discontinued. Low-dose dapsone therapy was continued. In October 1998, an upper respiratory tract infection developed, and the patient began taking an *Echinacea* supplement. He had never taken herbal supplements before. Within 1 week of beginning this supplement, blisters developed on his trunk, head, and oral mucosa. Stopping *Echinacea* and reinstituting prednisone, azathioprine, and dapsone resulted in partial disease control. However, the patient has not achieved complete remission again.

Conclusions.—In the 3 cases presented, *Echinacea* and the alga *Spirulina platensis* were implicated in 2 patients' flares of pemphigus vulgaris, and a supplement containing the alga *Spirulina platensis* and *Aphanizomenon flos-aquae* was implicated in the onset and a severe flare of dermatomyositis in a third. Thus, immunostimulatory herbal supplements may exacerbate pre-existing autoimmune disease or even precipitate such disorders in genetically predisposed individuals. Increased TNF-α production may play a role.

▶ This article by Lee and Werth confirms the importance of taking a complete drug history from all our patients. Intake of all prescription and nonprescription remedies should be recorded, as such preparations can effect both the expression of disease and the response to treatment. An excellent review of commonly used herbal medicines has recently been published.[1]

B. H. Thiers, MD

Reference

1. Bent S, Ko R: Commonly used herbal medicines in the United States: A review. *Am J Med* 116:478-485, 2004.

13 Drug Development and Promotion

Association of Funding and Findings of Pharmaceutical Research at a Meeting of a Medical Professional Society
Finucane TE, Boult CE (Johns Hopkins Bloomberg School of Public Health, Baltimore, Md)
Am J Med 117:842-845, 2004   13-1

Background.—Each year thousands of studies sponsored by the pharmaceutical industry are presented at meetings of medical professional societies. The extent to which the financial interests of a study's funder impact the study's findings was examined.

Methods.—The authors reviewed 520 abstracts presented at the annual scientific meeting of a clinically oriented US medical professional society. Of these, 48 studies examined the efficacy or safety of medications. Two raters independently classified each study's findings as either positive (ie, the drug was effective, safe, and/or superior to another drug) or negative (ie, the drug was ineffective, caused unacceptable adverse events, and/or was not superior to another drug). The raters also evaluated each study as either having pharmaceutical industry support (ie, receipt of a grant from a pharmaceutical company, or having an author affiliated with a pharmaceutical company or with a private research corporation supported by the pharmaceutical industry) or not having industry support.

Results.—Most of these 48 reports were nonrandomized observational studies (n = 20) or randomized clinical trials (n = 20). The 2 raters were in complete agreement (kappa = 1.0) about the results of the study and the funding source. Of these 48 studies, 30 (63%) were industry supported and 18 (37%) received no support from the pharmaceutical industry. All 30 of the industry-supported studies reported positive findings for the drug (100%), compared with only 12 of the studies that received no industrial support (67%). The association between pharmaceutical funding and positive findings was significant ($P < .0007$), both for the nonrandomized observational studies and for the randomized clinical trials.

Conclusion.—At this scientific meeting, pharmaceutical company funding was associated with study findings in support of drugs marketed by the sponsoring drug company. In contrast, about one third of the studies without pharmaceutical industry support reported negative findings. Conflict of interest could jeopardize the credibility of research results presented at scientific meetings. To avoid this, the authors suggest researchers presenting their studies at annual meetings should make full disclosure of funding sources. Furthermore, medical professional societies should adopt policies to avoid "outcome bias" (ie, accepting papers without regard for whether the findings are positive or negative) and to educate their members about how to recognize conflict of interest and scientific bias.

▶ In an accompanying editorial, Landefeld[1] suggests the creation of an independent funding mechanism to eliminate the link between sponsorship and research. The proposed National Institute of Pharmaceutical Research would, like the National Institutes of Health, award grants for clinical trials to investigators on the basis of independent peer review. Under the current system, these trials are conducted by for-profit contract research organizations. Funding under the proposed system would be accomplished by pooled resources from the pharmaceutical industry, and the Food and Drug Administration might be required to consider only evidence resulting from such independent funding mechanisms when evaluating a drug for approval. The creation of an independent grant-making agency would eliminate commercial bias and assure the highest scientific standards for pharmaceutical research, enhancing research credibility and quality. Whether such an agency ever becomes a reality can only be a matter of speculation.

B. H. Thiers, MD

Reference

1. Landefeld CS: Commercial support and bias in pharmaceutical research. *Am J Med* 117:876-878, 2004.

Does the Type of Competing Interest Statement Affect Readers' Perceptions of the Credibility of Research? Randomised Trial
Schroter S, Morris J, Chaudhry S, et al (BMA House, London; Wythenshawe Hosp, Manchester, England; Univ Hosp, Stoke-on-Trent, England)
BMJ 328:742-743, 2004   13–2

Introduction.—Financial relationships among industry and academic institutions can influence both the author's conclusions and the reader's opinions of published studies. The reader's perceptions of the credibility of medical research were investigated in a randomized trial.

Methods.—Participants were drawn from the membership of the British Medical Association. Two studies were sent to 900 members: 450 received a paper about the use of problem lists in letters between hospital doctors and general practitioners (problem lists paper), and 450 received a paper documenting the impact on daily functioning from pain related to herpes zoster (herpes paper). For each study, 150 readers received the paper with no competing interests indicated, 150 with a financial statement, and 150 with a statement that the author had received funding from research grants. Readers were asked to score the studies for interest, importance, relevance, validity, and believability.

Results.—Questionnaires were returned by 66% of those who received the problem lists paper and 52% of those sent the herpes paper. Overall ratings of importance, relevance, validity, and believability were significantly less for the "financial statement" group than those for the "no competing interests" group. Validity ratings were also significantly less for the "financial statement" group than those for the "grants statement" group. The problem lists paper scored significantly more on all measures than the herpes paper. Ratings for all 5 measures increased significantly with respondent's age, and women reported significantly higher ratings than men.

Conclusion.—Readers' perceptions of the credibility of published research was influenced by both the content of the study and the type of competing interest disclosed. Journal editors should include a declaration of authors' competing interest so that readers can make better-informed judgments.

▶ Perhaps not surprisingly, a declaration of competing interests affects readers' believability in the results of published studies.

B. H. Thiers, MD

Turning a Blind Eye: The Success of Blinding Reported in a Random Sample of Randomised, Placebo Controlled Trials

Fergusson D, Glass KC, Waring D, et al (Ottawa Health Research Inst, Ont, Canada; McGill Univ, Montreal)
BMJ 328:432-434, 2004   13–3

Introduction.—In a double-blind trial, the patient, investigators, and outcome assessors should be unaware of the patient's assigned treatment throughout the trial. If a placebo is used to assess effectiveness of an active treatment, valid results can be obtained only when blinding of the placebo arm is successful. A sample of randomized placebo-controlled trials was examined for the reporting and success of double blinding.

Methods.—Nine leading journals, 5 devoted to general medicine and 4 to psychiatry, were selected for the study. A MEDLINE search for the period between January 1, 1998, and October 1, 2001, yielded a random sample of 200 randomized, placebo-controlled clinical trials, half from the general medicine and half from the psychiatry literature. At least 2 researchers independently abstracted data from each study.

Results.—The inclusion criteria were met by 97 general medicine and 94 psychiatry articles. Most of the general medicine trial interventions were pharmacologic (83%); the most common placebo types were injection (27%), tablet (24%), and capsule (21%). Only 53% of these trials reported the matching characteristics of the placebo (46 of 51 trials), and only 7 assessed the success of blinding. More than 40% of psychiatry trials did not report the type of placebo used; only 8 of 94 trials reported evidence of successful blinding.

Conclusion.—Some aspects of the quality of reporting in clinical trials have improved, but the methods of blinding and the subsequent success of blinding are underreported. Overall, only 8% of sampled trials from leading general medicine and psychiatry journals provided information on the success of blinding. The findings of this review challenge the notion that placebo-controlled trials inherently possess assay sensitivity. Trials that will particularly benefit from assessment of blinding are those with patient-reported subjective outcomes or those where side effects are well known.

▶ Although the statement that a trial is "blinded" is often taken at face value, the authors demonstrate that the success of blinding is not well reported. Thus, a blinded trial may not be truly blinded. More efforts are needed to report such information and its potential effect on study results. As stated by the authors, the efficacy of blinding cannot be assumed on theoretical grounds.

B. H. Thiers, MD

Availability of Large-Scale Evidence on Specific Harms From Systematic Reviews of Randomized Trials
Papanikolaou PN, Ioannidis JPA (Univ of Ioannina, Greece; Tufts Univ, Boston)
Am J Med 117:582-589, 2004   13–4

Introduction.—Empirical evidence is needed concerning whether it is possible, on a large scale, to collect evidence on specific, well-defined harms from systematic reviews of randomized trials. These meta-analyses could generate accurate information on both common and uncommon risks of interventions. The frequency with which evidence on specific, well-defined adverse events is available in a quantitative manner from systematic reviews of large randomized trials was examined, along with whether common and uncommon harms may be assessed with this approach.

Methods.—The Cochrane Database of Systematic Reviews was searched for reviews that contained quantitative data regarding specific, well-defined harms for at least 4000 randomized research subjects, which was the minimum sample needed for adequate power to identify an adverse event caused by an intervention in 1% of research subjects. The primary outcome measures included the number of reviews with eligible large-scale data on adverse events, the number of ineligible reviews, and the magnitude of recorded harms (absolute risk, relative risk) based on large-scale evidence.

Results.—Of 1727 reviews, 138 included evidence regarding 4000 or more research subjects. However, only 25 (18%) had eligible data concerning adverse events; 77 had no harms data; and 36 had data on harms that were either nonspecific or applied to fewer than 4000 research subjects. Concerning 66 specific adverse events for which data were adequate in the 25 eligible reviews, 25 demonstrated statistically significant differences between comparison arms; most pertained to serious or severe adverse events and absolute risk differences less than 4%. In 9 of 31 (29%) of a sample of large trials in reviews with poor reporting of harms, specific harms were presented sufficiently in the trial reports yet were not included in the systematic reviews.

Conclusion.—Systematic reviews can provide useful large-scale information concerning adverse events. The importance of and difficulties in assessing harms is acknowledged, but the reporting of adverse effects needs to be improved in both randomized trials and systematic reviews.

▶ Unfortunately, randomized trials often concentrate more on collecting data on benefits than on adverse events. Papanikolaou and Ioannidis suggest that the reporting of adverse events must be improved in both randomized trials and systematic reviews.

B. H. Thiers, MD

Importance of Patient Pressure and Perceived Pressure and Perceived Medical Need for Investigations, Referral, and Prescribing in Primary Care: Nested Observational Study
Little P, Dorward M, Warner G, et al (Southampton Univ, England; Nightingale Surgery, Romsey, England; Three Swans Surgery, Salisbury, England)
BMJ 328:444-447, 2004   13–5

Objective.—To assess how pressures from patients on doctors in the consultation contribute to referral and investigation.

Design.—Observational study nested within a randomised controlled trial.

Setting.—Five general practices in three settings in the United Kingdom.

Participants.—847 consecutive patients, aged 16-80 years.

Main Outcomes Measures.—Patient preferences and doctors' perception of patient pressure and medical need.

Results.—Perceived medical need was the strongest independent predictor of all behaviours and confounded all other predictors. The doctors thought, however, there was no or only a slight indication for medical need among a significant minority of those who were examined (89/580, 15%), received a prescription (74/394, 19%), or were referred (27/125, 22%) and almost half of those investigated (99/216, 46%). After controlling for patient preference, medical need, and clustering by doctor, doctors' perceptions of patient pressure were strongly associated with prescribing (adjusted odds ratio 2.87, 95% confidence interval 1.16 to 7.08) and even more strongly associated with examination (4.38, 1.24 to 15.5), referral (10.72, 2.08 to 55.3), and investigation (3.18, 1.31 to 7.70). In all cases, doctors' perception of patient pressure was a stronger predictor than patients' preferences. Controlling for randomisation group, mean consultation time, or patient variables did not alter estimates or inferences.

Conclusions.—Doctors' behaviour in the consultation is most strongly associated with perceived medical need of the patient, which strongly confounds other predictors. However, a significant minority of examining, prescribing, and referral, and almost half of investigations, are still thought by the doctor to be slightly needed or not needed at all, and perceived patient pressure is a strong independent predictor of all doctor behaviours. To limit unnecessary resource use and iatrogenesis, when management decisions are not thought to be medically needed, doctors need to directly ask patients about their expectations.

▶ What factors determine how we treat our patients? Little et al found that a substantial number of examinations, tests, prescriptions, and referrals are considered by the physician to be of little value yet are ordered because of perceived patient pressure. They suggest that to limit the unnecessary use of resources, patients' expectations must be directly addressed and identified.

B. H. Thiers, MD

Marketing in the Lay Media and Prescriptions of Terbinafine in Primary Care: Dutch Cohort Study
't Jong GW, Stricker BHC, Sturkenboom MCJM (Erasmus Univ, Rotterdam, The Netherlands)
BMJ 328:931, 2004   13–6

Background.—In 2000, the Dutch company Novartis, which manufactures terbinafine, recommended for the treatment of onychomycosis, launched a nationwide information campaign in The Netherlands including television advertisements advising persons with onychomycosis to see their general practitioner about their condition. In July 2002, Novartis stopped the campaign. The changes in prescription rates of terbinafine and itraconazole during that time were determined.

Methods.—Data were obtained from a Dutch research database that included 150 general practitioners. Prescriptions written for onychomycosis between 1996 and 1999 and between 2000 and 2002 were recorded and divided by the amount of person-time in the population. The source population consisted of 470,775 patients with a total follow-up time of 1.5 million person-years.

Findings.—Between 1996 and 1999, the overall prescription rates of terbinafine and itraconazole were 6.5 and 6.84, respectively, per 1000 person-years. The terbinafine prescription rate increased from 7.7 in the month before the television campaign to 15.2 per 1000 person-years in the month after the start of the campaign. Between 2000 and 2002, the terbinafine prescription rate was 10.26 per 1000 person-years. The itraconazole prescription rate, however, decreased to 6.07 per 1000 person-years. Consultation rates for new onychomycosis were 5.9 per 1000 person-years in 1999, 8.2 in 2000 and 2001, and 4.9 in 2002.

Conclusion.—This analysis shows that the rate of terbinafine prescriptions increased markedly after the start of an information campaign about onychomycosis launched by the manufacturer of terbinafine in The Netherlands.

▶ Even without specifically mentioning the drug, Novartis was able to increase prescriptions for terbinafine, which was the treatment for onychomycosis recommended by the Dutch Society of General Practitioners' guidelines. The authors also made the provocative comment that "lay media marketing medicinal products for cosmetic indications...(increases) practitioners' workloads and costs. This may affect patients who need care for more serious problems."

B. H. Thiers, MD

14 Practice Management and Managed Care

Length of Patient's Monologue, Rate of Completion, and Relation to Other Components of the Clinical Encounter: Observational Intervention Study in Primary Care
Rabinowitz I, Luzzatti R, Tamir A, et al (Technion-Israel Inst of Technology, Haifa)
BMJ 328:501-502, 2004   14-1

Background.—The patient's opening statement is an important component of history taking. Physicians are encouraged not to interrupt the patient, but they often do so, most likely because the patient's opening statement is considered time consuming. However, several studies have shown that patients who are uninterrupted will conclude their opening statements in less than 30 seconds in primary care and in about 90 seconds in consultant settings. Primary care encounters were evaluated that included a new clinical problem. The length and rate of completion of patients' monologues were recorded before and after instructing physicians not to interrupt the patient.

Methods.—Consecutive encounters between 8 family physicians and their patients were recorded on 2 days in 6 family clinics in northern Israel. All of the physicians were videotaped on both days. The physicians had been told that the study focused on the doctor-patient interaction. Patients were also given this information. At the start of the second day, the physicians were instructed not to interrupt the patient when he or she started speaking until the physician was satisfied that the patient had finished the opening statement.

Results.—Of the 214 encounters evaluated, 112 (52%) involved a new clinical problem. The mean duration of the monologue was 26 seconds on day 1 and 28 seconds on day 2. However, the difference between the median duration of dialogues on days 1 and 2 is a better representation of the difference between baseline and postintervention (15 seconds before intervention vs 21 seconds after intervention). Twice as many monologues were completed after the intervention. A physical examination was performed in 88% of encounters, with an average duration of 1½ minutes.

Conclusions.—It takes little time to allow patients to complete their opening statements. The significant increase in the proportion of completed monologues was compatible with the observation that completed monologues are only marginally longer than interrupted ones. This findings is likely reflective of the natural brevity of patients' monologues.

▶ My mentor, Dr Richard Dobson, taught me decades ago never to interrupt the patient. His reasoning was quite simple; every interruption in effect resets the clock and starts the patient on a whole new monologue. If allowed to speak uninterrupted, most patients will, for lack of a better phrase, "run out of gas," at which time the physician can evaluate the problem and then begin his own monologue indicating his assessment of the condition and its appropriate treatment.

B. H. Thiers, MD

Health Related Virtual Communities and Electronic Support Groups: Systematic Review of the Effects of Online Peer to Peer Interactions
Eysenbach G, Powell J, Englesakis M, et al (Univ of Toronto; Univ of Southampton, England)
BMJ 328:1166-1171, 2004   14-2

Introduction.—The many virtual communities that focus on health issues often have the function and character of self-support groups. Eleven databases devoted to health, social sciences, communication, and informatics, including MEDLINE and PsycINFO, were searched for studies on the effectiveness of health-related electronic support groups.

Methods.—Articles of interest included before and after studies, interrupted time series, cohort studies, and studies with control groups. Eligible studies measured knowledge, health, psychological or social outcomes, or the use of health services. Included studies were abstracted into an electronic form consisting of 72 questions related to study characteristics and results.

Results.—Forty-five publications describing 38 distinct studies met inclusion criteria: 20 randomized trials, 3 meta-analyses, 3 nonrandomized controlled trials, 1 cohort study, and 11 before and after studies. Thirty-one studies evaluated complex interventions in which psychoeducational programs or one-to-one communication with health care professionals were often included. Outcomes frequently examined were depression and social support, and most studies yielded conflicting findings or nonsignificant effects associated with virtual community participation.

Conclusion.—Even after extensive searches, no strong evidence was found to confirm the health benefits of virtual communities and peer-to-peer online support. This does not mean that virtual communities have no effect, but quantitative research is needed to determine the conditions under which they are most effective.

▶ Patient support groups and electronic "chat rooms" are a 2-sided coin. They can be a valuable source of information and support for networked individuals. Unfortunately, many participants in such discussion groups tend to be patients who are not responding well to prescribed treatments and thus may impart an unduly pessimistic prognostic outlook to online information seekers.

B. H. Thiers, MD

Doctors' Experience With Handheld Computers in Clinical Practice: Qualitative Study
McAlearney AS, Schweikhart SB, Medow MA (Ohio State Univ, Columbus)
BMJ 328:1162-1166, 2004   14–3

Introduction.—Approximately 25% of physicians in the United States are reported to use handheld computers, and the proportion was expected to have doubled by 2005. Eight focus groups, which included clinicians from across the country with diverse training and practice patterns, were conducted to investigate doctors' perspectives on the use of handheld computers in their practice.

Methods.—Focus group sessions lasted 60 to 90 minutes and were held between April 2002 and September 2003. Two investigators conducted each session with an open-ended list of questions covering general use patterns, expectations, barriers, or challenges related to handheld computers, and organizational support.

Results.—One third of the 54 focus group participants were women, and three fourths of the participants were generalists. The group included both nonusers and users, representing a variety of levels and practice. Those who used handheld computers seemed generally satisfied, reporting increased productivity and improved patient care (Table). Barriers to use cited were comfort with present practice and a preference for paper. Participants suggested that organizations provide advice on purchase, training, and usage of the devices. Concerns were expressed about reliability, security, and overdependence on handheld computers in clinical practice.

Conclusion.—Doctors expect handheld computers to be increasingly helpful in everyday practice. Current users seem generally satisfied, and many see the devices as a means to develop their ability to access clinical information electronically.

▶ Ever the optimists, doctors expect handheld computers to become more useful in the future, with increased ease of input and options for wireless connectivity. Reliability and dependency of the devices remain a concern. Other articles in the same issue of the *BMJ* presented a comprehensive review of handheld computers[1] and a perspective on the effect on patient care of the electronic medical record.[2]

B. H. Thiers, MD

References

1. Al-Ubaydli M: Handheld computers. *BMJ* 328:1181-1184, 2004.
2. Walsh SH: The clinician's perspective on electronic health records and how they can affect patient care. *BMJ* 328:1184-1187, 2004.

TABLE.—Patterns and Characteristics of Users of Handheld Computers

Category	Non-Users	Niche Users	Routine Users	Power Users
Representation in focus groups	17%	20%	50%	13%
Use	Had never used or had used but abandoned	Regular use limited to single application; popular uses include ePocrates, MercuryMD, or scheduling function	Regular use integrated into clinical workflow and daily life; use of multiple applications for different purposes	Constant use characterised by desire to push device to its functional limits; often developed original programs or databases; described frequent upgrades
Usage replaces	Nothing	Some paper references: "It replaces the PDR"	Most paper references: "I no longer carry a calendar or most of my reference books"	All paper: It replaces "everything in my pocket"
User characteristics	Sceptical, uninterested in change, relatively uninterested in new technologies, perceive little or no value in handheld computers	Busy but list oriented, curious but hesitant, low or limited expectations, committed with one application	Willing to experiment gradually, open to new information about handheld computers, can be peer champions, recognise greater potential	Technophiles, peer champions, active promoters, like to show off latest devices and functions
Representative comments	"Paper references and nurses are quicker"; "I don't have time to figure that out"	"I don't have a lot of extra time"; "For ePocrates, it's great"	"I know it can do more"; "I think this is great"	"It's my life"; "I've always loved technology and gadgets"

(Courtesy of McAlearney AS, Schweikhart SB, Medow MA: Doctors' experience with handheld computers in clinical practice: Qualitative study. BMJ 328:1162-1166, 2004. Copyright 2004, with permission from the BMJ Publishing Group.)

Prescribing Safety Features of General Practice Computer Systems: Evaluation Using Simulated Test Cases

Fernando B, Savelyich BSP, Avery AJ, et al (Thames Avenue Surgery, Rainham, Kent, England; Univ of Nottingham, England)

BMJ 328:1171-1173, 2004   14–4

Introduction.—Computer systems containing drug interaction alerts are widely used by general practices in the United Kingdom (UK). However, a set of rules established by the National Health Service Information Authority for general practice computer systems contains only general references to safety and may not prevent contraindicated prescribing. A laboratory-based evaluation of safety features for prescribing was done, including the 4 main computing systems used in UK primary care.

Methods.—A list of 55 theoretically derived statements related to safety was circulated to 22 members of a selected multidisciplinary expert panel. Statements related to 8 broad themes covering key areas in the medicines management process. More than 90% of panel members judged 32 of the statements to be important. Eighteen scenarios were then developed from these statements (Table) and tested on the 4 computing systems, using dummy patient records. Two members of the project team independently evaluated each system.

Results.—None of the systems evaluated produced alerts for all 18 scenarios, and none warned for all 10 drug pairs considered in cases of drugs with similar names. The suppliers of each of the 4 systems agreed with the findings of this evaluation.

Conclusion.—Clinically important deficiencies were identified in the safety features of computing systems now used in about 75% of general practices in the UK. More explicit regulations are needed, and many of the observed problems could be resolved by manufacturers of the computer systems.

▶ The failure of the computer system to produce the expected alerts on a consistent basis is disconcerting but simply demonstrates that one cannot reduce the practice of medicine to a software program. On the other hand, such programs can bombard the user with warnings when alerts are really not indicated. For example, our VA prescribing system has a virtual seizure whenever ketoconazole cream is prescribed in conjunction with a drug, such as cyclosporine, that interacts with oral ketoconazole. Computer systems such as these should be viewed more as a safety net and not as a substitute for good clinical judgment.[1]

B. H. Thiers, MD

Reference

1. Ferner RE: Commentary: Computer-aided prescribing leaves holes in the safety net. *BMJ* 328:1172-1173, 2004.

TABLE.—Responses of Computer Systems Tested for Prescribing Scenarios

Test	Prescribing Scenario Tested	Alert Produced?			
		System A	System B	System C	System D
1	Aspirin prescribed for child of 8 years	No	No	No	No
2	Methotrexate prescribed in pregnancy	No	Yes	No	No
3	Penicillin prescribed in patient with penicillin allergy	No	Yes	Yes	Yes
4	Oxytetracycline prescribed in a patient with renal impairment	No	Yes	No	No
5	Enalapril prescribed in patient with renal impairment	No	No	No	No
6	Microgynon 30 (combined contraceptive pill) prescribed in patient with history of deep vein thrombosis	No	No	No	No
7	Oxytetracycline prescribed in patient with serum creatinine of 160 µmol/l	No	No	No	No
8	Propranolol prescribed in patient with history of heart failure	No	No	No	No
9	Sumatriptan prescribed in patient with history of coronary heart disease	No	No	No	No
10	Naproxen prescribed in patient with history of peptic ulcer disease	No	No	No	No
11	Propranolol prescribed in patient with history of asthma	No	No	No	No
12	Sildenafil prescribed to patient already taking isosorbide mononitrate	Yes	Yes	Yes	Yes
13	Methotrexate prescribed on a daily basis	No	Yes	No	No
14	When patient requests salbutamol inhaler it should be clear whether this has been authorised as a repeat item	Yes	No	No	No
15	Repeat prescription of salbutamol inhaler issued before it is scheduled	Yes	Yes	No	No
16	Atenolol prescribed to patient taking amiodipine*	No*	Yes	No*	No*
17	Amoxicillin prescribed to patient taking hormone replacement therapy*	No*	No*	No*	Yes
18	The 10 most frequently used drug pairs with similar names†	No	No	No	No
All	No of appropriate alerts	4	7	4	3

*In these situations "No" was the appropriate outcome since these interactions are clinically relevant (but appear as spurious alerts on some systems).

†"No" was recorded if systems failed to warn prescribers about all of these drugs with similar names.

(Courtesy of Fernando B, Savelyich BSP, Avery AJ, et al: Prescribing safety features of general practice computer systems: Evaluation using simulated test cases. *BMJ* 328:1171-1172, 2004. Copyright 2004, with permission from the BMJ Publishing Group.)

Medicare, Medicaid, and Access to Dermatologists: The Effect of Patient Insurance on Appointment Access and Wait Times

Resneck J Jr, Pletcher MJ, Lozano N (Univ of California, San Francisco)
J Am Acad Dermatol 50:85-92, 2004   14–5

Introduction.—Reductions in Medicare physician payments are raising concerns about the ability of Medicare beneficiaries to obtain physician services. An American Medical Association report published in July 2002 showed that 24% of physicians had either placed limits on the number of Medicare patients they treat or planned to institute limits in the next 6 months. To determine the impact of reduced Medicare payments on access to dermatologists, a survey gathered data on wait times for routine new-patient visits in 12 large and mid-sized communities.

Methods.—Dermatologists or members of their staff were contacted by telephone and asked whether they would be willing to participate in a study on appointment wait times. Hypothetical patients for whom appointments were sought were insured by Medicaid, Medicare, or fee-for-service private insurance. All calls were completed within a 10-day period in early December 2002. The insurance type specified for each office contact was selected in a randomized manner.

Results.—A total of 612 (97%) of 631 dermatology offices contacted agreed to participate. The vast majority of actual respondents were receptionists or schedulers. Response rates, proportion of physicians who were women (approximately 36%), and the mean age of participant physicians (51 years) were similar for each of the 3 insurance groups. Patient acceptance rates were similar for Medicare (85%) and private insurance (87%), but far lower for Medicaid (32%). The mean wait times were 37 days for patients with Medicare or private insurance versus 50 days for patients with Medicaid.

There was considerable geographic variation in acceptance rates and wait times. Both Medicare and Medicaid patients had higher rejection rates and longer wait times in areas with low payment rates relative to commercial payers. Wait times were also longer for women physicians and in communities with a low concentration of dermatologists.

Conclusion.—Patients with Medicare and private insurance appear to have comparable access to dermatologists, but Medicaid beneficiaries are clearly at a disadvantage. Medicare patients also experience access problems in areas where Medicare payments are low relative to private insurance, and this trend may increase with continued declines in Medicare physician reimbursement.

▶ The shortage of dermatologists has allowed many of us to be choosy about whom we agree to see. Access problems will likely continue until the dermatology workforce is expanded.

B. H. Thiers, MD

The Dermatology Workforce Shortage

Resneck J Jr, Kimball AB (Univ of California, San Francisco; Stanford Univ, Calif)

J Am Acad Dermatol 50:50-54, 2004   14–6

Introduction.—Previous forecasts of an oversupply of dermatologists in the United States appear to be flawed, for recent studies suggest that a shortage may exist. To more thoroughly examine the issue of a dermatology workforce shortage, anonymous surveys were administered to practicing dermatologists and recent training graduates.

Methods.—Surveys were mailed in 2002 to 4090 members of the American Academy of Dermatology Association, selected to obtain a geographic distribution that matched that of the general membership. A total of 1425 completed surveys (35%) were returned. The survey was designed to provide surrogate indicators of the supply and demand for dermatologic ser-

---

TABLE 2.—Mean Wait Time (Calendar Days) for New
Patient Appointments by Selected States

Pennsylvania	66
North Carolina	57
Minnesota	57
Wisconsin	48
Indiana	47
Virginia	43
Arizona	41
Ohio	40
Oregon	40
Connecticut	39
Illinois	39
Kansas	39
Michigan	39
Alabama	38
Tennessee	38
Massachusetts	37
Kentucky	36
Maryland	36
South Carolina	35
Utah	35
Texas	34
Florida	33
Georgia	31
Washington State	31
California	28
Colorado	27
Missouri	23
New Jersey	23
New York	23
Iowa	21
Louisiana	21
Oklahoma	21
Mississippi	18

Note: States with fewer than 10 respondents excluded from this analysis.

(Reprinted by permission of the publisher from Resneck J, Jr, Kimball AB: The dermatology workforce shortage. *J Am Acad Dermatol* 50:50-54, 2004. Copyright 2004 by Elsevier.)

---

vices. Most responders were men (70.3%) between the ages of 40 and 59 (62.6%); 52.2% practiced in a suburban area, 37.9% in an urban area, and 10.0% in a rural area. Another survey was administered in 1999, 2000, and 2002 to residency graduates attending board review courses.

Results.—The mean wait time for new patients to secure an appointment with a dermatologist was 36 calendar days. Wait times varied considerably by state, however, with means ranging from 9 to 120 days (Table 2). The overall mean wait time for established patients was 20 days. Only 20% of dermatologists described the local supply as too high; 49.9% believed that their community needed more dermatologists, especially medical and general dermatologists. A third of practices reported that they were looking for new associates. Most recent graduates (86%-93%) had no difficulty in finding desirable positions, and only 10% were not satisfied with their current job.

Conclusion.—The current supply of dermatologists appears to be inadequate, based upon findings of surveys that examined wait times, physician perceptions, openings at established practices, and the experience of recent graduates entering the workforce.

▶ Resneck and Kimball confirm that there is now a considerable undersupply of dermatologists. Ways to fill the gap include training more residents and increasing the use of physician extenders. As the authors conclude, if dermatologists do not provide dermatologic care, it will be provided by someone else.

B. H. Thiers, MD

Gender and Parenting Significantly Affect Work Hours of Recent Dermatology Program Graduates

Jacobson CC, Nguyen JC, Kimball AB (Stanford Univ, Calif)
Arch Dermatol 140:191-196, 2004   14-7

Background.—The proportion of female physicians has increased in the past 30 years. This fact may have important implications for future workforce needs. The roles of sex, marital status, and parenting in future dermatologist employment choices were investigated.

Methods.—An anonymous survey was distributed to recent dermatology residents taking a board examination review course between 1999 and 2002. The main outcome measures were the number of hours per weeks that respondents saw patients and number of hours per week spent in each field of dermatology.

Findings.—One hundred ninety-one residents responded to the survey in 2002, for a 54% response rate,. Fifty-seven percent were women. Women saw patients for a mean 26 hours per week, compared with a mean of 31 hours for men. Women spent more time practicing medical dermatology. Marital status had no significant effect on number of hours worked. Women and men without children worked a comparable number of hours per week.

However, men with children saw patients for a mean of 34 hours per week, compared with 24 hours for women with children. Men with children spent more hours a week seeing patients than men who did not have children. The opposite was true for women; that is, women parents spent less time seeing patients than women who were not parents.

Conclusions.—Gender alone had little impact on dermatologists' workforce choices. However, parenting and gender together do affect such choices.

▶ The data clearly show that neither sex nor marital status affects the number of hours a dermatologist works until children are thrown into the equation, at which time female parents work less time than male parents. This demonstrates that women still carry most of the child-rearing responsibilities, whereas men take on more of the economic obligations in the family structure.

B. H. Thiers, MD

Compensation and Advancement of Women in Academic Medicine: Is There Equity?
Ash AS, Carr PL, Goldstein R, et al (Boston Univ)
Ann Intern Med 141:205-212, 2004   14–8

Background.—Women have been entering academic medicine in numbers at least equal to men for several decades, but women do not appear to advance in academic rank as quickly and their salaries have not attained parity. Equity in promotion and salary for female and male medical school faculty nationwide was investigated.

Methods.—Twenty-four randomly selected US medical schools were mailed surveys. Data were obtained on a total of 1814 full-time medical school faculty in 1995 and 1996. Research subjects were stratified by sex, specialty, and graduation cohort.

Findings.—Female faculty with similar professional roles and achievement as men were less likely than men to be full professors. Sixty-six percent of men and only 47% of women with 15 to 19 years of seniority were full professors. Logistic models accounting for a broad range of other professional characteristics and achievements, such as total career publications, years of seniority, hours worked per week, department type, minority status, medical versus nonmedical final degree, and school, confirmed that large deficits existed in rank for senior faculty women. Similar multivariate modeling also indicated an inequity in compensation. The base salaries of nonphysician faculty were comparable for men and women, but female physician faculty salaries were a mean $11,691 less than male physician faculty salaries. Both physician and nonphysician women with greater seniority had larger deficits in salary.

Conclusions.—Despite similar professional roles and achievements, female medical school faculty do not advance as rapidly as their male colleagues, nor are the women compensated as well as are the men. Deficits are greater for female physician than for female nonphysician faculty. Among physicians and nonphysicians, women's deficits are most pronounced for faculty with more seniority.

▶ The authors conclude their article by stating that "medical schools should closely examine their environment for gender equity in promotion and compensation." An accompanying editorial[1] suggested ways to remedy this disparity.

B. H. Thiers, MD

Reference

1. Laine C, Turner BJ: Unequal pay for equal work: The gender gap in academic medicine. *Ann Intern Med* 141:238-240, 2004.

Medicaid Prior-Authorization Programs and the Use of Cyclooxygenase-2 Inhibitors
Fischer MA, Schneeweiss S, Avorn J, et al (Harvard Med School, Boston)
N Engl J Med 351:2187-2194, 2004   14–9

Introduction.—During the past 5 years, selective cyclooxygenase-2 inhibitors (coxibs) have been responsible for an increasing proportion of prescriptions for nonsteroidal anti-inflammatory drugs (NSAIDs). To control costs, Medicaid programs have implemented prior-authorization requirements in many states before coxibs can be prescribed. The effect of such programs on the use of coxibs by Medicaid beneficiaries was evaluated.

Methods.—State Medicaid agencies were surveyed to ascertain whether prescription of coxibs needed prior authorization and, if so, what were the criteria for authorization. For each program, these criteria were compared with those of evidence-based criteria for prescribing coxibs. With the use of data for all filled prescriptions in 50 state Medicaid programs from 1999 through the end of 2003, the proportion of defined daily doses of NSAIDs that were coxibs were calculated. Changes were evaluated in prescription patterns after implementation of each prior-authorization program.

Results.—By 2001, coxibs comprised half of all NSAID doses covered by Medicaid. This proportion varied widely according to state in 2003, from a low of 11% to a high of 70% of all NSAID doses. Twenty-two states implemented prior-authorization programs for coxibs during the evaluation period. Overall, the implementation of such programs diminished the proportion of NSAID doses that were coxibs by 15.0% (95% CI, 10.9%-19.2%), which corresponded to a reduction of $10.28 (95% CI, $7.56-$13.00) in spending per NSAID prescription. The effect of such programs was not impacted by the extent to which they incorporated evidence-based prescribing recommendations.

Conclusion.—Implementation of Medicaid prior-authorization programs was linked with a marked reduction in the use of coxibs and consequent large reductions in spending by state Medicaid programs.

▶ Dermatologists are quite familiar with prior authorization programs for prescription drugs; the one that comes first to mind is topical tretinoin. Such policies clearly result in substantial cost savings, but the questions that remain are whether they are clinically appropriate and whether they compromise patient care. The most effective policies will be those that can contain escalating pharmaceutical costs while preserving appropriate clinical decision making.

B. H. Thiers, MD

Utilization of Nonsteroidal Anti-inflammatory Drugs and Antisecretory Agents: A Managed Care Claims Analysis
Ofman JJ, Badamgarav E, Henning JM, et al (Cedars-Sinai Med Ctr, Los Angeles; Zynx Health-A Cerner Company, Beverly Hills, Calif; TAP Pharmaceutical Products Inc, Lake Forest, Ill; et al)
Am J Med 116:835-842, 2004   14–10

Purpose.—To describe patients initiating nonsteroidal anti-inflammatory drug (NSAID) therapy with regard to gastrointestinal and cardiac risks and patterns of antisecretory agent use, and to explore the relation between therapy type and subsequent outcomes.

Methods.—We studied patients aged 18 years or older who had continuous coverage from 1998 to 2001 and who had initiated treatment with cyclooxygenase-2 (COX-2) selective inhibitors or nonselective NSAIDs. Patients were categorized with respect to gastrointestinal and cardiac risk profiles. Proton pump inhibitor use within 15 days of initiating NSAID therapy was considered prophylactic. Logistic regression analysis was used to evaluate associations between treatment and hospitalization events, cardiac events, and health care costs.

Results.—We identified 106,564 eligible NSAID initiators: 65.2% used COX-2 inhibitors and 34.8% used traditional NSAIDs. Users of COX-2 inhibitors were more likely to be at higher risk of gastrointestinal bleeding and cardiac events than were NSAID users. Proton pump inhibitor prophylaxis was most common among users of COX-2 inhibitors, but was only 11% in patients at high risk of gastrointestinal bleeding. There were no differences among treatment groups in terms of gastrointestinal or cardiac events. Initiation of COX-2 inhibitor therapy was associated with greater total health care costs.

Conclusion.—Although we found that COX-2 inhibitors were used more frequently than were traditional NSAIDs in certain groups of patients with varying cardiac or gastrointestinal risk, we did not find that their use resulted in reductions in clinical events, cotherapy with proton pump inhibitors, or costs, suggesting that a better understanding of the relation between NSAID treatment strategies and outcomes in patients with differing risk characteristics is needed.

▶ Although COX-2 inhibitors were used more frequently than traditional NSAIDs in patients fitting various cardiac or gastrointestinal risk profiles, their use did not result in decreases in adverse effects, fewer prescriptions of proton pump inhibitors, or reduced costs. This suggests that the clinical benefits of these drugs may be more perceived than real.

B. H. Thiers, MD

Cost-Lowering Strategies Used by Medicare Beneficiaries Who Exceed Drug Benefit Caps and Have a Gap in Drug Coverage
Tseng C-W, Brook RH, Keeler E, et al (Univ of Hawaii, Honolulu; Pacific Health Research, Honolulu; University of California, Los Angeles; et al)
JAMA 292:952-960, 2004   14–11

Introduction.—A gap in the new national Medicare drug benefit means that individuals with high medication expenditures will face a period without coverage. When total drug costs exceed $2500 in a given year, no further coverage is provided for the rest of the year unless total drug costs exceed $5100. Patients may reduce medication use during the period in which they are responsible for the entire cost of prescriptions. Medicare + Choice beneficiaries, 65 years or older, were surveyed about their financial burden and strategies adopted to lower prescription costs.

Methods.—Participants were drawn from Medicare enrollees in a single state's Medicare + Choice plan. All had filled at least 1 prescription in 2001. A total of 665 patients exceeded a $750 or $1200 yearly cap and had coverage gaps of 75 to 180 days in 2001. The 643 control participants had $2000 caps, which they did not exceed. Study group members and control subjects were matched for age and average monthly drug costs (patient plus plan costs). All participants were asked about their strategies for lowering out-of-pocket medication costs. Financial burden was measured by self-reported ease or difficulty in paying for prescriptions.

Results.—Multivariate analysis revealed that, compared with control subjects, a higher proportion of patients who exceeded caps reported using less of their prescribed medications (18% vs 10%, respectively). Eight percent of both groups, however, reported stopping medications completely, and similar proportions did not start prescribed medications (6% and 5%, respectively). Compared with control subjects, patients with coverage gaps were more likely to call pharmacies to find the best price, to switch medications, to use samples, and to report difficulty paying for prescriptions (62% vs 37% for control subjects). Many of the drugs that were either not started or were reduced or discontinued had been prescribed for serious chronic conditions.

Conclusion.—Gaps in coverage may lead many Medicare beneficiaries to decrease dosage or stop essential medications for the treatment of disabling and potentially life-threatening illnesses. Even when they increased their efforts to obtain drugs at lower cost, half of the participants experienced difficulty in paying for prescriptions.

Clinician Identification of Chronically Ill Patients Who Have Problems Paying for Prescription Medications

Heisler M, Wagner TH, Piette JD (Dept of Veterans Affairs Ctr, Ann Arbor, Mich; Univ of Michigan, Ann Arbor; Dept of Veterans Affairs, Palo Alto, Calif; et al)
Am J Med 116:753-758, 2004   14–12

Purpose.—Little is known about whether health care providers are effectively identifying patients who have difficulty covering the costs of out-of-pocket prescription medications. We examined whether and how providers are identifying chronically ill adults who have potential problems paying for prescription medications.

Methods.—We conducted a cross-sectional survey of a national sample of 4050 adults aged 50 years or older who use prescription medications for at least one of five chronic health conditions. The primary outcome measure was patient report of being asked by a doctor or nurse in the prior 12 months whether the patient could afford the prescribed medication. The measures of prescription cost burden were cost-related underuse of medications, cutting back on other necessities to pay for medications, and worries about medication costs. We adjusted for patient income, education, race/ethnicity, age, sex, health status, number of prescribed medications, pharmacy benefits, frequency of outpatient visits, having a regular health care provider, and sampling weights.

Results.—In the weighted analyses, 16% (547/4050) of respondents reported that they had been asked about potential problems paying for a prescribed medication. Only 360 (24%) of the 1499 respondents who reported one or more burdens from out-of-pocket medication costs reported being asked this question. After adjusting for potential confounders, patients who had cut back on medication use or other necessities to cover payments were no more likely than other patients to be asked about the ability to pay for prescription medications. Concerns about medication costs, being a racial/ethnic minority, taking seven or more prescription medications, and having no prescription coverage were independently associated with a greater likelihood of being asked about possible problems with prescription costs.

Conclusion.—Few chronically ill patients who are at risk of or experiencing problems related to prescription medication costs report that their clinicians had asked them about possible medication payment difficulties.

▶ The new, much-touted national Medicare prescription drug benefit plan will pay 75% of prescription drug costs for beneficiaries until their total drug costs exceed $2250; subsequently, there is no further coverage for the remainder of the year until total drug costs exceed $5100. Thus, a gap in coverage is created during which patients must pay the entire cost of their medications. Tseng et al (Abstract 14–11) studied the impact of this coverage gap on prescription drug use. Not surprisingly, they showed that Medicare beneficiaries often had difficulty in paying for prescriptions and decreased their use of essential medications for potentially life-threatening illnesses such hypertension and diabetes when they fell into the "donut hole" in the drug benefit plan. As noted by Heisler et al (Abstract 14–12), physicians need to be more aware of the financial impact of the prescriptions they prescribe and discuss with their patients possible medication payment difficulties. Clinicians, insurance companies, and the public need to be more sensitive in designing prescription drug plans that appropriately balance costs and benefits.

B. H. Thiers, MD

15 Miscellaneous Topics in Clinical Dermatology

Treatment of Cutaneous Sarcoidosis With Thalidomide
Nguyen YT, Dupuy A, Cordoliani F, et al (Hôpital Saint Louis, Paris)
J Am Acad Dermatol 50:235-241, 2004   15–1

Background.—Some evidence suggests that thalidomide may be effective against cutaneous sarcoidosis. The authors added 12 cases to reports of thalidomide use in patients with cutaneous sarcoidosis.

Methods.—The medical records of 5 men (mean age, 31 years) and 7 women (mean age, 41 years) with cutaneous sarcoidosis who were treated between 2000 and 2002 were reviewed.

Results.—Patients were treated with oral thalidomide, 50 to 200 mg/d, for 2 to more than 17 months. Four patients (33%) had a complete response (disappearance of all cutaneous lesions), 6 (50%) had a partial response (skin lesions improved without complete regression), and 2 (17%) had stable disease during treatment. The average time for cutaneous lesion regression was 2 to 3 months (Fig 1).

Symptoms in other systems (nasopharynx, lungs, nervous system, liver) improved in some patients as well. Three patients relapsed after discontinuing thalidomide. The drug was well tolerated, but 3 patients had paresthesias, 3 had constipation, and 3 had diurnal drowsiness while taking the drug. Additionally, 1 patient had a deep venous thrombosis while taking thalidomide.

Conclusion.—Thalidomide appears to be effective and safe for treating cutaneous sarcoidosis. Further study is required to optimize its use in this population.

▶ A larger controlled investigation is needed to confirm these results. The data presented here suggest that thalidomide only temporary alleviates, rather than eradicates, the cutaneous disease, as relapses occur in most patients when the drug is discontinued.

B. H. Thiers, MD

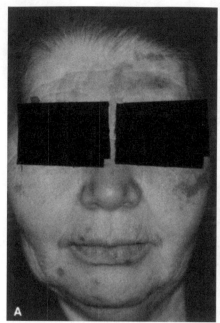 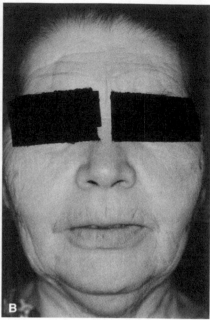

FIGURE 1.—Patient with infiltrated plaques and papules before (**A**) and after (**B**) 2 months of treatment with thalidomide (100 mg/d). (Reprinted by permission of the publisher from Nguyen YT, Dupuy A, Cordoliani F, et al: Treatment of cutaneous sarcoidosis with thalidomide. *J Am Acad Dermatol* 50:235-241, 2004. Copyright 2004 by Elsevier.)

A Prospective Proof of Concept Study of the Efficacy of Tacrolimus Ointment on Uraemic Pruritus (UP) in Patients on Chronic Dialysis Therapy

Kuypers DR, Claes K, Evenepoel P, et al (Univ Hosps Leuven, Belgium)
Nephrol Dial Transplant 19:1895-1901, 2004   15–2

Background.—Many patients receiving chronic dialysis therapy have uremic pruritus (UP), which can cause serious skin damage and can disrupt sleep. Some evidence suggests that UP may be an inflammatory systemic disease rather than a local skin disorder. The effects of topical tacrolimus on the incidence and severity of UP in patients receiving chronic dialysis were examined.

Methods.—The research subjects were 21 patients receiving chronic dialysis therapy who had UP (8 men and 13 women; mean age, 61.6 years). First, patients applied 0.1% tacrolimus ointment for 3 weeks, then they applied 0.03% tacrolimus ointment for 3 weeks (total of 6 weeks of uninterrupted active treatment). Patients were evaluated at baseline, during tacrolimus application, and at week 8 (ie, after a 2-week washout) to evaluate their UP symptoms. UP was assessed according to a modified score that considered the severity and distribution of pruritus and sleep disturbance and a 10-point visual analog scale (VAS).

Results.—The modified pruritus assessment score at baseline (median, 11) decreased significantly during 6 weeks of tacrolimus therapy (median score, 2; decrease of 81.8%) then returned toward baseline values at week 8 (median score, 8). Results were similar with the VAS ratings: the median VAS score decreased by 42.9% between baseline and week 6 (from 7 to 4) then returned toward baseline values at week 8 (median VAS score, 6). No systemic reactions to tacrolimus ointment were noted, but 4 patients reported transient stinging and burning during the first week of treatment; 1 patient had a mild skin rash. No serious adverse events occurred, and tacrolimus ointment was well tolerated.

Conclusion.—This prospective, open-label, single-center, proof-of concept study indicates that 6 weeks of treatment with tacrolimus ointment significantly reduces the severity of UP in patients receiving chronic dialysis. It is also well tolerated.

▶ Although the results are encouraging, larger, randomized, placebo-controlled trials are necessary for confirmation. The financial implications of tacrolimus treatment are considerable, as the itching that affects patients with UP is often severe and involves a large portion of the body surface area.

B. H. Thiers, MD

A Comparative Study on the Effects of Naltrexone and Loratadine on Uremic Pruritus

Legroux-Crespel E, Clèdes J, Misery L (Univ Hosp, Brest, France)
Dermatology 208:326-330, 2004   15–3

Background.—Research has yielded inconsistent findings on the efficacy of naltrexone in patients with uremic pruritus. The efficacy and tolerance of naltrexone and loratadine were compared in this patient population.

Methods.—Fifty-two patients with uremic pruritus undergoing hemodialysis participated in the study. Treatment consisted of 50 mg/d naltrexone or 10 mg/d loratadine for 2 weeks after a 48-hour washout period. The intensity of pruritus was scored on a visual analog scale (VAS).

Findings.—The mean posttreatment VAS scores did not differ between the 2 groups. However, in 7 patients, naltrexone administration resulted in a dramatic decline in VAS scores. The main adverse events associated with naltrexone were nausea and sleep disturbances, occurring in 10 of the 26 recipients of the drug.

Conclusions.—Naltrexone seems to be effective only in a subset of patients. In addition, adverse effects were common with naltrexone. Thus, this agent may be considered for second-line treatment of uremic pruritus. A difference in naltrexone efficacy and tolerance among patients may be related to individual differences in metabolism.

▶ Previous published studies on naltrexone for the relief of uremic pruritus have yielded contradictory results. Peer et al[1] found a significant decrease in pruritus in all of their 15 treated patients, whereas Pauli-Magnus et al[2] could not confirm these results in a similar study involving 23 patients.

B. H. Thiers, MD

References

1. Peer G, Kivity S, Agami O: Randomized crossover trial of naltrexone in uremic pruritus. *Lancet* 348:1552-1554, 1996.
2. Pauli-Magnus C, Mikus G, Alscher D, et al: Naltrexone does not relieve uremic pruritus: Results of a randomized, double-blind, placebo-controlled crossover study. *J Am Soc Nephrol* 11:514-519, 2000.

Palifermin for Oral Mucositis After Intensive Therapy for Hematologic Cancers

Spielberger R, Stiff P, Bensinger W, et al (City of Hope Natl Med Ctr, Duarte, Calif; Loyola Univ, Maywood, Ill; Fred Hutchinson Cancer Research Ctr, Seattle, Wash; et al)

N Engl J Med 35:2590-2598, 2004

15–4

Introduction.—Oral mucositis, a common complication of high-dose chemotherapy and radiation, can produce potentially life-threatening complications in severe cases. No standard therapy is available, however, to prevent or treat severe oral mucositis. Patients with hematologic cancers participated in a trial that tested the safety and efficacy of palifermin (recombinant human keratinocyte growth factor) in the treatment of oral mucosal injury induced by cytotoxic therapy.

Methods.—In a double-blind manner, 106 patients were randomly assigned to palifermin (60 µg/kg of body weight per day) and 106 to placebo. Treatment was given IV for 3 consecutive days immediately before the initiation of conditioning therapy (fractionated total-body irradiation plus high-dose chemotherapy) and after autologous hematopoietic stem-cell transplantation. Patients were evaluated daily for 28 days after transplantation.

Results.—The 2 patient groups were similar in baseline characteristics. World Health Organization (WHO) grade 3 or 4 oral mucositis developed in 63% of patients in the palifermin group versus 98% of those in the placebo group. The median duration of oral mucositis of grade 3 or 4 was 6.0 days for affected patients in the palifermin group and 9.0 days for those in the placebo group. Both the incidence and duration of WHO grade 4 oral mucositis were significantly reduced when palifermin recipients were compared with placebo recipients. Palifermin was similarly beneficial and superior to placebo when median scores for soreness of the throat and mouth, use of opioid analgesics, and need for total parenteral nutrition were compared. Adverse events associated with palifermin included rash, pruritus, erythema, mouth and tongue disorders, and taste alteration. These effects ranged from mild to moderate in severity but were temporary.

Conclusion.—Palifermin was safe and effective when used to reduce the severity and duration of oral mucositis in patients treated with intensive chemotherapy and radiotherapy for hematologic cancers. The most debilitating form of oral mucositis, WHO grade 4, occurred in 62% of the placebo group versus 20% in the palifermin group.

▶ Spielberger et al report the use of palifermin, a recombinant keratinocyte growth factor, to decrease oral mucositis induced by cytotoxic therapy. As noted by Garfunkel[1] in an accompanying editorial, rapid advances are being made in the understanding of the pathogenesis, prevention, and treatment of this condition. Mucositis induced by chemotherapy is not simply an epithelial process, but involves microvascular injury as well. Keratinocyte growth factor will likely be only 1 component of a multifaceted approach to this troublesome condition.

B. H. Thiers, MD

Reference

1. Garfunkel AA: Oral mucositis—The search for a solution. *N Engl J Med* 351:2649-2650, 2004.

Bilateral Diagonal Earlobe Crease and Coronary Artery Disease: A Significant Association
Evrengül H, Dursunoğlu D, Kaftan A, et al (Pamukkale Univ, Denizli, Turkey; Ege Univ, Izmir, Turkey; Cag Hosp, Ankara, Turkey)
Dermatology 209:271-275, 2004   15–5

Background.—The debate continues as to whether the presence of a diagonal earlobe crease (ELC) is associated with an increased risk of coronary artery disease (CAD). These authors evaluated the incidence of bilateral ELC in patients with proven CAD, and a possible association between ELC and other risk factors for coronary atherosclerosis.

Methods.—The subjects were 415 patients (72.5% men; mean age, 58.9 years) undergoing coronary angiography for angina pectoris, prior acute myocardial infarction, atypical cardiac complaints, or a positive treadmill exercise test. The incidence of bilateral ELC (defined as a deep crease or wrinkle present bilaterally on free or attached earlobes that descended obliquely and posterolaterally across at least half of the earlobe) was compared between the 119 patients (28.7%) with no angiographic evidence of CAD and the 296 patients (71.3%) with angiographically confirmed CAD. Possible correlations between bilateral ELC and traditional coronary risk factors (sex, age, family history of CAD, hypertension, diabetes mellitus, cigarette smoking, lipidemia, obesity) were also examined.

Results.—Bilateral ELC was significantly more common in the patients with CAD than in the patients without CAD (51.4% vs 15.1%). Bilateral ELC was also significantly correlated with hypertension, older age, being male, cigarette smoking, and a family history of CAD. Multivariate regression analyses showed bilateral ELC was a significant and independent predictor of CAD. The presence of bilateral ELC had a sensitivity of 51.3%, specificity of 84.8%, positive predictive value of 89.4%, and negative predictive value of 41.2% in predicting the presence of CAD.

Conclusion.—In these patients undergoing coronary angiography, the presence of bilateral diagonal ELC was significantly associated with the presence of CAD and many traditional coronary risk factors. Dermatologists could play an important role in identifying patients with possible CAD on the basis of the presence of bilateral diagonal ELC.

▶ The authors found the diagonal ELC to be an independent predictive variable for CAD. The cohort studied included patients admitted for coronary angiography. A similar study based on an unselected group of patients would help to confirm the predictive value of this finding.

B. H. Thiers, MD

Photokeratitis and UV-Radiation Burns Associated With Damaged Metal Halide Lamps
Kirschke DL, Jones TF, Smith NM, et al (Ctrs for Disease Control and Prevention, Atlanta, Ga; Tennessee Dept of Health, Nashville; Vanderbilt Univ, Nashville, Tenn)
Arch Pediatr Adolesc Med 158:372-376, 2004   15–6

Introduction.—Mercury-vapor or metal halide lamps, often used to light gymnasiums, can cause photokeratitis and UV-radiation (UVR) burns when the lamps' outer glass envelope is broken. Although the Food and Drug Administration requires warning labels on these lamps and has published recommendations to prevent injuries, outbreaks of photokeratitis and UVR burns continue to be reported. Three outbreaks involving 273 potentially exposed individuals were investigated.

Methods.—The initial outbreak was reported to the Tennessee Department of Health, Nashville, in February 2003. Publicity about 8 individuals who experienced severe eye symptoms after attending an event in a gymnasium led to the identification of 2 subsequent outbreaks. Questionnaires were administered to those attending the initial event, and measurements were taken in the gymnasium with the use a radiometer–photometer to estimate the hazard created by the damaged lamp.

Results.—An estimated total of 600 individuals attended the fund-raiser and were seated at tables arranged throughout the gymnasium. Eighteen attendees met the case definition for photokeratitis: acute characteristic eye symptoms and onset within 12 hours of the event, affecting individuals with no pre-existing eye symptoms. Thirteen (72%) of these patients had UVR burns, most commonly on the forehead or eyelids. The high-risk area for photokeratitis and UVR burns was the back of the gymnasium, where 46% of attendees were affected. Two attendees who were wearing UVR protective eyeglasses had face burns but no eye symptoms. None of the 3 facilities had complied with preventive recommendations.

Conclusion.—Damaged metal halide lamps in the second outbreak created an intensity of UVR radiation that would limit occupational exposure to 10 to 15 minutes. Actual exposure times, however, ranged from 2 to 3 hours. The Centers for Disease Control and Prevention advises minimizing UVR exposure, especially in children. Because damage to the metal halide lamps in facilities such as gymnasiums may go unrecognized, self-extinguishing lamps or enclosed fixtures are recommended by the Food and Drug Administration. The National Electric Code may need to be amended to ensure compliance.

▶ Erythema, edema, and subsequent desquamation of the eyelids and the skin adjacent to the eyes, along with keratitis, may result from UVR burns associated with damaged metal halide lamps. The authors suggest that the condition is underrecognized and that the symptoms are often misdiagnosed as an infectious process. Because of the involvement of the skin surrounding the eyes, patients could potentially present to the dermatologist. Although the injury generally resolves spontaneously, recognition might lead to the discovery of a damaged lamp as the source of the injury and prevent harm to other individuals.

S. Raimer, MD

Systematic Review: Surveillance Systems for Early Detection of Bioterrorism-Related Diseases

Bravata DM, McDonald KM, Smith WM, et al (Univ of California, San Francisco; Stanford Univ, Calif; Veterans Affairs Palo Alto Healthcare System, Calif; et al)
Ann Intern Med 140:910-922, 2004   15–7

Background.—The threat of bioterrorism and the availability of electronic data for surveillance have prompted a multitude of surveillance systems. The goal of a surveillance system, according to the Centers for Disease Control and Prevention, is to "collect and analyze morbidity, mortality, and other relevant data and facilitate the timely dissemination of results to appropriate decision makers." A systematic review was undertaken to investigate surveillance systems for detecting illness and syndromes potentially associated with bioterrorism-related pathogens.

Methods.—The authors searched electronic databases of peer-reviewed articles (MEDLINE, GrayLIT, National Technical Information Service), government Web sites and reports, commercial and academic Web sites and reports, relevant reference lists, and conference proceedings to identify candidates for inclusion in their analyses. Only studies describing or evaluating systems for collecting, analyzing, or presenting surveillance data for illnesses or syndromes potentially related to bioterrorism were eligible for inclusion.

Results.—Of the 17,510 articles and 8088 Web sites reviewed, the authors identified 192 reports of 115 systems eligible for inclusion. Of these

115 surveillance systems, 29 systems were designed explicitly for bioterrorism-related surveillances, including 9 designed to monitor the incidence of bioterrorism-related syndromes and 20 designed to monitor environmental samples for possible bioterrorism agents. The remaining 86 systems were designed to monitor naturally occurring illnesses that could be relevant to bioterrorism surveillance (ie, collection of antimicrobial resistance data or food-borne illness data).

Only 2 of the 9 syndromic surveillance systems, and non of the 20 environmental monitoring systems, were evaluated in peer-reviewed studies. Furthermore, data on sensitivity and specificity were available for only 3 of these systems. The 9 surveillance systems collecting syndrome reports have been used for continuous bioterrorism surveillance and for event-based surveillance (eg, at the 1999 World Trade Organization Summit). However, there have been no published reports of the efficacy of event-based surveillance systems.

Conclusion.—Only a few systems have been designed specifically to collect and analyze data for the early detection of bioterrorism-related illnesses or syndromes. Furthermore, there are few data available on the sensitivity and specificity of these surveillance systems and their ability to facilitate decision making in a bioterrorist attack. Thus, decisions based on these systems may be compromised.

▶ Bioterrorism surveillance systems monitor either the incidence of bioterrorism-related syndromes or perform environmental sampling for bioterrorism agents. The authors argue that existing surveillance systems for detecting bioterrorism have not been sufficiently evaluated to judge their effectiveness.

B. H. Thiers, MD

DERMATOLOGIC SURGERY AND CUTANEOUS ONCOLOGY

16 Nonmelanoma Skin Cancer

Mice With Genetically Determined High Susceptibility to Ultraviolet (UV)-Induced Immunosuppression Show Enhanced UV Carcinogenesis
Noonan FP, Muller HK, Fears TR, et al (George Washington Univ, Washington, DC; Univ of Tasmania, Hobart, Australia; Natl Cancer Inst, Bethesda, Md; et al)
J Invest Dermatol 121:1175-1181, 2003   16–1

Introduction.—Ultraviolet (UV) B is known to initiate selective immuno-suppression in both humans and experimental animals, and this form of im-munosuppression appears to be a critical step in UV carcinogenesis. The in-duction of UV skin cancer was studied in 2 strains of mice to examine the premise that genetically determined differences in susceptibility to UV-induced immunosuppression are reflected in UV carcinogenesis.

Methods.—Animals used in the study were male $CB6F_1$ hybrid and $B6CF_1$ hybrid mice, which differed approximately 2-fold in their susceptibility to UV immunosuppression. Four experimental groups were treated 3 times weekly with 2 UV regimens, with daily doses increasing from 2.25 to 6 or 4.5 to 12 kJ per m^2. The mice were monitored weekly for tumor development and were euthanized before tumors reached 1 cm in any dimension. Speci-mens of tumors were obtained for histologic examination.

Results.—The mean number of tumors per mouse was 1.5 for all groups. Unirradiated mice in a control group showed no tumor development over the course of 365 days. In the 4 treatment groups, survival without a skin tumor differed by group and according to UV regimen within each strain. The differences between strains were significant for the higher dose only, suggesting a dose-strain interaction.

Tumor-free survival in animals receiving the higher UV dose was reduced significantly more in the $CB6F_1$ strain than in the $B6CF_1$ strain. Histologic examination identified fibrosarcomas, squamous carcinomas, and mixed tu-mors. There was a significantly greater proportion of mixed tumors in the $CB6F_1$ males that received the higher UV protocol, indicative of their en-hanced susceptibility to UV carcinogenesis. This dose-strain interaction ap-peared only in the development of mixed tumors.

Conclusion.—Within both strains of mice, the higher UV dose resulted in a significantly faster development of tumors than did the lower UV dose. But when both strains received the higher dose, mice with higher susceptibility to UV-induced immunosuppression showed much faster tumor development than mice with lower susceptibility when both strains received the higher dose.

▶ The results support the importance of UV-induced immunosuppression in the pathogenesis of skin cancer.

B. H. Thiers, MD

Changing Patterns of Sun Protection Between the First and Second Summers for Very Young Children
Benjes LS, Brooks DR, Zhang Z, et al (Boston Univ; Massachusetts Dept of Health, Boston; Falmouth Hosp, Mass)
Arch Dermatol 140:925-930, 2004   16–2

Background.—Many skin cancers are caused by excessive and unprotected exposure to the sun. Painful sunburns during childhood are a significant factor in the development of melanoma, and yet at least two thirds of children in the United States are not adequately protected from the sun despite numerous federal recommendations for safe sun practices. Whether an intensive intervention directed at mothers of newborns would increase levels of sun protection practices and decrease the rates of sunburning for their children was determined. In addition, the changes in sun protection practices and burning rates experienced between the first and second summers of life were assessed.

Methods.—This randomized study was conducted among mothers of infants living in a coastal town in Massachusetts. The mothers were randomly selected to receive hospital education alone or hospital education plus tailored materials and telephone counseling. The main outcome measures were sun protection practices for children and the degree of skin damage at mean ages of 6 and 18 months, as reported by the mother.

Results.—Baseline surveys were completed by 108 mothers, and 92 (85%) completed posttests. Few differences were observed between the intervention and control groups in the use of sun protection for infants from the first summer to the second summer. The child's routine use of hats, shirts, and shade decreased significantly from the first to the second summer, while sunscreen use increased from 34% to 93% for the same period. In the first summer, 22% of children received a sunburn or tan compared with 54% during the second summer.

Conclusions.—The decline in comprehensive sun protection for children occurs at a much earlier age than has been previously reported. A need exists for more studies that focus on parental attitudes regarding the necessity and practice of vigilant sun protection as children grow from infant to toddler.

▶ This study demonstrated an increase in the use of sunscreens but a decrease in physical barrier protection between the first and second years of life among 92 predominantly fair-skinned children. This was associated with increased evidence of solar damage. It is surprising that sun protection decreased so early when, except for frequently not being able to keep a hat on a toddler, parents can generally control the kind of clothing worn and the amount of time children are exposed to sun at this age. Parents were good about sunscreen use; it is likely that they have a misperception about how complete protection is achieved with sunscreen use. Therefore, as physicians, we need to continue to emphasize the importance of shade and physical barriers for sun protection.

S. Raimer, MD

Imiquimod 5% Cream for the Treatment of Actinic Keratosis: Results From Two Phase III, Randomized, Double-blind, Parallel Group, Vehicle-controlled Trials
Lebwohl M, Dinehart S, Whiting D, et al (Mount Sinai School of Medicine, New York; Univ of Arkansas, Little Rock; Bressinck, Gibson, Parker, Dinehart and Sangster Dermatology, Little Rock, Ark; et al)
J Am Acad Dermatol 50:714-721, 2004   16–3

Background.—Suppression of the cutaneous immune response plays a critical role in the pathogenesis of actinic keratosis (AK). Imiquimod is an immune system stimulator approved for the treatment of external genital warts. Two phase III trials were undertaken to evaluate the efficacy and safety of topical 5% imiquimod cream in the treatment of AKs on the face and balding scalp.

Methods.—Data from 2 phase III trials involving 436 patients at 24 centers in the United States and Canada were pooled. All patients had 4 to 8 AKs located on the face or balding scalp. Patients (87% men; mean age, about 66 years) were randomly assigned to apply either vehicle or 5% imiquimod cream to their AKs once per day, 2 days per week for 16 weeks. Patients were evaluated 8 weeks after the end of treatment to assess the clinical response. A complete response was defined as the absence of clinically visible AKs in the treatment area. A partial response was defined as a 75% or greater reduction in the number of AKs in the treatment area compared with baseline.

Results.—Significantly more patients in the imiquimod group had complete clearance (45.1% vs 3.2%; Fig 2) and partial clearance (59.1% vs 11.8%). The median percent reduction in AKs was also significantly higher in the imiquimod group (83.3% vs 0%). Overall, imiquimod was well tolerated. Drug-related adverse events were more common with imiquimod than with vehicle (34.4% vs 14.9%), but none was serious. The imiquimod group had significantly more patients with itching (20.5% vs 6.8%), burning (5.6% vs 1.8%), or bleeding (3.3% vs 0.5%) at the application site. Erythema at the treatment site was also more common with imiquimod (17.7% vs 2.3%).

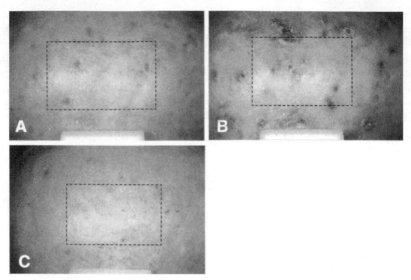

FIGURE 2.—**A,** Baseline count of 4 AKs in treatment area (an approximation of the treatment area is outlined). **B,** Treatment area with 6 AKs, mild flaking/scaling/dryness, and moderate erythema after 4 weeks of treatment. **C,** Complete clearance at 8 weeks posttreatment (0 lesions). (Reprinted by permission of the publisher from Lebwohl M, Dinehart S, Whiting D, et al: Imiquimod 5% cream for the treatment of actinic keratosis: Results from two phase III, randomized, double-blind, parallel group, vehicle-controlled trials. *J Am Acad Dermatol* 50:714-721, 2004. Copyright 2004 by Elsevier.)

Conclusion.—Topical 5% imiquimod cream used once daily twice a week for 16 weeks is effective and safe for the treatment of AKs on the face and balding scalp.

▶ While not as striking as the results reported in preliminary studies utilizing different protocols,[1,2] the efficacy data are quite competitive with that previously reported for topical 5-fluorouracil and diclofenac sodium preparations. A somewhat better response is observed when imiquimod is applied 3 times per week.[3]

B. H. Thiers, MD

References

1. Stockfleth E, Meyer T, Benninghoff B, et al: A randomized, double-blind, vehicle-controlled study to assess 5% imiquimod cream for the treatment of multiple actinic keratoses. *Arch Dermatol* 138:1498-1502, 2002.
2. Stockfleth E, Meyer T, Benninghoff B, et al: Successful treatment of actinic keratosis with imiquimod cream 5%: A report of six cases. *Br J Dermatol* 144:1050-1053, 2001.
3. Szeimies SM, Gerritsen MJ, Gupta G, et al: Imiquimod 5% cream from the treatment of actinic keratosis: Results from a phase III, randomized, double-blind, vehicle-controlled, clinical trial with histology. *J Am Acad Dermatol* 51:547-555, 2004.

Photodynamic Therapy With Aminolevulinic Acid Topical Solution and Visible Blue Light in the Treatment of Multiple Actinic Keratoses of the Face and Scalp: Investigator-Blinded, Phase 3, Multicenter Trials

Piacquadio DJ, Chen DM, Farber HF, et al (Univ of California, San Diego; Northwestern Univ, Chicago; Univ of California, Irvine; et al)
Arch Dermatol 140:41-46, 2004   16–4

Background.—Actinic keratoses are the most common epithelial precancerous lesions among light-complexioned persons. A small percentage of actinic keratoses may progress to invasive squamous cell carcinoma, and some authors have speculated that an actinic keratosis is in fact a squamous cell carcinoma in the early stage of development. Among the current treatments for actinic keratoses are cryosurgery, curettage, electrosurgery, excision, dermabrasion, laser surgery, and topical chemotherapy. Photodynamic therapy is a cytotoxic process that depends on the simultaneous presence of a photosensitizing agent, light, and oxygen. The efficacy of photodynamic therapy was determined by using 20% wt/vol aminolevulinic acid hydrochloride (ALA) and visible blue light for the treatment of multiple actinic keratoses of the face and scalp.

Methods.—A randomized, placebo-controlled, uneven parallel group study was conducted among 243 patients who were randomly assigned to receive vehicle or ALA followed within 14 to 18 hours by photodynamic therapy. Follow-up examinations were conducted at 24 hours and at 1, 4, 8, and 12 weeks after photodynamic therapy. Any target lesions remaining at week 8 were re-treated. The main outcome measure was clinical response based on lesion clearing by week 8.

Results.—Most of the patients in both groups had 4 to 7 lesions. Response rates (ie, patients with 75% or more of the treated lesions clearing) at weeks 8 and 12 were 77% and 89%, respectively, for the drug group and 18% and 13%, respectively, for the vehicle group. The week 12 response rate included 30% of patients who received a second treatment. Most of the patients had erythema and edema develop at the treated site, which resolved or improved within 1 to 4 weeks after therapy. Most patients also had stinging or burning during light treatment, which decreased or resolved within 24 hours.

Conclusions.—Phototherapy with topical ALA is a safe and effective treatment for multiple actinic keratoses of the face and scalp.

▶ This is another study demonstrating the efficacy of topical ALA in combination with a blue light source for the management of multiple actinic keratoses. The response rate at 12 weeks was 89%, but to achieve this 30% of the patients had to receive a second treatment and there was no long-term follow-up to assess the relapse rate. The investigators did admit that most patients had significant discomfort during treatment, which was in part ameliorated by interventions such as topical anesthetics or a fan. Although supposedly this was a study to assess the efficacy of photodynamic therapy to treat multiple actinic keratoses, most patients had only 4 to 7 lesions, which certainly is not typical of the usual patient treated with topical 5-fluorouracil. A drawback to the treatment protocol is having the patient return the day after ALA application for light treatment. Short contact therapy in conjunction with a pulsed dye laser appears to be a more expedient approach for those with access to this device.

P. G. Lang, Jr, MD

A Trial of Short Incubation, Broad-Area Photodynamic Therapy for Facial Actinic Keratoses and Diffuse Photodamage

Touma D, Yaar M, Whitehead S, et al (Boston Univ)
Arch Dermatol 140:33-40, 2004   16–5

Introduction.—Actinic keratoses (AKs) are a common finding, especially among fair-skinned, elderly, white individuals. These lesions are precursors of squamous cell carcinoma and their presence indicates a higher risk for all forms of skin cancer. Because none of the treatments now offered for multiple AKs is completely satisfactory, a protocol using photodynamic therapy (PDT) was evaluated in 18 patients with at least 4 nonhypertrophic facial AKs and mild to moderate diffuse photodamage.

Methods.—During a 7-day period, patients (11 women, 7 men; age range, 41-76 years) applied 40% urea cream or vehicle to half of the treatment area to enhance penetration and then applied δ-aminolevulinic acid (δ-ALA) to the total area for 1, 2, or 3 hours. Topical 3% lidocaine hydrochloride (to decrease discomfort) or vehicle cream was also applied to the entire area 45 minutes before exposure to 10 J/cm^2 of blue light. Patients were evaluated for pain, phototoxic reactions, AK counts, and an improvement in the photodamage at 1 day, 1 week, 1 month, and 5 months.

Results.—Seventeen patients completed the study, and 10 were available for the 5-month follow-up visit. There were no adverse reactions to urea versus vehicle cream pretreatment or to lidocaine versus vehicle cream as a topical anesthetic. All patients acknowledged at least mild to moderate discomfort after exposure to PDT. Reported pain levels were not influenced by urea cream pretreatment nor the length of δ-ALA incubation. Application of 3% lidocaine hydrochloride 45 minutes before light exposure was only slightly superior to vehicle for pain control. Patients generally required analgesia with acetaminophen for up to 3 days. Moderate phototoxic effects continued for 1 week. All treatment groups showed a significant reduction in AKs and a significant improvement in several photodamage variables at the 1- and 5-month follow-up visits. Satisfaction was generally high, and most patients commented on the decreased roughness of their skin.

Conclusion.—Patients with multiple AKs responded well to broad-area δ-ALA–PDT. The protocol was at least as effective as conventional fluorouracil therapy and far better tolerated.

▶ The clinical trials resulting in the US Food and Drug Administration approval of PDT used incubation times of 14 to 18 hours. This study shows an equivalent efficacy with contact times as low as 1 hour. This significantly improves the ease of use of this effective method of treating AKs.

J. Cook, MD

Basal Cell Carcinoma and Its Development: Insights From Radiation-Induced Tumors in *Ptch1*-Deficient Mice
Mancuso M, Pazzaglia S, Tanori M, et al (ENEA-Ente per le Nuove Tecnologie, Rome; Univ of Goettingen, Germany; GSF-Natl Research Ctr for Environment and Health, Munich)
Cancer Res 64:934-941, 2004   16–6

Background.—Inactivation of the tumor suppressor gene *Patched (Ptch1)* is involved in the pathogenesis of basal cell nevus syndrome, an autosomal dominantly inherited disorder characterized by multiple basal cell carcinomas (BCCs) resulting from hypersensitivity to ionizing radiation. Knockout mice heterozygous for *Ptch1* (*Ptch1*[neo67/+]) were studied to explore the effects of ionizing radiation-induced BCC tumorigenesis.

Methods.—Mice lacking 1 *Ptch1* allele were generated by disruption of exons 6 to 7 and were phenotyped with the use of polymerase chain reaction. Animals heterozygous for *Ptch1*[neo67/+] and their wild-type littermates were either left untreated (52 controls with each phenotype) or were exposed to 3 Gy of whole-body irradiation as newborns (age, 4 days) or as adults (age, 90 days) or to 4 Gy of local irradiation at age 2 months (152 heterozygotes, 142 wild-type mice). Animals were examined daily and were killed for histologic analysis and tumor quantification at the first sign of morbidity.

Results.—When irradiated as adults, tumor-free survival of irradiated *Ptch1*[neo67/+] mice was similar to that of unirradiated heterozygotes. When irradiated as neonates, however, by 28 weeks, mortality rates were significantly higher in the irradiated than in the unirradiated heterozygotes (80% vs 13%, respectively). Histologic examination showed that both irradiated and unirradiated heterozygotes, but not wild-type mice, had hyperproliferation of basaloid cells. However, lesions progressed to nodular and infiltrative BCCs only in the irradiated heterozygotes. Data on the incidence, multiplicity, and latency of BCCs in these irradiated *Ptch1*[neo67/+] mice add further support to the notion that epidermal hyperproliferation, nodular BCC, and infiltrative BCC represent different stages of tumor development. Staining for p53 increased significantly from the epidermal (0% staining) to the infiltrative (100% staining) subtypes. Also, the normal remaining *Ptch1* allele was present in all nodular, circumscribed BCCs, whereas the normal *Ptch1* allele was absent in all infiltrative BCCs.

Conclusion.—BCC seems to progress in a step-like fashion, from basaloid hyperproliferation, to nodular BCC, and then to infiltrative BCC, as sequential genetic alterations accumulate. This model provides an opportunity to examine the molecular events leading from precursor lesions to full BCC.

▶ Activation of the hedgehog pathway (resulting from loss-of-function mutations in *Ptch1*) has been demonstrated in human BCC, and inhibitors of this pathway are under investigation as a possible treatment for this condition.

B. H. Thiers, MD

Ornithine Decarboxylase Is a Target for Chemoprevention of Basal and Squamous Cell Carcinomas in *Ptch1*$^{+/-}$ Mice

Tang X, Kim AL, Feith DJ, et al (Columbia Univ, New York; Penn State College of Medicine, Hershey, Pa; Univ of California, San Francisco; et al)
J Clin Invest 113:867-875, 2004   16–7

Background.—Basal cell carcinoma (BCC) is the most common form of cancer in humans, affecting approximately 1 million Americans annually. Patients who are affected by the rare, dominantly inherited disorder nevoid basal cell carcinoma syndrome (NBCCS), or Gorlin syndrome, develop dozens to hundreds of BCCs as well as various extracutaneous tumors. These patients are known to have *PTCH1* mutations, and mutations in *PTCH1* and smoothened (SMO) have been identified in sporadic BCCs. Solar ultraviolet B (UVB) radiation induces cutaneous ornithine decarboxylase (ODC), which is the first enzyme in the polyamine-biosynthesis pathway. ODC prompts continued proliferation and clonal expansion of initiated (mutated)

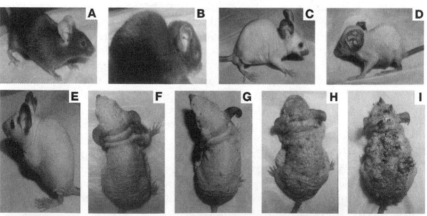

FIGURE 1.—*Ptch1*$^{+/+}$ heterozygous mice overexpressing ODC (*Ptch1*$^{+/-}$/ODC TgN mice). **A**, *Ptch1*$^{+/-}$ heterozygous mouse. **B**, *Ptch1*$^{+/-}$ heterozygous mouse showing skull abnormality. **C**, *Ptch1*$^{+/-}$/ODC TgN mouse. **D**, *Ptch1*$^{+/-}$/ODC TgN mouse showing skull abnormality. **E**, *Ptch1*$^{+/-}$/ODC TgN mouse at week 10. **F**, *Ptch1* +/−/ODC TgN mouse at week 30. **G**, UVB-irradiated *Ptch1*$^{+/-}$/ODC TgN mouse at week 10. **H**, UVB-irradiated *Ptch1*$^{+/-}$/ODC TgN mouse at week 20. **I**, UVB-irradiated *Ptch1*$^{+/-}$/ODC TgN mouse at week 30. (Republished with permission of the *Journal of Clinical Investigation* from Tang X, Kim AL, Feith DJ, et al: Ornithine decarboxylase is a target for chemoprevention of basal and squamous cell carcinomas in *Ptch1*$^{+/-}$ mice. *J Clin Invest* 113:867-875, 2004. Reproduced by permission of the publisher via Copyright Clearance Center, Inc.)

cells, which results in tumorigenesis. ODC is therefore a potentially significant target for chemoprevention of BCCs, most of which have mutations in the tumor-suppressor gene *PTCH*. The suitability of ODC as a target for chemoprevention of BCCs was assessed.

Methods.—ODC was first overexpressed in the skin of $Ptch1^{+/-}$ mice using a keratin 6 (K6) promoter that directs constitutive ODC expression in the outer root sheath of the hair follicle. Further verification of the role of ODC in BCC tumorigenesis was obtained through use of an antienzyme (AZ) approach to inhibit ODC activity in the $Ptch1^{+/-}$ mice.

Results.—Mice with K6-enhanced ODC expression showed accelerated induction of BCCs (Fig 1; see color plate XVIII). The $Ptch1^{+/-}$ mice with AZ overexpression driven by the K6 promoter were resistant to the induction of BCCs by UVB . In addition, oral administration of the suicidal ODC inhibitor α-difluoromethylornithine reduced UVB-induced BCCs in $Ptch1^{+/-}$ mice.

Conclusions.—The significance of ODC for the induction of BCCs is underscored by these results. Chemopreventive strategies directed at inhibiting ODC may be useful in the reduction of BCCs in humans.

▶ The enzyme ornithine decarboxylase catalyzes the conversion of ornithine to putrescine, which is the essential building block required for the production of the higher polyamines, including spermidine and spermine, within the cell. These molecules are critical for normal and neoplastic cell growth. Excessive activity of ornithine decarboxylase was a popular theory for the pathogenesis of psoriasis in the 1980s. Tang and colleagues suggest a role for this enzyme in the pathogenesis of BCC, and speculate that it might be a viable target for inhibiting tumor development.

B. H. Thiers, MD

The Effect of Skin Examination Surveys on the Incidence of Basal Cell Carcinoma in a Queensland Community Sample: A 10-Year Longitudinal Study
Valery PC, Neale R, Williams G, et al (Queensland Inst of Medical Research, Australia; Univ of Queensland, Australia; Princess Alexandra Hosp, Brisbane, Australia)
J Investig Dermatol Symp Proc 9:148-151, 2004   16–8

Background.—The incidence of skin cancer has increased throughout the world over the past few decades. Skin cancers are not suitable for routine cancer registration, so monitoring of the burden of skin cancer and the success of skin cancer control strategies depends on ad hoc community or population surveys. One such study has been ongoing in a community sample in Queensland, Australia. A previous report described the incidence rates of clinically and histologically diagnosed basal cell carcinoma (BCC) and squamous cell carcinoma (SCC) in this population from 1986 to 1992. The results of monitoring the incidence of BCC and SCC from 1992 to 2001 were presented.

Methods.—The incidence of BCC and SCC in a Queensland community was prospectively monitored over a 10-year period by recording newly treated lesions, supplemented by skin examination surveys.

Results.—The age-standardized incidence rates of people with new, histologically confirmed BCC were 2787 per 100,000 person-years at risk (PYAR) among men and 1567 per 100,000 PYAR among women. The corresponding tumor rates were 5821 per 100,000 PYAR and 2733 per 100,000 PYAR, respectively. The incidence rates for new SCC were 944 per 100,000 PYAR in men and 675 per 100,000 PYAR in women, whereas tumor rates were 1754 per 100,000 PYAR and 846 per 100,000 PYAR, respectively. A notable variation in the incidence rates of BCC but not SCC was present according to the method of surveillance; the BCC incidence rates based on skin examination surveys were approximately 3 times higher than background treatment rates. This finding was attributable mainly to an increase in diagnosis of new BCC on sites other than the head and neck, arms, and hands associated with skin examination surveys and was not strongly related to advancing the time of diagnosis of BCC on these sites, as evidenced by a return to background rates after the examination surveys.

Conclusion.—BCCs that might otherwise go unreported are detected during skin examination surveys; thus, skin cancer screening can influence the apparent burden of skin cancer.

Imiquimod 5% Cream for the Treatment of Superficial Basal Cell Carcinoma: Results From Two Phase III, Randomized, Vehicle-Controlled Studies

Geisse J, Caro I, Lindholm J, et al (Solano Dermatology Associates, Vallejo, Calif; Harvard Med School, Boston; Dermatopathology Associates, Fridley, Minn; et al)
J Am Acad Dermatol 50:722-733, 2004   16–9

Background.—Imiquimod is an immune response modifier that stimulates monocytes/macrophages and dendritic cells to produce interferon-α and other cytokines involved in cell-mediated immunity. Phase 2 studies suggest imiquimod can promote histologic clearance of basal cell carcinoma (BCC) and has slightly more efficacy for superficial BCC (sBCC) than for nodular tumors. Two phase 3 trials were undertaken to assess the efficacy and safety of 5% imiquimod cream applied either 5 or 7 times a week for 6 weeks in patients with sBCC.

Methods.—Two identical multicenter, randomized, double-blind, vehicle-controlled phase 3 studies were performed, and their results were pooled. Overall, 724 patients with sBCC (61% men; mean age, 58.8 years) were divided into 4 equal treatment groups. Two groups were treated on a 5-times-per-week (5×/wk) schedule with either 5% imiquimod cream or placebo, and the other 2 groups were treated on a 7-times-per-week (7×/wk) schedule with either active drug or placebo. All drugs were applied once daily to the same target lesion for 6 weeks. Clinical and histologic responses were examined 12 weeks after the end of treatment. Complete composite clearance was defined as the absence of both clinical and histologic evidence of BCC or as the presence of clinically suspicious BCC but no histologic evidence of BCC in patients in whom histologic findings explained the false-positive clinical finding.

Results.—Composite clearance rates were 75% in the 5×/wk group, 73% in the 7×/wk group, and 2% in the combined vehicle group. Histologic clearance rates were 82% in the 5×/wk group, 79% in the 7×/wk group, and 3% in the vehicle group. During treatment, drug-related adverse events were experienced by 58% of the 5×/wk group, 64% of the 7×/wk group, and 36% of the vehicle group. In the posttreatment period, 33% of the 5×/wk group and 31% of the 7×/wk group had drug-related adverse events. Only 11 patients in the combined imiquimod groups discontinued treatment because of adverse events or a local skin reaction. The only adverse events significantly more common in the 7×/wk group than in the 5×/wk group were application site reactions. Composite clearance rates and histologic clearance rates correlated significantly and positively with the severity of erythema, erosions, and scabbing/crusting.

Conclusion.—With each dosing regimen, imiquimod was significantly more effective than vehicle in inducing clinical and histologic clearance of sBCCs. The 2 active treatments were equally effective, but the 7×/wk regimen was associated with more application site reactions. Thus, the 5×/wk imiquimod regimen for 6 weeks is recommended for patients with sBCC.

▶ The data reported by Geisse et al are similar to that reported in previous studies of 5% imiquimod cream in the treatment of sBCC. Clearance rates, as well as local adverse reactions, are directly correlated with the frequency of application. Application of the cream 5 times per week appears to represent the best compromise between favorable response rates and tolerability of the treatment regimen. The mechanism of action of imiquimod seems to involve increased apoptosis of tumor cells.[1,2]

B. H. Thiers, MD

References

1. Schon M, Bong AB, Drewniok C, et al: Tumor-selective induction of apoptosis and the small-molecule immune response modifier imiquimod. *J Natl Cancer Inst* 95:1138-1149, 2003.
2. Urosevic M, Maier T, Benninghoff B, et al: Mechanisms underlying imiquimod-induced regression of basal cell carcinoma in vivo. *Arch Dermatol* 139:1325-1332, 2003.

Topical Imiquimod Treatment for Nodular Basal Cell Carcinomas: An Open-Label Series

Huber A, Huber JD, Skinner RB Jr, et al (Univ of Tennessee, Memphis; Univ of Oklahoma, Oklahoma City)
Dermatol Surg 30:429-430, 2004   16–10

Background.—Imiquimod is a new immunomodulator with reported efficacy in treating basal cell carcinoma (BCC). The first open-label study of topical imiquimod in the treatment of nodular BCC, with confirmation of tumor elimination by Mohs micrographic surgery, is described.

Methods.—Research subjects were 15 patients with nodular BCC 3 to 25 mm in diameter. Patients applied topical 5% imiquimod cream to the tumor 3 times a week for 12 weeks; occlusion was not used. At week 15, all treatment sites were excised with the use of Mohs micrographic surgery and were examined to determine tumor clearance.

Results.—Treatment with imiquimod resulted in 100% clearance of all nodular BCCs. None of the patients had a recurrence at the 18-month visit. Adverse events were erythema, ulceration, and mild pain at the treatment site.

Conclusion.—These results bolster claims that 5% imiquimod cream is effective for nodular BCC. Nonetheless, more studies are needed before this off-label use can be routinely recommended.

▶ In the current article, application of imiquimod 3 times per week for 12 weeks yielded a clearance rate of 100% in patients with nodular BCC. In a previous investigation,[1] only 76% of patients with nodular BCC cleared after *daily* application of the drug for a similar duration of time. Interestingly, the current study was an open-label series, whereas the previously reported data were generated from a randomized, vehicle-controlled, double-blind dose-response protocol. Go figure!

B. H. Thiers, MD

Reference

1. Shumack S, Robinson J, Kossard S, et al: Efficacy of topical imiquimod 5% cream for the treatment of nodular basal cell carcinoma: Comparison of dosage regimens. *Arch Dermatol* 138:1165-1171, 2002.

Safety and Efficacy of Dose-Intensive Oral Vitamin A in Subjects With Sun-Damaged Skin

Alberts D, Ranger-Moore J, Einspahr J, et al (Univ of Arizona, Tucson, Ariz; Univ of Texas, Houston)
Clin Cancer Res 10:1875-1880, 2004   16–11

Background.—In an earlier phase III trial, the authors showed that 25,000 IU/d of oral vitamin A reduced the risk of cutaneous squamous cell carcinoma by 32% in patients with moderately severe actinic keratoses. The effects of higher doses of vitamin A (up to 75,000 IU/d) on skin cancer chemoprophylaxis were investigated.

Methods.—The subjects were 129 patients (64% men; mean age, approximately 63.5 years) with severely sun-damaged skin on their lateral forearms. Patients were randomly assigned to 1 of 4 groups for 12 months of oral therapy with either placebo or 25,000, 50,000, or 75,000 IU/d of vitamin A. Clinical and laboratory parameters, quantitative karyometric image analysis, and expression of retinoid receptors in the sun-damaged skin were assessed at baseline and at the end of therapy.

Results.—The incidence and the severity of adverse clinical and laboratory events were similar in the 3 active drug groups. Compared with quantitative karyometric images at baseline, patients taking 25,000, 50,000, or 75,000 IU/d of vitamin A had significantly decreased actinic damage compared with patients taking placebo (64.5%, 80.8%, and 78.6%, respectively, vs 25.0%). Vitamin A treatment also significantly upregulated retinoic acid receptors α and β and retinoid X receptor αlevels, with an increased effect at larger doses.

Conclusion.—Oral vitamin A at dosages of 50,000 and 75,000 IU/d for 12 months were as safe and effective as a lower dose of 25,000 IU/d. Higher dosages were associated with greater upregulation of retinoid receptors, however. These findings suggest that dosages of up to 75,000 IU/d should be used in future studies of the chemoprophylactic effect of vitamin A on skin cancer.

▶ These authors previously reported a large placebo-controlled study involving more than 2000 randomized participants with moderately severe actinic keratoses.[1] In it, intake of 25,000 IU/d vitamin A was associated with a 32% risk reduction for cutaneous squamous cell carcinoma. In the current study, karyometric features of basal cell layer cells were examined in patients receiving higher doses (50,000 IU/d or 75,000 IU/d) of vitamin A. The authors found the results encouraging enough to recommend that these higher doses be used in future skin cancer chemoprevention studies.

B. H. Thiers, MD

Reference

1. Moon TE, Levine N, Cartmel B, et al: Effect of retinol in preventing squamous cell skin cancer in moderated-risk subjects: A randomized, double-blind, controlled trial. *Cancer Epidemiol Biomark Prev* 6:949-956, 1997.

Retinoic Acid Increases the Expression of p53 and Proapoptotic Caspases and Sensitizes Keratinocytes to Apoptosis: A Possible Explanation for Tumor Preventive Action of Retinoids

Mrass P, Rendl M, Mildner M, et al (Med Univ of Vienna; Centre de Recherches et d'Investigation Epidermiques et Sensorielles, Neuilly, France)
Cancer Res 64:6542-6548, 2004   16–12

Introduction.—Retinoids are an important therapy for dermatologic disorders and can also inhibit the development of nonmelanoma skin cancer (NMSC) in patients with defects of DNA repair and those receiving immunosuppressive agents after a transplant. However, the mode of action by which retinoids prevent NMSC is unclear. Retinoids induce keratinocyte (KC) proliferation when applied topically in vivo and have only moderate effects on KC proliferation in vitro. The effect of all-*trans*-retinoic acid (ATRA) on KC apoptosis was investigated in an effort to explain the tumor preventive action of retinoids.

Methods and Results.—Keratinocytes that were cultured in confluent monolayers for several days acquired resistance against UVB-induced apoptosis. However, when the cells were treated with 1 μmol/L ATRA for 6 days, then irradiated with varying doses of UVB, massive apoptosis was confirmed by morphological analysis, by expression of activated caspase-3, and by DNA fragmentation. The substitution of doxorubicin for UVB yielded the same effect. Real-time polymerase chain reaction and Western blot analyses demonstrated that ATRA treatment substantially increased the messenger RNA and protein expression of p53 and caspase-3, -6, -7, and -9 (key regulators of apoptosis). UVB irradiation of ATRA-treated cells (but not of control cells) resulted in the accumulation of p53 protein and of its target gene *Noxa*. The inhibition of p53 and caspases with α-pifithrin and z-Val-Ala-Asp-fluoromethyl ketone, respectively, blocked UVB- and doxorubicin-induced apoptosis in ATRA-treated KCs. Similar to the ATRA effects in monolayer cultures, the effects on in vitro-generated organotypic skin cultures included upregulation of p53 and proapoptotic caspases and an increased sensitivity to UVB-induced apoptosis.

Conclusion.—The finding that ATRA treatment upregulates central elements of the proapoptotic machinery in human primary KCs and sensitizes them to DNA damage-induced apoptosis suggests that sensitization to apoptosis by retinoids may be involved in the prevention of UV-associated NMSC in patients on immunosuppressive therapy or with DNA-repair defects.

▶ The authors demonstrate a possible mechanism for the chemopreventive effect of retinoids against the development of NMSC.

B. H. Thiers, MD

Evidence of Increased Apoptosis and Reduced Proliferation in Basal Cell Carcinomas Treated With Tazarotene

Orlandi A, Bianchi L, Costanzo A, et al (Tor Vergata Univ of Rome)
J Invest Dermatol 122:1937-1041, 2004   16–13

Background.—Tazarotene is a new acetylenic retinoid approved to treat psoriasis, acne, and photoaging. Some evidence suggests that it may also be effective for treating basal cell carcinoma (BCC). Thus, both the in vitro and in vivo effects of topical tazarotene on BCC were examined.

Methods.—For in vitro studies, immortalized basal keratinocyte and squamous epidermal tumor cell lines were incubated with different concentrations of tazarotene or dimethyl sulfoxide and examined to determine cell viability. Some cells were transfected with a luciferase reporter plasmid, incubated for 48 hours with 1 or 5 µmol/L tazarotene, and examined under fluorescence microscopy for features of apoptosis. Cells were also examined by sodium dodecyl sulfate–polyacrylamide gel electrophoresis, western blotting, and polymerase chain reaction to measure changes in expression of retinoic acid receptors (RARs), Ki-67, p53, bcl-2, and bax. For in vivo studies, 20 superficial and 10 nodular BCCs from 26 patients were treated with 0.1% tazarotene gel once a day for 24 weeks; another 10 BCCs from age-matched patients were left untreated to serve as controls. Biopsy samples were taken at 12 and 24 weeks and underwent histologic, immunohistochemical, and TdT-mediated dUTP-biotin nick-end labeling analysis to determine the expression of the aforementioned proteins.

Results.—In vitro, tazarotene induced a dose-dependent increase in RAR-β and bax expression in the basaloid tumor cells but not the squamous tumor cells. The associated increases in apoptosis and growth inhibition were also significant in the basaloid tumor cells. In vivo, apoptosis was apparent after 12 weeks of treatment. Overall, 76.7% of treated tumors had a greater than 50% reduction in both diameter and thickness. Almost half the treated lesions (46.7%) had complete healing, which has been maintained without recurrence for at least 2 years. Regression was significantly associated with reduced proliferation and increased apoptosis in both superficial and nodular BCCs. Both RAR-β and bax expression were significantly greater in the treated BCCs than in controls.

Conclusion.—Tazarotene has both in vitro and in vivo antiproliferative and proapoptotic effects in BCC. RAR-β may mediate the drug's action by modulating growth in basaloid cells.

▶ The suggestion that topical tazarotene might be useful in the treatment of BCC was first made in a letter to the editor by Peris et al.[1] The current observation of increased apoptosis of tumor cells in tazarotene-treated lesions is reminiscent of the same phenomenon reported with imiquimod and discussed in the 2004 YEAR BOOK OF DERMATOLOGY AND DERMATOLOGIC SURGERY.[2,3]

B. H. Thiers, MD

References

1. Peris K, Fargnoli MC, Chimenti S: Preliminary observations on the use of topical tazarotene to treat basal-cell carcinoma. *N Engl J Med* 341:1767-1768, 1999.
2. Schon M, Bong AB, Drewniok C, et al: Tumor-selective induction of apoptosis and the small-molecule immune response modifier imiquimod. *J Natl Cancer Inst* 95:1138-1149, 2003.
3. Urosevic M, Maier T, Benninghoff B, et al: Mechanisms underlying imiquimod-induced regression of basal cell carcinoma in vivo. *Arch Dermatol* 139:1325-1332, 2003.

High Recurrence Rates of Basal Cell Carcinoma After Mohs Surgery in Patients With Chronic Lymphocytic Leukemia

Mehrany K, Weenig RH, Pittelkow MR, et al (Mayo Clinic, Rochester, Minn)
Arch Dermatol 140:985-988, 2004   16–14

Introduction.—The use of micrographic surgery routinely provides the highest cure rates while maximizing the preservation of normal adjacent tissue for reconstruction of the defect and may be an option in patients with basal cell carcinoma (BCC) and chronic lymphocytic leukemia (CLL), a population known for aggressive nonmelanoma skin cancers. The recurrence rates for BCC after Mohs surgery were evaluated in patients with CLL.

Methods.—Twenty-four patients with CLL who underwent Mohs surgery for 33 BCCs of the head and neck and 66 controls matched for gender, age, and surgical year when Mohs surgery was performed (May 1988 through September 1998) were evaluated.

Results.—There were 4 recurrences of BCC among the 24 patients with CLL who underwent Mohs surgery for 33 BCCs. The cumulative incidence of recurrence on a per tumor basis was 3%, 12%, and 22%, respectively at 1 year, 3 years, and 5 years. Compared with controls, BCC was 14 times as likely to recur in patients with CLL ($P = .02$). Overall, there were no significant differences between patients with CLL and controls in preoperative tumor size (median, 1.6 cm vs 1.4 cm; $P = .18$) or the proportion of aggressive histologic subtypes of BCC (58% vs 41%; $P = .12$).

Conclusion.—Recurrence rates of BCC are 14-fold higher after Mohs surgery in patients with CLL compared to rates in controls. It does not appear that patients with CLL have significantly larger BCCs or more aggressive histologic subtypes of BCC compared with controls. Close surveillance to detect recurrent BCCs is recommended in these patients.

▶ This study demonstrates that even Mohs surgery struggles to achieve the expected high success rate when treating basal cell carcinoma in patients with CLL. Such patients manifest significant immune dysregulation and have a propensity for aggressive nonmelanoma skin cancer much like solid organ transplant recipients. The dense lymphocytic infiltrates commonly seen in the Mohs specimens in these patients may make histologic interpretation more difficult, thus increasing recurrence rates. The use of immunohistochemical staining may improve the utility of Mohs surgery.

J. Cook, MD

Variation in Care for Nonmelanoma Skin Cancer in a Private Practice and a Veterans Affairs Clinic

Chren M-M, Sahay AP, Sands LP, et al (Univ of California, San Francisco)
Med Care 42:1019-1026, 2004   16–15

Background.—Tumor destruction, local excision, and Mohs micrographic surgery are each effective options for treating nonmelanoma skin cancer. Many factors influence a physician's choice of treatment, and one of these factors may be the difference in practice settings. Differences in the treatment of nonmelanoma skin cancer between a Veterans Administration (VA) medical center and a university-affiliated private dermatology practice were examined.

Methods.—The medical records of 1375 patients given diagnoses of nonmelanoma skin cancer in 1999-2000 were reviewed. Of these, 839 patients (1111 tumors) were treated in a private dermatology practice and 536 patients (666 tumors) were treated at a VA medical center's dermatology clinic. Demographic and clinical factors and treatment characteristics were compared between the 2 groups.

Results.—Compared with patients treated at the VA medical center, patients treated in the private practice were significantly younger (mean age, 62.7 vs 72.0 years), significantly more likely to be women (43.3% vs 3.2%), and significantly less likely to be poor (72.1% vs 21.6% had annual incomes of ≥$30,000). Also, patients treated in private practice had significantly smaller tumors (mean, 10.2 vs 11.2 mm in diameter), and the tumors were significantly less likely to be on visible areas of the body. The treatment differed significantly at the 2 sites. Specifically, local excision was more frequent at the VA medical center (48% of cases vs 25% in private practice), and Mohs surgery was more common in private practice (37% of cases vs 25% in the VA setting). The proportions of tumors treated by destruction in private practice and in the VA setting were similar: 23% and 19%, respectively. Even after an adjustment was made for clinical features that can influence the treatment choice, Mohs micrographic surgery was twice as common in the private practice setting as in the VA medical center (adjusted odds ratio, 2.39).

Conclusion.—Treatment choices for patients with nonmelanoma skin cancer differ markedly depending on the site of treatment. Mohs micrographic surgery is more commonly performed in private practice, whereas almost half of all patients treated in the VA setting undergo local excision. Understanding differences in many aspects of care (eg, practice setting, patient preferences, type of insurance) may help improve the quality of care that patients receive.

▶ In this era of cost containment, the increasing incidence of nonmelanoma skin cancer is proving to be a significant strain on health care delivery systems. In this country, skin cancer is the fifth most expensive cancer to treat in the Medicare population. This article attempts to compare the delivery of care within a VA clinic setting with an academically affiliated private practice site. Patients at the VA center were more likely to undergo standard excision, whereas patients in the private setting were more likely to have Mohs surgery. Although the authors state that "these findings raise questions not only about overuse or underuse of procedures at the 2 sites, but also about systematic differences in patient preferences and/or physician incentives," the variability in the 2 patient populations may prohibit a more precise comparison.

Many factors influence a physician's choice of prescribed therapy, including tumor and patient characteristics, patient age, patient preferences, and many other variables. For this reason, it is unfair to suggest that financial incentive is the sole cause of many of these differences. Moreover, the authors fail to consider prior studies, which have shown nearly equivalent utilization of Mohs micrographic surgery in settings in which financial incentives do not drive the use of this procedure. The authors also state that "the charge for Mohs surgery is generally significantly higher than that for other therapies." They do not cite prior studies that clearly document the cost-effectiveness of Mohs micrographic surgery compared with conventional surgical excision. Because of the lower recurrence rates and bundling of pathology charges, Mohs surgery represents a cost-effective treatment for primary and recurrent melanoma and nonmelanoma skin cancers in all anatomical areas.

When treating a nonmelanoma skin cancer, the physician must choose a prescribed therapy that yields an acceptable cure rate and that causes minimal morbidity. The cost-effectiveness of this treatment certainly must be considered. Because of the known high cure rate of Mohs surgery, the documented tissue preservation, and the repeatedly demonstrated cost-effectiveness of Mohs surgery, can one simply suggest that the choice of Mohs surgery rests solely on potential financial benefit? This study certainly raises questions about differences in the delivery of care in 2 quite different clinical settings. In my experience, there are many differences between "private practice" patients and our nation's veterans. As a physician who cares for both groups, I believe that the differences in these 2 patient populations may largely explain the differences in prescribed therapies.

J. Cook, MD

Randomized, Controlled Surgical Trial of Preoperative Tumor Curettage of Basal Cell Carcinoma in Mohs Micrographic Surgery

Huang CC, Boyce S, Northington M, et al (Univ of Alabama, Birmingham)
J Am Acad Dermatol 51:585-591, 2004   16–16

Background.—Many surgeons use preoperative tumor curettage before Mohs micrographic surgery to reduce the tumor load and to better define clinical tumor margins. Others, however, believe preoperative curettage is detrimental because it makes tumor-containing skin more friable and may result in falsely large erosions. The wound surface area and other variables were prospectively compared among patients with basal cell carcinoma (BCC) after Mohs micrographic surgery who either did or did not undergo preoperative tumor curettage.

Methods.—The research subjects were 166 patients (75% men; mean age, 64 years) with BCC less than 2 cm in diameter on the head or neck. Patients were randomly assigned to either a control group that did not undergo tumor curettage before Mohs micrographic surgery or to the treatment group, which underwent tumor curettage immediately before surgery. Changes in tumor surface area and wound surface area and operative characteristics (ie, number of tissue layers removed and postoperative complications) were compared between the 2 groups.

Results.—The mean percentage increase in tumor-to-wound surface area was significantly greater in the patients undergoing preoperative tumor curettage (399% increase) than in the control subjects (263% increase). The mean absolute increase in tumor surface area was also significantly greater in the preoperative curettage group than in the control subjects (1.78 vs 1.40 cm²). Preoperative curettage was associated with the removal of fewer tissue layers, but this advantage was not statistically significant. Neither the type of repair performed (primary vs secondary) nor the number or type of postoperative complications differed significantly according to the preoperative treatment.

Conclusion.—Tumor curettage before Mohs micrographic surgery significantly increased the absolute and relative tumor surface area in patients with BCC of the head and neck. Thus, preoperative curettage often causes an erosion that is larger than the tumor margin, which results in the removal of excess normal skin and a larger-than-necessary surgical wound. Preoperative tumor curettage may, however, reduce the number of stages needed to complete surgery; thus, it might have a benefit in select patients undergoing the Mohs procedure.

▶ The debate continues over the utility of preoperative curettage before Mohs micrographic surgery. In theory, curettage may allow the surgeon to better judge the true extent of the neoplasm. This may yield fewer stages of Mohs surgery and may reduce the rate of false-positive results on histologic examination. However, opponents of preoperative curettage have suggested that the procedure is unnecessary and may, in fact, enlarge the surgical defect, especially in actinically damaged skin. This study showed that preoperative curettage resulted in significantly larger postoperative wounds. The curettage group had a tendency toward fewer stages required for successful extrication. In my practice, I have largely discontinued preoperative curettage as I believe that it inordinately increases the size of surgical defects, findings similar to those reported in this study. Nevertheless, I appreciate the value of preoperative curettage in the hands of the experienced Mohs surgeon.

J. Cook, MD

Mohs Micrographic Surgery vs Traditional Surgical Excision: A Cost Comparison Analysis
Bialy TL, Whalen J, Veledar E, et al (Emory Univ, Atlanta, Ga; Univ of Connecticut, Farmington)
Arch Dermatol 140:736-742, 2004   16–17

Introduction.—Among the accepted treatment approaches for nonmelanoma skin cancers (NMSCs) are traditional surgical excision (TSE), radiation therapy, cryosurgery, electrodesiccation and curettage, photodynamic therapy, topical chemotherapy agents, and Mohs micrographic surgery (Mohs). The dermatologic community has made several published requests for definitive cost analysis investigations for use of Mohs in patients with NMSC that meet established criteria warranting such surgery. The cost and margin adequacy of Mohs and TSE in the treatment of facial and auricular NMSC were examined in a prospective cost analysis in which each patient acted as his or her own control.

Methods.—A total of 98 consecutive patients age 18 years and older with a primary diagnosis of NMSC of the face and ears were enrolled. A cost comparison for Mohs and TSE was conducted using the American Medical Association 2002 *Current Procedural Terminology*, which was converted into dollar amounts using the Connecticut Medicare reimbursement rates for 2002.

Results.—The cost of Mohs was comparable to that of TSE when the subsequent procedure for inadequate TSE margin after permanent section was Mohs ($937 vs $1029; $P = .16$) or a subsequent TSE ($937 vs $944; $P = .53$). When facility-based frozen sections were used for TSE, Mohs cost significantly less ($956 vs $1399; $P < .001$). The cost difference between Mohs and TSE was sensitive to the type of repair selected.

Conclusion.—If the end point is clear margins, Mohs is comparable in cost to TSE conducted by an otolaryngologic surgeon. When assessing the cost of facial and auricular NMSC treatment, caution is necessary because the choice of repair can significantly impact the cost conclusions.

▶ This study echoes the findings of a study this reviewer published with John Zitelli in 1998.[1] Mohs surgery is a cost effective method for addressing skin cancer in a variety of locations. Because of documented tissue conservation (not duplicated in this study), preservation of critical anatomic structures, and the theoretical potential for more simple repairs, Mohs surgery yields unsurpassed cure rates as the initial treatment modality obviating, in many cases, the need for subsequent procedures. This results in savings of both time and money.

J. Cook, MD

Reference

1. Cook J, Zitelli J: Mohs micrographic surgery: A cost analysis. *J Am Acad Dermatol* 39:698-703, 1998.

Interventions for Basal Cell Carcinoma of the Skin: Systematic Review
Bath-Hextall F, Bong J, Perkins W, et al (Queen's Med Centre, Nottingham, England)
BMJ 329:705-708, 2004   16–18

Introduction.—The first line of treatment for basal cell carcinoma (BCC) is typically surgical excision. Several alternative approaches are available, including curettage, cryosurgery, laser treatment, surgical excision with predetermined margins of clinically normal tissue, excision under frozen-section control, Mohs micrographic surgery, radiotherapy, topical treatment, intralesional treatment, photodynamic therapy, immunomodulators, and chemotherapy. Data that compare the various treatment modalities and different types of tumors are sparse. The effects of treatments for BCC were evaluated.

Methods.—A systematic review of randomized controlled trials of interventions for histologically verified BCC was performed with the use of published and unpublished material. There were no language restrictions. The primary outcome measure was clinical recurrence of BCC at 3 years or beyond.

Results.—Seven trials were identified that addressed 7 therapeutic categories. Only 1 trial that evaluated surgical excision versus radiotherapy contained primary outcome data, which demonstrated significantly more persistent tumors and cases of recurrence in the radiotherapy group than in the surgery group (odds ratio, 0.09; 95% CI, 0.01-0.67). One trial that compared cryotherapy with surgery had inconclusive findings at 1 year. One comparison of radiotherapy versus cryotherapy revealed significantly more cases of recurrence at 1 year in the cryotherapy group. Preliminary trials indicated a short-term success rate of 87% to 88% for imiquimod cream for treatment of superficial BCCs; this cream has not been compared with surgery. No consistent evidence of benefits was identified for the other treatment modalities.

Conclusion.—Little good quality research has been performed concerning the treatments used for the most common human cancer. Simple long-term trials that document the site, size, and type of BCC are necessary to compare the various available treatment approaches with excisional surgery.

▶ Although the cure rate of BCC is high, some tumors recur years after apparent initial clearance, and most are locally destructive. Although most dermatologists believe that excisional surgery with frozen-section control is the best treatment for these tumors, good long-term studies to compare this treatment's efficacy with other modalities are lacking.

B. H. Thiers, MD

▶ This review of the literature on the treatment of BCC tells us what we already know: there are no well-matched controlled studies comparing the various modalities used to treat BCC. Moreover, it is difficult to control for those modalities that are very operator dependent, for example, cryosurgery. Unfortunately, this article does not give the reader a feel for the effectiveness of some of these approaches nor a better understanding of the indications and limitations of the various modalities.

P. G. Lang, Jr, MD

Human Papillomavirus and Extragenital In Situ Carcinoma
Quéreux G, N'Guyen JM, Dreno B (CHU, Nantes, France; Hôpital Saint-Jacques, Nantes, France)
Dermatology 209:40-45, 2004   16–19

Introduction.—The few studies on the relationship between human papillomavirus (HPV) and extragenital Bowen's disease (BD) in immunocompetent and immunocompromised patients have varied in their findings. An in situ hybridization method was used to determine the rate of HPV detection and the roles of immune status and sun exposure in a large series of patients with extragenital BD.

Methods.—Included in the study group were all patients with histologically confirmed extragenital BD seen at a single institution in 1999. The 50 patients, all of whom were white, ranged in age from 40 to 98 years (mean, 72.3 years); 33 were men and 17 were women. Twenty patients (40%), including 12 who had received renal grafts, had immunosuppression. Samples from a total of 69 BD lesions underwent analysis by 2 independent interpreters.

Results.—HPV DNA was detected in 58% of the samples. Four of 69 samples contained 3 different types of HPV, and 12 contained 2 types. Rates of HPV detection did not differ significantly between immunosuppressed (60%) and immunocompetent (55%) patients. In addition, the percentage of HPV detection was not significantly higher in exposed versus unexposed areas (55% and 65%, respectively).

Conclusion.—Both oncogenic and nononcogenic types of HPV are a common finding in extragenital BD, even in immunocompetent patients and outside acral or light-exposed sites. However, HPV 6/11 was detected more often in immunosuppressed patients (37% vs 11% in immunocompetent patients.)

▶ The article by Quéreux et al adds to other articles documenting the presence of HPV in extragenital nonmelanoma skin cancers in immunocompetent as well as immunosuppressed patients.[1-3]

B. H. Thiers, MD

References

1. Harwood CA, Surentheran T, Sasieni P, et al: Increased risk of skin cancer associated with the presence of epidermodysplasia verruciformis human papillomavirus types in normal skin. *Br J Dermatol* 150:949-957, 2004.
2. Iftner A, Klug SJ, Garbe C, et al: The prevalence of human papillomavirus genotypes in nonmelanoma skin cancers of nonimmunosuppressed individuals identifies high-risk genital types as possible risk factors. *Cancer Res* 63:7515-7519, 2003.
3. Masini C, Fuchs PG, Gabrielli F, et al: Evidence for the association of human papillomavirus infection and cutaneous squamous cell carcinoma in immunocompetent individuals. *Arch Dermatol* 139:890-894, 2003.

Dermoscopy of Bowen's Disease
Zalaudek I, Argenziano G, Leinweber B, et al (Univ of Graz, Austria; Second Univ of Naples, Italy; Univ Tor Vergata, Rome; et al)
Br J Dermatol 150:1112-1116, 2004   16–20

Background.—A variety of differential diagnoses must be considered in many pigmented and nonpigmented skin tumors because they may present overlapping clinical features. Dermoscopy has been shown to improve the accuracy of diagnosis of pigmented skin lesions and is also useful in the evaluation of nonpigmented skin tumors because it permits recognition of vascular structures not visible to the naked eye. Bowen's disease (BD) is a squamous cell carcinoma in situ that is usually nonpigmented but may rarely be pigmented. The dermoscopic features in a series of pigmented and nonpigmented BD were described.

Methods.—The dermoscopic images of 21 histopathologically confirmed cases of BD were evaluated for the presence of various dermoscopic features. The patients included 14 women and 7 men with a median age of 71 years (range, 54-85 years). Each lesion was photographed at 10-fold magnification, and the color slides were scanned to digital format.

Results.—Most of the BD cases showed a peculiar pattern characterized by glomerular vessels (90%) and a scaly surface (90%). The pigmented lesions demonstrated small brown globules that were regularly packed in a patchy distribution (90%). Structureless grey to brown pigmentation was observed in 80% of the pigmented lesions (Table 1).

Conclusions.—Dermoscopy can aid in the diagnosis of BD because of the presence of repetitive morphologic findings, such as glomerular vessels and a scaly surface. In addition, small brown globules or homogeneous pigmentation can also be seen.

TABLE 1.—Clinical and Dermoscopic Characteristics Observed in Pigmented and Nonpigmented BD

Patient	Age (Years)	Sex	Location	Clinical Diagnosis	Glomerular Vessels	Scale	Brown Globules	Structureless (Homogeneous) Pigmentation	Pigmented Streaks	Pigment Network	Ulceration
1	79	F	Leg	AK, AMM, BD	+	+					+
2	74	M	Back	BCC, LAK	+	+					
3	85	F	Leg	AMM, SCC	+	+					
4	82	F	Leg	BCC, SCC, MM	+	+	+	+			+
5	64	M	Leg	SK	+	+	+	+			
6	72	F	Back	SK, AN		+	+	+			
7	75	M	Leg	SK	+				+		
8	55	M	Leg	SL, PAK, AN		+	+	+			
9	67	F	Leg	AMM	+	+	+	+			
10	75	F	Leg	BCC, SK	+	+				+	+
11	65	F	Leg	BD, AMM, BCC	+	+					
12*	68	M	Leg	AMM, BCC, AK	+	+	+	+			
13	65	F	Leg	AN, MM, SK	+	+	+				
14	65	F	Hand	BD, BCC, AK	+	+					
15	62	F	Leg	BCC, AMM	+	+	+	+			
16	54	F	Leg	AK, SCC, BD, BCC	+	+					+
17	67	M	Leg	SK, LAK	+	+	+	+			
18	75	F	Leg	BCC, AK	+	+					
19	73	M	Back	BCC, AMM	+	+					+
20	81	F	Leg	BCC, AMM	+	+					+
21	81	F	Leg	BCC	+	+					
Total					19 90%	19 90%	9 90%†	8 80%†	1 10%†	1 10%†	6 28·6%

*This case also showed atypical vessels (linear irregular and dotted vessels).
†Percentage related to the cases of pigmented BD (10 of 21).
Abbreviations: AK, Actinic keratosis; *AMM,* amelanotic melanoma; *AN,* atypical nevus; *BCC,* basal cell carcinoma; *LAK,* lichenoid actinic keratosis; *MM,* melanoma; *PAK,* pigmented actinic keratosis; *SK,* seborrheic keratosis; *SL,* solar lentigo; *SCC,* squamous cell carcinoma; *F,* female; *M,* male.
(Courtesy of Zalaudek I, Argenziano G, Leinweber G, et al: Dermoscopy of Bowen's disease. *Br J Dermatol* 150:1112-1116, 2004. Reprinted by permission of Blackwell Publishing.)

Keratoacanthoma Observed
Griffiths RW (Northern Gen Hosp, Sheffield, England)
Br J Plast Surg 57:485-501, 2004   16–21

Introduction.—Most studies of keratoacanthoma recommend complete excision because of concern that the lesion may be an invasive squamous cell carcinoma or may result in a poor quality scar if left to involute. Nevertheless, the condition can regress spontaneously. Fourteen of 19 patients in the author's practice underwent observational management only, and their outcomes are reported.

Methods.—All patients were given diagnoses over an 11-year period (1992-2002) and had photographic records and case notes available for review. The observational management program included assessment of the lesion, frequent follow-up, and excision, if warranted by the growth pattern (Table 2). Patients were warned that the scar quality after excision could not be predicted and that they might experience a recurrence if the excision were performed in the phase of proliferation.

Results.—Patients were 10 men and 4 women who ranged in age from 42 to 86 years (mean, 65 years). The growth pattern of the keratoacanthoma was regressing in 8 cases, static in 4, proliferating in 1, and uncertain in 1 (Table 4). The mean duration of the lesion at referral was 9 weeks, and the mean time from appearance to resolution was 27 weeks. With a mean follow-up period of 3 years and 5 months after regression, no recurrence and no need for surgical revision of scars had been noted.

Conclusion.—In this series of keratoacanthomas managed by observation, the largest published to date, resolved lesions did not leave poor quality scars in need of surgical revision (Fig 17; see color plate XVIII). A recurrence after an intervention, however, may be protracted and resistant to treatment. Patients should accept the policy of observation if there are signs of resolution. Likewise, the consequences of surgical revision should be explained. Progression to invasive squamous cell carcinoma is rare.

▶ This very nicely illustrated study demonstrates the natural history of keratoacanthoma. Nevertheless, conservative excision might still be the best approach for most patients.

B. H. Thiers, MD

TABLE 2.—Principles of Management by Observation

Initial question—has the growth plateaued and is the lesion regressing
No biopsy
Close personal follow-up every 2 weeks
Photograph at each attendance
Be prepared to excise if patient and/or surgeon are concerned at growth
   pattern i.e. failure to regress

(Reprinted by permission of the publisher from Griffiths RW: Keratoacanthoma observed. *Br J Plast Surg* 57:485-501, 2004. Copyright 2004 by Elsevier.)

TABLE 4.—Patient Characteristics

Number	Sex	Age (Years)	Previous Trauma	Growth Pattern	Previous Intervention	History (Weeks)	Site	Time to Resolution (Weeks)	Follow-up Years/Months
1	M	83	No	Regressing	No	8	Cheek	16	6 year 9 months
2	M	42	Paint spray	Proliferating	Curette/cautery at 5/7 weeks	7	Nose	19	8 year
3	F	61	Spectacles	Unsure	No	7	Nose	15	6 year 10 months
4	M	66	No	Static	No	6	Lower lip	16	4 year 10 months
5	F	51	No	Regressing	Biopsy at 4 weeks	11	R hand	31	4 year
6	M	52	No	Regressing	No	28	R hand	48	3 year 10 months
7	M	57	Paraffin/work	Regressing	No	8	R hand	28	3 year 8 months
8	M	75	No	Regressing	Biopsy at 2 weeks	12	Eyebrow	64	2 year 7 months
9	F	86	No	Regressing	No	6	Upper lip	26	2 year 2 months
10	M	70	No	Static	No	8	Cheek	16	2 year 4 months
11	F	50	No	Regressing	No	6	Alar base	32	1 year 7 months
12	M	74	No	Static	No	4	Nose	12	1 year 1 months
13	M	72	Pinched on metal	Regressing	Biopsy 5 weeks	8	R hand	23	9 months
14	M	80	Rotivator injury	Static	No	8	R ring finger	24	11 months

(Reprinted by permission of the publisher from Griffiths RW: Keratoacanthoma observed. Br J Plast Surg 57:485-501, 2004. Copyright 2004 by Elsevier.)

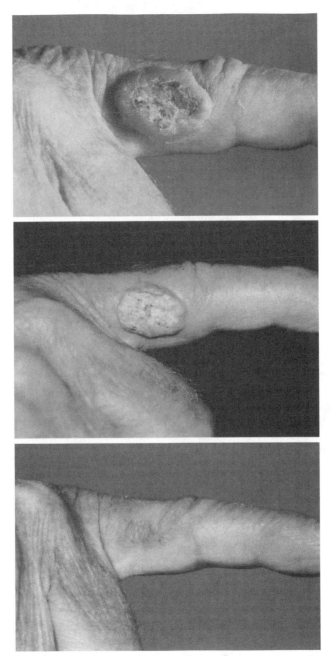

FIGURE 17.—Male age 80 years. Right index finger lesion, views 8, 12, and 24 weeks after initial appearance. (Reprinted by permission of the publisher from Griffiths RW: Keratoacanthoma observed. *Br J Plast Surg* 57:485-501, 2004. Copyright 2004 by Elsevier.)

Sentinel Node Biopsy for High-Risk Nonmelanoma Cutaneous Malignancy

Wagner JD, Evdokimow DZ, Weisberger W, et al (Indiana Univ, Indianapolis)
Arch Dermatol 140:75-79, 2004   16–22

Introduction.—There currently is no adequate noninvasive technique for identification of occult metastases in regional nodes in most malignancies. The feasibility of sentinel node biopsy in selected high-risk skin cancers was examined by ascertaining its false-negative rate and sensitivity for identifying occult regional lymph node metastases.

Methods.—The cumulative experience with sentinel node staging in nonmelanoma cutaneous malignancies was reviewed in a consecutive series of clinically node-negative patients evaluated between 1997 and 2002. Sentinel node biopsies were performed using preoperative lymphoscintigraphy, blue dye, and intraoperative radiolocalization, after which patients underwent either complete lymphadenectomy for all basins identified by lymphoscintigraphy or definitive radiation therapy. The sentinel nodes were step sectioned at 1-mm intervals and examined by light microscopy using hematoxylin-eosin stain. The sensitivity of the procedure was ascertained by comparing the incidence of micrometastasis in the sentinel node with the histologic findings of the complete lymphadenectomy in 12 patients.

Results.—Twenty-nine nodal basins identified by lymphoscintigraphy underwent sentinel node biopsy in 24 patients. The primary diagnoses were squamous cell carcinoma, Merkel cell carcinoma, and adenocarcinoma, respectively, in 17, 5, and 2 patients. A tumor-positive sentinel node was identified in 7 patients (29%). Sentinel node biopsy followed by complete lymphadenectomy was performed in 12 patients; 12 patients underwent sentinel lymph node biopsy alone. Tumor-positive lymph nodes were observed in 8 patients, 7 of whom also had positive sentinel nodes. There was 1 false-positive finding (1/8 [12%]) in a patient who had squamous cell carcinoma of the scalp. At a median follow-up of 10 months, there were no recurrences in a sentinel node-negative basin. The sensitivity of sentinel node staging was 88%; the negative predictive value was 0.94.

Conclusion.—Sentinel node biopsy was useful in identifying occult regional lymph node disease in selected patients with non-melanoma cutaneous malignancies.

▶ Lymphatic mapping and sentinel lymph node biopsy (SLNB) have become commonplace in the management of cutaneous melanoma and breast cancer; however, experience with these techniques in nonmelanoma skin cancer is more limited. Included in this study were high-risk squamous cell carcinoma (SCC) of the skin and genitalia, recurrent SCC, SCC in immunosuppressed patients, Merkel cell carcinoma (MCC), and primary adenocarcinoma of the skin. As in most series, only a relatively small number of patients were studied. However, lymphatic mapping and SLNB do appear to be feasible in the staging in high-risk nonmelanoma skin cancer. As with melanoma, false-negative results occasionally may be observed.

P. G. Lang, Jr, MD

Surgical Management of Metastatic Inguinal Lymphadenopathy
Swan MC, Furniss D, Cassell OCS (Radcliffe Infirmary, Oxford, England)
BMJ 329:1272-1276, 2004   16–23

Background.—Inguinal lymphadenectomy is important in the management of patients with penile, vulval, anal, or cutaneous malignancies. However, groin dissection is associated with a high rate of complications. The key aspects of inguinal lymphadenectomy were summarized.

Methods.—The MEDLINE and Cochrane Library databases were searched to identify relevant articles concerning inguinal lymphadenectomy, groin dissection, or sentinel lymph node biopsy, combined with melanoma or cancer of the vulva, penis, or anus.

Results.—The most common tumors metastasizing to the inguinal lymph nodes are squamous cell carcinoma of the penis, vulva, anus, or skin of the legs and trunk. Malignant melanoma also often metastasizes to the inguinal lymph nodes. Patients with these cancers can readily be taught how to rec-

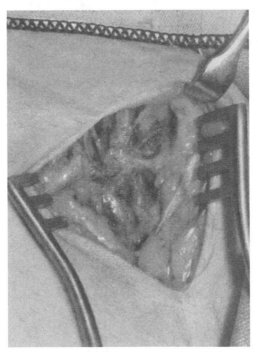

FIGURE 2.—Intraoperative appearance of a left groin sentinel lymph node stained with blue dye. (Courtesy of Swan MC, Furniss D, Cassell OCS: Surgical management of metastatic inguinal lymphadenopathy. *BMJ* 329: 1272-1276, 2004. Copyright 2004, with permission from the BMJ Publishing Group.)

ognize inguinal metastasis. Still, many patients with penile or vulval cancer elect prophylactic inguinal lymphadenectomy; therapeutic bilateral lymphadenectomy is indicated when lymph node involvement is confirmed on pathologic examination. In patients with anal squamous cell carcinoma, inguinal lymphadenectomy is generally performed only in those with clinically evident disease in the inguinal nodes after chemotherapy has been completed. Routine prophylactic lymphadenectomy, however, has not been shown to improve survival in patients with malignant melanoma, although some patient subgroups can benefit from the procedure. Given the high morbidity associated with prophylactic inguinal lymphadenectomy, many surgeons choose sentinel lymph node biopsy before proceeding with surgery. In the authors' experience, the use of a radiolabeled nanocolloid combined with blue dye injection allows for identification of 98% of sentinel lymph nodes (Fig 2). As experience with sentinel inguinal lymph node biopsy increases, prophylactic lymphadenectomy may be rendered obsolete. After inguinal lymphadenectomy, patients must be closely monitored for complications such as lymphedema (which occurs in up to 80% of patients), wound dehiscence (up to 65%), seroma or lymphocele (up to 40%), wound infection (up to 20%), and hematoma (up to 4%). Meticulous attention to surgical technique is required to reduce postoperative complications.

Conclusion.—Inguinal lymphadenectomy is a key component of treatment for squamous cell carcinoma of the penis, vulva, anus, and skin. Prophylactic lymphadenectomy is often used, but may be supplanted by the use of sentinel lymph node biopsy. Postoperative morbidity is high, but can be improved by meticulous attention to technique.

▶ Dermatologists are well aware that sentinel lymph node biopsy is a technique that has refined the indications for lymphadenectomy, and may provide better prognostic information and reduce morbidity.

B. H. Thiers, MD

The Influence of Resection and Aneuploidy on Mortality in Oral Leukoplakia
Sudbø J, Lippman SM, Lee JJ, et al (Univ of Oslo, Norway; Univ of Texas, Houston; Norwegian Univ of Science and Technology, Trondheim)
N Engl J Med 350:1405-1413, 2004   16–24

Background.—The treatment of oral leukoplakia varies widely, from watchful waiting to complete resection. Aneuploid oral erythroplakia is more aggressive than the more common oral leukoplakia, suggesting that aneuploidy may increase the risk of poor outcomes. The impacts of resection margins and ploidy status on the risks of new cancer and cancer-specific death in patients with oral leukoplakia were investigated.

Methods.—The subjects were 103 patients (56% men; mean age, 69.6 years) with diploid dysplastic oral leukoplakia, 20 patients (50% men; mean age, 64.5 years) with tetraploid lesions, and 27 patients (56% men; mean age, 69.6 years) with aneuploid lesions. Patients were monitored for a median of 80 months to determine the incidence of primary oral cancer, new or recurrent oral cancer, and death from oral cancer as a function of resection margins and ploidy status. Only squamous cell carcinoma was considered in analyses.

Results.—After resection of the leukoplakia, 37 patients (24.7%) had positive margins and 113 patients (75.3%) had negative margins. Margin status at the initial leukoplakia resection did not correlate significantly with the subsequent development of oral cancer. During follow-up, 47 patients (31%) had primary oral cancer develop; initial leukoplakia lesions were diploid in 5 patients, tetraploid in 16 patients, and aneuploid in 26 patients. Oral cancers in patients with aneuploid leukoplakia were at a significantly more advanced stage than were oral cancers occurring in patients with diploid or tetraploid leukoplakia.

In the 47 patients in whom cancer developed, recurrence was noted in 26 patients (55%); initial leukoplakia lesions were tetraploid in 4 patients and aneuploid in 22 patients. Thus, recurrences were seen in 0% of patients with diploid leukoplakia, 25% of patients with tetraploid leukoplakia, and 85% of patients with aneuploid leukoplakia. Also, recurrences in the patients with aneuploid leukoplakia were more likely to be multiple and to occur at distant sites within the oral cavity compared with recurrences in patients with tetraploid leukoplakia.

All 47 patients with oral cancer underwent surgery and radiation therapy, and the 26 patients with recurrences underwent chemotherapy. None of the 21 patients with diploid or tetraploid leukoplakia died of oral cancer, compared with 21 of 26 patients with aneuploid leukoplakia ($P < .001$).

Conclusion.—Even complete resection of oral leukoplakia does not prevent oral squamous cell carcinoma. The risk is especially high for patients with aneuploid leukoplakia. Furthermore, standard treatment for oral cancer did not prevent death for the patients with oral cancer arising in aneuploid leukoplakia, which indicates that more effective treatments for this subgroup are urgently needed.

▶ Sudbø et al show that complete resection of aneuploid leukoplakia does not prevent the subsequent development of aggressive oral carcinoma and a possible fatal outcome. This suggests that aneuploidy should be considered an important prognostic indicator in the study of oral cancer. From a more practical standpoint, the data also raise the question of what effective treatment can be offered to patients with aneuploid dysplastic leukoplakia. The same authors have shown that the enzyme, cyclooxygenase-2, is more frequently overexpressed in aneuploid oral dysplasia than in diploid or tetraploid dysplasia, and inhibitors of this enzyme deserve study for their possible therapeutic benefit.[1,2]

B. H. Thiers, MD

References

1. Greenspan D, Jordan RCK: The white lesion that kills—Aneuploid dysplastic oral leukoplakia. *N Engl J Med* 350:1382-1384, 2004.
2. Sudbø J, Ristimaki A, Sondresen JE, et al: Cyclooxygenase-2 (COX-2) expression in high-risk premalignant oral lesions. *Oral Oncol* 39:497-505, 2003.

Quantification of Plasma Epstein-Barr Virus DNA in Patients With Advanced Nasopharyngeal Carcinoma

Lin J-C, Wang W-Y, Chen KY, et al (Taichung Veterans Gen Hosp, Taiwan; Natl Yang-Ming Univ, Taipei, Taiwan; Natl Cheng Kung Univ, Tainan, Taiwan; et al)
N Engl J Med 350:2461-2470, 2004   16–25

Introduction.—Advances in radiation oncology have improved local control of nasopharyngeal carcinoma, but the outcome is poor for patients with recurrence. Because this tumor is associated with Epstein-Barr virus (EBV) infection and EBV is present in cells from almost every primary and metastatic nasopharyngeal carcinoma, the prognostic significance of the plasma EBV DNA load was investigated in a group of previously untreated patients.

Methods.—All 99 patients in the study had biopsy-proven disease and no evidence of distant metastasis. A control group consisted of 79 individuals as follows: 40 healthy volunteers, 20 patients who had survived more than 5 years after radiotherapy with no signs of recurrence, and 19 patients with distant metastasis. Patients in the study group underwent 10 weeks of chemotherapy followed 1 week later by radiotherapy, with total doses of 70 Gy to 74 Gy according to disease stage. Plasma EBV DNA loads were measured by real-time quantitative polymerase chain reaction.

Results.—Ninety-four of the 99 patients in the study group had plasma EBV DNA detected before treatment. Plasma samples were negative, however, in all healthy control subjects and cured patients. The median concentration of plasma EBV DNA correlated with disease stage. The number of copies per milliliter was higher in stage IV disease (1703) than in stage III disease (681), and patients with distant metastasis had a median concentration of 291,940 copies/mL. Patients with complete clinical remission had plasma EBV DNA concentrations that were persistently low or undetectable.

Paired samples of plasma and primary tumor showed consistent genotyping, suggesting that circulating cell-free EBV DNA may originate from the primary tumor. The 99 prospectively studied patients were monitored for a median of 30 months. Rates of both overall survival and relapse-free survival were significantly lower among patients with higher pretreatment EBV DNA concentrations (at least 1500 copies/mL).

Conclusion.—Plasma EBV DNA concentrations can be used as a molecular marker for screening, monitoring, and prediction of relapse in patients with nasopharyngeal carcinoma. After adjustment for other variables, a persistently detectable concentration of EBV DNA in plasma after radiotherapy was the most important prognostic factor.

▶ Nasopharyngeal carcinoma is endemic in Taiwan, and EBV has been shown to be a pathogenetic factor. Lin et al demonstrate that the plasma EBV load correlates with the response to treatment, the likelihood of relapse, and survival in patients with this disease.

B. H. Thiers, MD

Human Papillomavirus in Oral Exfoliated Cells and Risk of Head and Neck Cancer

Smith EM, Ritchie JM, Summersgill KF, et al (Univ of Iowa, Iowa City; Veterans Affairs Med Ctr, Iowa City, Iowa; Univ of Pittsburgh, Pa)
J Natl Cancer Inst 96:449-455, 2004   16–26

Background.—Recent studies have reported an association between human papillomavirus (HPV) and the development of head and neck cancers. This association is strengthened by the detection of the same oncogenic HPV types in cervical carcinomas and in head and neck cancers. There is also evidence that the viral oncoproteins E6 and E7 of HPV high-risk types, which inactivate tumor suppressor gene pathways and promote genomic instability in cervical cancer, also perform the same activities in head and neck cancer. Infection with HPV types and use of alcohol or tobacco, the other major risk factors for head and neck cancer, may be alternative pathways for the development of head and neck cancers. The purpose of this study was to describe risk factors for head and neck cancers associated with oncogenic HPV detection and to determine whether HPV detected in oral exfoliated cells is an independent predictor of head and neck cancer risk.

Methods.—A case-control study was conducted in 201 head and neck cancer patients and 333 control subjects, frequency matched for age and gender. Oral exfoliated cells and tumor tissue were evaluated for HPV using polymerase chain reaction and DNA sequencing to type HPV. Odds ratios for head and neck cancer with HPV infection and 95% confidence intervals were calculated with logistic regression, with adjustment for age, tobacco use, and alcohol consumption.

Results.—Oncogenic, or high-risk (HR), HPV types were detected in oral cells from 22.9% of case patients and 10.8% of control subjects. The most frequently detected type was HPV16 (19% of cases and 10% of control subjects). After adjustment of for age, tobacco use, and alcohol consumption, the risk of head and neck cancer was statistically significantly greater in persons with HPV-HR types but not in persons with nononcogenic HPV types compared with HPV-negative persons. In a comparison of persons who were HPV-negative and did not use alcohol or tobacco, there was a statistically significant synergistic effect between detection of HPV-HR and heavy alcohol consumption but an additive effect between the detection of HPV-HR and tobacco use. HPV-HR types detected in oral exfoliated cells were predictive of HPV-HR types in tumor tissue.

Conclusions.—Infection of oral exfoliated cells with HPV-HR types is a risk factor for head and neck cancer. This association is independent of alcohol and tobacco use and is synergistic with consumption of alcohol. HPV testing of an oral rinse may be predictive of HPV-related head and neck cancer.

Age, Sexual Behavior and Human Papillomavirus Infection in Oral Cavity and Oropharyngeal Cancers

Smith EM, Ritchie JM, Summersgill KF, et al (Univ of Iowa, Iowa City)
Int J Cancer 108:766-772, 2004 16–27

Background.—A growing number of studies have pointed to a causal link between human papillomavirus (HPV) infections and the development of head and neck carcinomas (HNCs), particularly in the oropharynx. However, several unanswered questions remain, and few patient risk factors associated with HPV infection in cancers of the oral cavity and oropharynx have been well established. Whether there are significant differences in the risk factors and tumor characteristics for HPV-positive and HPV-negative cancer cases was investigated.

Methods.—Patients who presented between 1994 and 1997 with cancer of the oral cavity or oropharynx were recruited into the study. HPV was evaluated in cancer tissue and exfoliated oral cells of 193 oral cavity/oropharynx cancer patients using polymerase chain reaction and direct DNA sequencing. A patient questionnaire was used to collect information about risk factors, sexual practices, and medical history.

Results.—The prevalence of HPV high-risk (HR) types was 20% in cancer cases. Three types of HPV-HR were identified: HPV-16 (87%), HPV-18 (3%), and HPV-33 (11%). The risk factors for HPV-HR included younger age (55 years or younger vs over 55 years of age) and younger age-cases who had more lifetime sex partners and practiced oral-genital or oral-anal sex. Compared with HPV-negative cancers, HPV-HR cancers were more likely to have a positive HPV-HR exfoliated oral cytology test, later stage, nodal involvement, and advanced grade.

Conclusions.—These findings are more evidence that the prevalence of oncogenic mucosal HPV is higher in younger-age oral cavity/oropharynx cancer patients whose sexual practices are typically associated with the virus. HPV detection may be indicative of characteristics of advanced disease, and different clinical treatment may be required for this subset of patients. This study found a positive exfoliated oral cytology test for HPV to be a significant predictor of high-risk types in these cancers, which suggests the feasibility of an oral rinse as an early biomarker of infected tumors.

▶ In what appears to be an oral mucosal variant of the Pap smear, Smith and colleagues (Abstracts 16–26 and 16–27) show that detection of HR HPV types in oral exfoliated cells is associated with an increased risk of head and neck cancer. Others have advocated using polymerase chain reaction–based assays for HPV in exfoliated cervical cells to identify women at risk for cervical cancer.[1] The similarity of the HPV types detected in both locations suggests the possibility of sexual transmission of the virus during orogenital contact.[2,3]

B. H. Thiers, MD

References

1. Wright TC Jr. Adding a test for human papillomavirus DNA to cervical-cancer screening. *N Engl J Med* 348:489-490, 2003.
2. Bosch FX, Manos MM, Munoz N, et al: Prevalence of human papillomavirus in cervical cancer: a worldwide perspective. International biological study on cervical cancer (IBSCC) Study Group. *J Natl Cancer Inst* 87:796-802, 1995.
3. Schwartz SM, Daling JR, Doody DR, et al: Oral cancer risk in relation to sexual history and evidence of human papillomavirus infection. *J Natl Cancer Inst* 90:1626-1636, 1998.

Postoperative Concurrent Radiotherapy and Chemotherapy for High-Risk Squamous-Cell Carcinoma of the Head and Neck

Cooper JS, for the Radiation Therapy Oncology Group 9501/Intergroup (New York Univ; et al)

N Engl J Med 350:1937-1944, 2004   16–28

Background.—High-risk squamous-cell carcinoma of the head and neck often recurs in the original tumor bed, despite treatment with resection and postoperative radiotherapy. Whether concurrent postoperative administration of cisplatin and radiotherapy would increase local and regional control rates was investigated.

Methods.—The study included 459 patients who were enrolled between 1995 and 2000. Total resection of all visible and palpable disease was performed in all patients. Patients were then assigned randomly to radiotherapy alone (60 to 66 Gy in 30 to 33 fractions during 6 to 6.6 weeks) or to this treatment plus concurrent IV cisplatin, 100 mg per square meter of body-surface area on days 1, 22, and 43. The median follow-up time was 45.9 months.

Findings.—Local and regional control rates were significantly greater for patients receiving combined therapy than for those given radiotherapy alone. The estimated 2-year rate of local and regional control was 82% for the combined treatment group and 72% for the radiotherapy only group. Disease-free survival was also significantly longer in the former group, even though overall survival was comparable between groups. Severe adverse effects of grade 3 or worse occurred in 77% of the combined therapy group and in 34% of the radiotherapy only group. Four patients died as a direct result of combined therapy.

Conclusions.—Concurrent chemotherapy and radiotherapy after resection significantly improves local and regional control and disease-free survival rates among high-risk patients with head and neck cancer. However, this combined approach is associated with a marked increase in adverse effects, some potentially fatal.

Postoperative Irradiation With or Without Concomitant Chemotherapy for Locally Advanced Head and Neck Cancer

Bernier J, for the European Organization for Research and Treatment of Cancer Trial 22931 (Oncology Inst of Southern Switzerland, Bellinzona; et al)
N Engl J Med 350:1945-1952, 2004   16–29

Background.—Among patients with stage III or IV squamous cell carcinoma of the head and neck, postoperative local or regional recurrences and distant metastases are common. The efficacy of concomitant cisplatin and irradiation was compared with that of radiotherapy alone as adjuvant therapy in this patient population.

Methods.—The study included 334 patients who had undergone surgery with a curative intent and were assigned randomly to radiotherapy alone (66 Gy during a 6.5-week period) or to the same radiotherapy plus cisplatin (100 mg per square meter of body-surface area on days 1, 22, and 43). The median follow-up time was 60 months.

Findings.—The combined therapy group showed a significantly greater progression-free survival rate than did the radiotherapy only group. The 5-year Kaplan-Meier estimates of progression-free survival were 47% and 36%, for the combined therapy and radiotherapy only groups, respectively. In addition, the overall survival rate was significantly higher for patients receiving combined treatment than for those receiving radiotherapy alone: 5-year Kaplan-Meier estimates were 53% and 40%, respectively. The cumulative incidence of a local or regional recurrence in the combined treatment group was significantly less than in the radiation only group; the estimates of 5-year cumulative incidence was 31% after radiotherapy and 18% after combined treatment. Adverse effects of grade 3 or higher occurred in 41% of the patients receiving combined therapy compared with the same adverse effects occurring in only 21% of those receiving radiotherapy alone. The types of severe mucosal adverse effects and the incidence of late adverse effects were comparable in the 2 groups.

Conclusions.—In patients with locally advanced head and neck cancer, postoperative concurrent administration of high-dose cisplatin with radiotherapy is more effective than radiotherapy alone. However, severe adverse effects were more common after combined therapy than after radiotherapy alone.

▶ These protocols (Abstracts 16–28 and 16–29) were designed to test the hypothesis that the addition of concurrent cisplatin to postoperative radiotherapy increases survival rates among patients with high-risk resected head and neck cancer. Both trials demonstrated that concurrent chemotherapy reduces the rate of failure of postoperative radiotherapy; nevertheless, the disease recurs locally in approximately 30% of patients. Further studies are needed to investigate the optimal dose, time frame, and regimen of fractionation for the radiotherapy. Although most trials of concurrent chemotherapy and radiotherapy have used conventional radiotherapy regimens of 6 or 7 weeks, recent phase 3 trials have suggested that the use of shorter than conventional overall treatment times for postoperative radiotherapy can improve tumor control and survival rates.[1,2] Thus, the impact of added chemotherapy may be reduced if it is given in conjunction with an accelerated radiotherapy regimen.[3] A possible causative role of human papillomavirus infection in head and neck cancer has been a topic of intense debate.[4]

B. H. Thiers, MD

References

1. Awwad HK, Lotayef M, Shouman T, et al: Accelerated hyperfractionation (AHF) compared to conventional fractionation (CF) in the postoperative radiotherapy of locally advanced head and neck cancer: Influence of proliferation. *Br J Cancer* 86:517-523, 2002.
2. Ang KK, Trotti A, Brown BW, et al: Randomized trial addressing risk features and time factors of surgery plus radiotherapy in advanced head-and-neck cancer. *Int J Radiat Oncol Biol Phys* 51:571-578, 2001.
3. Saunders MI, Rojas AM: Management of cancer of the head and neck—A cocktail with your PORT? *N Engl J Med* 350:1997-1999, 2004.
4. Gillison ML, Lowy DR: A causal role for human papillomavirus infection in head and neck cancer. *Lancet* 363:1488-1489, 2004.

Dermatofibrosarcoma Protuberans: Reappraisal of Wide Local Excision and Impact of Inadequate Initial Treatment
Khatri VP, Galante JM, Bold RJ, et al (Univ of California, Davis)
Ann Surg Oncol 10:1118-1122, 2003   16–30

Introduction.—The degree of local invasion in dermatofibrosarcoma protuberans (DFSP) can often be clinically difficult to appreciate, leading to inadequate resections. The effect of inadequate initial treatment and the efficacy of wide resection in patients with DFSP were investigated to ascertain their effect on the local aggressiveness of recurrent tumors and recurrence-free survival rate.

Methods.—A retrospective medical records analysis was performed on 35 patients with DFSP treated at a single institution between 1985 and 2001. Patients were classified into primary or recurrent disease groups. Data from pathology reports and operative reports were analyzed to determine lesion location, anatomical site, tumor size, and depth in relation to the investing fascia.

Results.—Of 24 eligible patients, 11 had definitive wide resection after diagnostic excision elsewhere (primary group) and 13 had recurrent tumors after prior surgical treatment elsewhere (recurrent group). Twenty-three patients underwent wide resection only. One patient with fibrosarcoma underwent treatment with adjuvant radiation. Five patients underwent Mohs surgery. At a median follow-up of 54 months, patients who underwent definitive treatment had a 100% recurrence-free survival rate. Eleven (85%) of the 13 recurrent tumors were deep (invading the underlying fascia or lying beneath the fascia), compared with 3 (27%) for primary DFSPs ($P = .011$). Bone involvement was observed in the recurrent group only (4/13 cases).

Compared with those of the primary group, recurrent DFSPs were significantly larger and deeper and were located in the head and neck region.

Outcomes of Surgery for Dermatofibrosarcoma Protuberans

Chang CK, Jacobs IA, Salti GI (Naples Community Hosp, Fla; St Mary's Hosp, Hoboken, NJ; Univ of Illinois, Chicago)

Eur J Surg Oncol 30:341-345, 2004   16–31

Introduction.—Dermatofibrosarcoma protuberans (DFSP), a rare soft-tissue sarcoma, usually appears as a nodular cutaneous mass on the trunk and extremities. Reported rates of local regional recurrence after wide surgical resection have ranged from 24% to 60%. Data for patients treated at a single institution between February 1968 and June 2001 were analyzed to determine disease-free survival (DFS) rate and time to recurrence of DFSP.

Methods.—All 60 patients (23 men, 37 women; mean age, 36 years) in the study underwent wide local excision with at least a 3-cm margin incorporating the underlying deep fascia and overlying skin. Three patients with microscopic margins or high-grade DFSP received adjuvant radiation therapy. The median follow-up was 59 months. Clinicopathologic variables were analyzed for their impact on DFSP recurrence.

Results.—The location of the primary tumor was the trunk in 23 patients, the head and neck in 16, the upper extremity in 11, and the lower extremity in 10. Tumor size was 5 cm or less in 56 patients. The 5- and 10-year disease-free survival rates of DFSP were 86% and 76%, respectively. The overall recurrence rate was 16.7%, and the mean time to recurrence was 38 months. No deaths were attributed to DFSP.

Conclusion.—DFSP is a locally aggressive tumor that rarely metastasizes. When metastases do occur, they often appear in the lung. Wide margins are required to prevent recurrence, and long-term follow-up is advised. Adjuvant radiotherapy is useful for cases in which adequate surgical margins cannot be obtained.

Modified Mohs Micrographic Surgery in the Therapy of Dermatofibrosarcoma Protuberans: Analysis of 22 Patients

Wacker J, Khan-Durani B, Hartschuh W (Univ of Heidelberg, Germany)

Ann Surg Oncol 11:438-444, 2004   16–32

Introduction.—Extensive resection is the primary treatment for dermatofibrosarcoma protuberans (DFSP), a rare fibrohistiocytic soft-tissue tumor. Systemic metastasis is rare, yet rates of local recurrence are high. Mohs micrographic surgery (MMS), with precise margin control, is the established surgical management. Outcomes are reported for 22 patients treated with modified MMS between 1987 and 2002.

Methods.—The patients were 15 women and 7 men with a mean age of 41 years at surgery. Eighteen tumors were on the trunk and neck, 3 were on the upper or lower limbs, and 1 was parietal. Thirteen tumors were primary, and 9 were recurrences. The visible or palpable tumor or residual scar tissue was excised with an approximately 1- to 2-cm lateral excision margin of clinically unaffected skin from the visible tumor margin. Specimens representing the entire outer surface of the resection margins were paraffin-embedded and cut for histologic evaluation.

Results.—The tumor size ranged from 1.5 to 15 cm, and excised scar areas were up to 15 cm in length. One to 3 stages of micrographic surgery were required to achieve histologically tumor-free margins. Ten of 22 tumors were completely excised after the first stage of surgery, including an initial lateral excision margin of 1 to 2 cm. Ten tumors were excised en bloc after 2 stages, and 2 required a third excision because of extensive spread (periosteal and osseous infiltration of the cortical bone of the scalp in 1 case; deep infiltration into the pectoral muscle in the other). During a mean follow-up of 54 months, none of the patients showed recurrent disease or distant metastasis.

Conclusion.—The study confirms that to ensure the successful and recurrence-free treatment of DFSP, MMS should be the treatment of choice. Use of MMS allows a more comprehensive microscopic examination of the surgical margin, thereby preserving a maximum amount of normal skin while achieving clear margins. Complete 3-dimensional histologic evaluation on paraffin sections including immunohistochemical analysis for CD34 is also recommended, especially for widespread or recurrent DFSP.

▶ DFSP is a low-grade fibrosarcoma with a high tendency for local recurrence but a limited potential for metastasis. If neglected or inadequately treated, it can invade widely and deeply and be quite destructive. Tumors with a significant (>5%) fibrosarcomatous component on histologic examination appear to be at higher risk for developing metastases. As these 3 articles (Abstracts 16–30 to 16–32) illustrate, there have been varying degrees of success in the surgical management of this tumor, despite the use of wide surgical margins. In this series of articles, 1 group (Khatri et al, Abstract 16–30) reported a 100% cure rate, even for recurrent tumors, with margins of 1.78 to 4.24 cm (mean, 2.5 cm for primary tumors and 3.3 cm for recurrent tumors). In contrast, another group (Chang et al, Abstract 16–31) reported an overall recurrence rate of 16.7%, despite achieving microscopically clear margins of more than 1 cm. As has been true of previous series and reviews, MMS (Wacker et al, Abstract 16–32) proved to be effective for managing this tumor (100% cure rate with a mean follow-up of 54 months). The take-home message from these articles is obvious: (1) to achieve a high cure rate when treating DFSP, one must achieve tumor-free margins; and (2) these margins must be reliable, that is, the recurrence rate with "clear" margins will reflect how thoroughly the margins were examined by the pathologist. Several other observations that can be made regarding these articles are (1) postoperative radiation may have a role in managing incompletely excised tumors or those with a significant fibrosarcomatous component; (2) when performing MMS, one may wish to begin with a wide margin (>1 cm) to expedite the surgery, since the probability of achieving clear margins with anything less is low; and (3) true MMS does not appear to have been performed on the 22 patients reported by Wacker et al; instead, a modified approach was used in an attempt to decrease the number of specimens to be examined. Obviously, this modification was successful, as reflected by the 100% cure rate, but this reviewer has some concerns regarding the handling of the initially excised specimens. While the authors may be correct in stating that paraffin-embedded specimens are preferable to frozen sections to ensure optimal quality and cellular detail, it is not clear if they systematically examined the entire deep margin since a combination of vertical and horizontal sections was used to decrease the amount of tissue that needed microscopic evaluation. Further study may indicate that in an effort to decrease the amount of tissue that must be processed, it may be reasonable to compromise between examining the entire deep margin and examining it "adequately"; however, a controlled study should be done that compares traditional MMS using paraffin-embedded sections with this modified approach. Moreover, much more detail on the processing of the specimens should be given; for example, the authors should indicate what proportion of the deep margin is subjected to horizontal sectioning and how many vertical sections are examined. In addition, as a final observation, even though immunostains using CD34 are helpful in distinguishing DFSP from scar tissue and other fibrohistiocytic tumors, they may be negative in transitional zones as one goes from obvious DFSP to obvious scar tissue and in the fibrosarcomatous component of DFSP.

P. G. Lang, Jr, MD

Conversion to Sirolimus: A Successful Treatment for Posttransplantation Kaposi's Sarcoma
Campistol JM, Gutierrez-Dalmau A, Torregrosa JV (Univ of Barcelona)
Transplantation 77:760-762, 2004   16–33

Background.—Immunosuppressive therapy for solid organ transplant recipients dramatically increases their risk of Kaposi's sarcoma (KS). Unlike other immunosuppressants such as cyclosporine, tacrolimus, azathioprine, and mycophenolate mofetil, sirolimus has potent antitumor activity in vitro and in vivo. Two patients who had posttransplantation KS while taking cyclosporine but whose lesions regressed after conversion to sirolimus were described.

Case Report.—Man, 68, with diabetic nephropathy, had cadaveric renal transplantation. His immunosuppressive regimen consisted of basiliximab (20 mg, 2 doses), cyclosporine (8 mg/kg/d), mycophenolate mofetil (1 gm twice a day), and prednisone (15 mg/d). The posttransplant period was uneventful, and the patient's serum creatinine level gradually decreased to 2.8 mg/dL. Three months later, however, he was seen with cutaneous KS lesions in the hands, legs, ears, neck, and abdomen. Cyclosporine and mycophenolate mofetil were withdrawn, and the patient was switched to sirolimus

(3 mg/d). After 3 months of sirolimus therapy, most of the KS lesions had disappeared.

At last report, the renal graft had remained stable during sirolimus therapy (serum creatinine level 2.7 mg/dL), and the patient was maintained on sirolimus (5 mg/d) and prednisone (10 mg/d). The other patient, a 67-year-old man with chronic glomerulonephritis, had similar success after switching from cyclosporine to sirolimus, with no adverse events and with excellent graft function.

Conclusion.—For patients with posttransplantation KS, switching from cyclosporine to sirolimus can lead to KS regression without increasing the risk of graft rejection. Sirolimus may thus offer a new approach to managing malignancies in organ transplant recipients.

▶ Traditional immunosuppressants—including the macrolides cyclosporine and tacrolimus, as well as other drugs—may promote tumor development. In contrast, sirolimus has potent antitumor activity in vitro and in vivo. This report describes 2 patients who developed KS in the context of potent immunosuppressive therapy. When they were converted from cyclosporine to sirolimus, their KS lesions regressed. The mechanism of the antiangiogenic activity of sirolimus may involve impaired vascular endothelial growth factor production.[1]

B. H. Thiers, MD

Reference

1. Guba M, von Breitenbuch P, Steinbauer M, et al: Rapamycin inhibits primary and metastatic tumor growth by antiangiogenesis: Involvement of vascular endothelial growth factor. *Nat Med* 8:128-135, 2002.

17 Nevi and Melanoma

Use of Topical Sunscreens and the Risk of Malignant Melanoma: A Meta-analysis of 9067 Patients From 11 Case-Control Studies
Huncharek M, Kupelnick B (Marshfield Clinic Cancer Ctr, Wis; Meta-Analysis Research Group, Stevens Point, Wis)
Am J Public Health 92:1173-1177, 2002   17–1

Purpose.—Exposure to sunlight and ultraviolet-B radiation is likely an important contributor to the rising incidence of malignant melanoma. Sunscreen use is widely recommended to prevent sunburn and other consequences of sun-induced skin damage, but little is known about its effect on melanoma prevention. In fact, some studies have suggested that sunscreen use may actually be associated with an increased risk of melanoma. A meta-analysis was performed to analyze the effects of sunscreen use on risk of malignant melanoma.

Methods and Findings.—Review of the literature and screening of identified articles revealed 11 case-control studies of the risk of malignant melanoma associated with sunscreen use. The studies included a total of 9067 patients. Eight of the studies had odds ratios greater than 1.0, suggesting a higher risk of melanoma among sunscreen users. Combined data from all 11 studies yielded a nonsignificant summary relative risk of 1.11 but also had a Q value suggesting that the pooled studies were heterogeneous. Further analysis of studies using nonheterogeneous data suggested a summary relative risk of 1.01, again suggesting no association between sunscreen use and risk of melanoma.

Conclusions.—Detailed analysis of previous studies does not support the conclusion that use of topical sunscreens is associated with an increased risk of malignant melanoma. Studies reaching this conclusion appear to reflect bias associated with the inclusion of hospital-derived data.

Sunscreen Use and the Risk for Melanoma: A Quantitative Review
Dennis LK, Freeman LE, VanBeek MJ (Univ of Iowa, Iowa City)
Ann Intern Med 139:966-978, 2003   17–2

Introduction.—The incidence of melanoma in the United States is increasing at a faster rate than that of other cancers. Sunscreen use during childhood can significantly reduce the lifetime risk for nonmelanoma skin cancers, but several recent reports suggest that sunscreen use may increase the risk of melanoma. Relevant studies were identified through a MEDLINE search and analyzed for evidence of an association between sunscreen use and melanoma.

Methods.—Articles eligible for analysis were cohort and case-control studies that measured sunscreen use in relation to melanoma in humans. The references of identified studies and bibliographies of review articles were checked for additional reports. Independent reviewers who were blinded to the authors, journal titles, and the introduction and discussion of each article abstracted data. The articles were also scored for quality.

Results.—Twenty studies were included in the meta-analysis, but 2 were subsequently judged ineligible. The remaining 18 studies were 9 population-based case-control studies, 7 nonpopulation-based studies, and 2 case-control studies. Odds ratios were pooled across studies with the use of standard meta-analysis techniques. Pooled odds ratios for every use among 18 heterogeneous studies provided no support for an association between sunscreen use and melanoma. In addition, the lack of a dose-response effect with frequency of sunscreen use (never, sometimes, or always) supported a null association. A few studies reported a protective relationship between sunscreen use and melanoma.

Conclusion.—A meta-analysis of studies published from 1966 through April 2003 yielded no evidence of an association between melanoma and sunscreen use. Previous reports of a positive association may not have controlled for variations in protection afforded by different products, sunscreen use patterns, and sun sensitivity of the study participants.

▶ There is little question that ultraviolet light (UVL) exposure plays a significant role in the pathogenesis of cutaneous melanoma. However, other factors are also associated with its development, eg, a family history of melanoma and the presence of numerous nevi. Thus, when designing a study that examines the effect of sunscreen use on the incidence of melanoma, these other factors must be controlled for. Moreover, the relationship of melanoma to sun exposure appears to be more complex than for nonmelanoma skin cancer. For example, some investigators believe that UVA exposure may be more important than UVB in causing melanoma. Moreover, melanoma appears to be more closely associated with intermittent rather than chronic sun exposure. Thus, the type of sun exposure needs to be documented when studying the value of sunscreens in melanoma prevention.

Studies have suggested that sunscreen use may be more common in patients who have sunburned or who have a history of melanoma. This latter observation could explain why some investigators have linked the development of melanoma to sunscreen use. It is therefore important to examine sunscreen use and sun exposure habits before the diagnosis of melanoma rather than after it. Studies have also suggested that individuals who use higher SPF sunscreens are more likely to expose themselves to the sun for longer periods of time. If such individuals are using sunscreens that provide minimal UVA protection, this could increase their risk of developing melanoma. Based on these observations it is clear that simply looking at sunscreen use by melanoma patients is too simplistic an approach and many other factors need to be taken into account when examining the role of sunscreen use in the cause or prevention of melanoma. This is, in essence, what the authors of these 2 studies concluded. Both groups found considerable heterogeneity among the studies reviewed which could have biased the conclusions of the original authors. Most importantly, they found no evidence to suggest that sunscreen use is associated with the development of melanoma. Thus, we need to continue to encourage our patients to use sunscreens in combination with judicious sun exposure and protective clothing.

P. G. Lang, Jr, MD

The Diameter of Melanomas
Fernandez EM, Helm KF (Penn State Univ, Hershey)
Dermatol Surg 30:1219-1222, 2004   17–3

Background.—The mnemonic ABCD—which stands for asymmetry, border irregularity, color variation, and diameter greater than 6 mm—was developed to help both physicians and patients diagnose melanoma and is used to alert physicians to a lesion suspicious for melanoma. Some authors have suggested the addition of "E" features, standing for elevation of the lesion above the skin surface or evolution or enlargement. The addition of "F" (representing flat) has also been suggested. These ABCD features are guidelines for diagnosis, but melanomas that do not follow the ABCD rule may be overlooked by the clinician. The sensitivity of the diameter portion of the ABCD rule was therefore examined.

Methods.—A retrospective study of the pathology reports of 383 melanomas was conducted. Data on the diameter, depth, and anatomic location of each melanoma and patient age and sex were compiled. A 95% confidence interval was used to identify the proportion of melanomas 6 mm or less in diameter. A 2-tailed *P* value analysis was used when evaluating 2 independent populations—lesions 6 mm or less and lesions greater than 6 mm in diameter.

Results.—Thirty-eight percent of melanomas were 6 mm or less in diameter after processing. Melanomas greater than 6 mm in diameter occurred in significantly older patients and at a greater Breslow thickness than smaller melanomas.

Conclusions.—A significant proportion of melanomas may be smaller than 6 mm. Patients should continue to be taught the ABCD rule, but the ABCD criteria are not absolute, and educators and dermatologists should emphasize that melanoma may have many different appearances and may start as small lesions. Any unusual lesions should undergo biopsy.

Early Diagnosis of Cutaneous Melanoma: Revisiting the ABCD Criteria

Abbasi NR, Shaw HM, Rigel DS, et al (New York Univ; Royal Prince Alfred Hosp, Sydney, Australia)
JAMA 292:2771-2776, 2004   17–4

Background.—The incidence of cutaneous melanoma has increased over the past several decades, and the early diagnosis of this disease has become a continuing public health priority. The ABCD acronym (for *a*symmetry, *b*order irregularity, *c*olor variegation, and *d*iameter >6 mm), has been widely used since 1985 in medical education and in the lay press to provide easy-to-understand parameters for assessment of pigmented cutaneous lesions that may need to be further examined by a specialist. However, reexamination of these criteria is necessary in light of recent data regarding the existence of small-diameter (≤6 mm) melanomas.

Methods.—A search was conducted of the Cochrane Library and PubMed from 1980 to 2004 for relevant English-language studies involving the ABCD criteria, melanomas, and small-diameter melanoma. Additional relevant information was obtained from bibliographies of the retrieved materials. The articles selected were retrospective clinicopathologic reports and case series describing and quantifying small-diameter melanomas in adult patients.

Results.—The available data do not support lowering the diameter criterion of ABCD from the current 6 mm or greater guideline. However, the data do support adding an "E" element to the acronym to emphasize the significance of evolving pigmented lesions in the natural history of melanoma. Physicians and patients with nevi should be attentive to changes in size, shape, symptoms (such as itching and tenderness), surface features (particularly bleeding), and shades of color.

Conclusions.—The ABCD criteria for evaluation of pigmented skin lesions and early diagnosis of cutaneous melanoma should be expanded to ABCDE to include the element "evolving." However, change to the existing diameter criterion is not needed at present.

▶ The ABCD criteria for the early clinical diagnosis of cutaneous melanoma, formulated in 1985 by Friedman et al, have stood the test of time. However, like all diagnostic tools or aids, it deserves periodic reassessment and refinement. As noted by many clinicians, not all melanomas are more than 6 mm in diameter. The article by Fernandez and Helm (Abstract 17–3) addressed the reliability of the diameter component of the ABCD criteria. Of 383 lesions, 38% were less than 6 mm in diameter. However, this study was flawed by the fact that this diameter was usually obtained at the time of acquisition of the specimen and did not take into account shrinkage during processing. Nevertheless, this study and similar ones reinforce what clinicians have known for years—one cannot use a cutoff of 6 mm as an absolute criterion for the clinical diagnosis of melanoma. Moreover, as the authors acknowledge, larger lesions tend to be more invasive; thus, if one can diagnose a melanoma when it is less than 6 mm in diameter, at least theoretically the prognosis should be better.

In contrast, Abbasi et al (Abstract 17–4) argue that the prevalence of invasive melanomas less than 6 mm in diameter is not high enough to justify changing the criteria for D, and that by not doing so would not increase the risk of patients presenting with advanced disease. Moreover, by not changing the criteria this would probably save many patients the cost and pain of undergoing unnecessary biopsies. The authors do emphasize that in using the ABCD criteria one should realize that any given melanoma may not meet all the criteria. The other issue addressed by these authors was adding the letter "E" to the ABCD criteria, with "E" standing for an evolving or changing lesion. For years we have told our patients to come in for evaluation if a mole was changing (in shape, size, or color) or was bleeding or symptomatic. This criterion alone has brought many patients to their physician's office, where a diagnosis of melanoma was made. A number of investigators have for this reason suggested adding "E" to the ABCD criteria. The authors of this article, on the basis of their own experience and the literature, agree that this would be a valuable addition that likely would facilitate the early diagnosis of melanoma.

P. G. Lang, Jr, MD

Diagnostic Accuracy of Patients in Performing Skin Self-Examination and the Impact of Photography
Oliveria SA, Chau D, Christos PJ, et al (Memorial Sloan-Kettering Cancer Ctr, New York; Univ of Miami, Fla)
Arch Dermatol 140:57-62, 2004   17–5

Introduction.—Because lesion thickness is the most important prognostic factor for primary cutaneous melanoma, early identification and excision of thin lesions could reduce the mortality rate from the disease. Skin self-examination (SSE) is the most common way skin cancer is currently detected. For patients with large numbers of dysplastic nevi, photographs of the skin can provide a baseline against which changes can be measured, and new lesions identified. The value of baseline photography to the practice of SSE was evaluated in 50 patients with 5 or more dysplastic nevi. Participants in the study were highly motivated; 65.8% had a history of malignant melanoma.

Methods.—Patients who had baseline digital photography and mole counts of their back, chest, and abdomen were instructed to perform a baseline SSE and were provided with print copies of the images. After the baseline SSE, the appearance of existing moles was altered, and new moles were created using cosmetic eyeliner. The results of SSEs completed with access to the baseline photos were compared with those completed without access to the baseline photos.

Results.—Patients were blindfolded while new and altered moles were created. Full-length and handheld mirrors were used during the SSEs. The median number of moles per patient was 50, and 10% of each patient's moles had been altered. The sensitivity and specificity of SSE for detection of both new and altered moles without photography were 60.2% and 96.2%, respectively; SSE with photography increased sensitivity and specificity to 72.4% and 98.4%, respectively. Men performed better than women without the aid of photography, but women had a higher sensitivity and specificity when SSE was performed with photographs. The results were similar when stratified by mole site.

Conclusion.—Baseline digital photography as an adjunct to SSE can improve the diagnostic accuracy of patients performing SSE.

▶ Total-body digital photography (TBDP) has been shown to be a useful adjunct for managing patients with many moles who are at significant risk for melanoma. TBDP potentially allows for the earlier detection of melanoma and can decrease the number of unnecessary biopsies. In addition, TBDP patients are encouraged to perform monthly SSEs, again in hope of detecting a melanoma in its earliest growth phase. Patients with numerous atypical nevi often find SSE to be overwhelming and anxiety provoking, since it is difficult for them to remember what a mole looked like previously or even if it is new. We have found, as this article substantiates, that giving the patient a compact disk of their TBDP allows their total-body skin examination to be more reliable and less frustrating. In this study, the baseline photographs were more helpful for detecting changes in size and preexisting markers as opposed to color, and for detecting new moles.

P. G. Lang, Jr, MD

Risk of Melanoma Arising in Large Congenital Melanocytic Nevi: A Systematic Review
Watt AJ, Kotsis SV, Chung KC (Univ of Michigan, Ann Arbor)
Plast Reconstr Surg 113:1968-1974, 2004   17–6

Background.—Large congenital melanocytic nevi are regarded by many clinicians as premalignant conditions, and these clinicians have advocated complete resection when possible. However, the risk of subsequent melanoma has not been adequately quantified in the literature. Published estimates have placed this risk in a range from 0% to 42%. The resection and reconstruction of large congenital melanocytic nevi are complex and often extensive, and the risk of malignant transformation is a crucial factor that must be weighed by surgeons and families when deciding whether to excise the lesion. A literature review was used as a basis for recommendations into further investigations.

Methods.—A systematic data analysis was conducted to critically evaluate published studies and to establish a crude incidence rate for the risk of malignant melanoma transformation in large congenital melanocytic nevi. Original studies published between 1966 and 2002 were included, and the following key words were applied to the English language search in PREMEDLINE and MEDLINE: "congenital nevus," "melanocytic nevus," "giant hairy nevus," and "bathing trunk nevus."

Results.—A comprehensive search of the literature yielded 8 studies that met the inclusion criteria. These studies included 432 patients with large congenital melanocytic nevi. Of those patients, 12 (2.8%) had cutaneous malignant melanoma develop during the reported follow-up periods. Comparison of these incidence rates to those of the Surveillance, Epidemiology, and End Results population-based database showed that patients with large congenital melanocytic nevi had an increased risk of melanoma compared with the general population. In terms of treatment before melanoma developed in the 12 patients, 6 were observed (ie, no treatment) before diagnosis, 2 had partial excision, 1 had dermabrasion, 1 had a chemical peel, and 2 did not have any treatment information.

Conclusions.—There is a significantly increased risk of melanoma in patients with large congenital melanocytic nevi. There is also a need for a standardized definition of large congenital melanocytic nevi and a long-term prospective study to determine the actual lifetime risk of melanoma in patients with and without surgical excision.

▶ This report represents a systematic review of the literature pertaining to the development of melanoma in large congenital nevi. Although it is generally agreed that there is an increased risk of melanoma in these lesions, there is no uniform agreement on how significant this risk is. In the series reviewed by these authors, 8 were deemed suitable for inclusion. Among the 8 series, the incidence of melanoma varied from 0% to 8.3%, with an overall incidence of 2.8%. The length of follow-up in the various series was often inadequate (ranging from 0.7-10.5 years, with an average of 6.2 years) and could have influenced the findings.

Another unanswered question in these patients is whether treatment prevents the development of melanoma. These children often have extensive lesions that cannot be totally excised. Although it has been suggested that partial removal may decrease the risk for melanoma development, there is no well-controlled study that addresses this issue. Although studies in recent years have given us a better idea of how to manage patients with congenital nevi, we still need more information regarding their natural history and the impact of treatment.

P. G. Lang, Jr, MD

Number of Satellite Nevi as a Correlate for Neurocutaneous Melanocytosis in Patients With Large Congenital Melanocytic Nevi
Marghoob AA, Dusza S, Oliveria S, et al (Memorial Sloan-Kettering Cancer Ctr, New York)
Arch Dermatol 140:171-175, 2004   17–7

Introduction.—Patients with large congenital melanocytic nevi (LCMN) are at a significantly high risk of neurocutaneous melanocytosis (NCM), and the risk is greatest among those with LCMN on the posterior axis and with many satellite nevi. The database of the first Internet patient support–

advocacy group-based registry of patients with LCMN was analyzed to determine the relationship between LCMN location, number of satellite nevi, and the risk of NCM.

Methods.—The registry is maintained by a support group, Nevus Outreach Inc. Individuals with LCMN or their guardians who visited the Nevus Outreach website were asked to complete a 6-page questionnaire that included information on the main nevus, satellite nevi, neurologic symptoms, surgical treatments, MRI findings, and personal and family history of melanoma.

Results.—Final analyses were based on responses from 379 patients with LCMN from 26 countries. At the time of the analysis, the median age of the group was 3 years, and the median diameter of the LCMN was 24.7 cm; 58% of the patients were female, and 42% were male. The LCMN were on the posterior axis in 72% of patients, on the chest or abdomen in 21%, and on an extremity in 7%. The median number of satellite nevi was 20 (range, 0-2500). Twenty-six registry members (7%) had a diagnosis of NCM, which was symptomatic in 22. A significantly higher percentage of patients with NCM had their LCMN on the posterior axis compared with those without NCM (96% vs 70%, respectively). The median number of satellite melanocytic nevi was markedly greater in patients with NCM than in patients without NCM (68.5 vs 18). In logistic regression analysis, the number of satellite nevi was the only significant risk factor for NCM.

Conclusion.—The most important risk factor for the development of NCM in patients with LCMN proved to be the presence of large numbers of satellite nevi. The location of LCMN on the posterior axis was a less important factor on multivariate analysis. Any anomaly in early embryogenesis that results in formation of LCMN and widespread satellites may also produce a deposit of excess melanocytes in the leptomeninges, leading to NCM.

▶ This is a self-reported study of the size and location of LCMN and the number of satellite nevi present in patients with and without NCM registered with an Internet patient support–advocacy group, Nevus Outreach Inc. A strong correlation was found between the number of satellite nevi and the presence of NCM. In this study, the number of nevi was of greater significance than a posterior axis location of the patient's LCMN. The authors suggest that a reasonable criterion for obtaining an MRI study of the CNS in asymptomatic children would be the presence of a large number of satellite nevi, specifically 20 or more lesions, regardless of the LCMN location.

S. Raimer, MD

Toenail Arsenic Content and Cutaneous Melanoma in Iowa

Beane Freeman LE, Dennis LK, Lynch CF, et al (Natl Cancer Inst, Bethesda, Md; Univ of Iowa, Iowa City)
Am J Epidemiol 160:679-687, 2004 17–8

Background.—Many epidemiologic studies and case reports suggest a link between arsenic and the development of skin cancer. This case–control study examined the association between environmental arsenic exposure (as measured in toenail clippings) and cutaneous melanoma in adults in Iowa.

Methods.—The case patients were 386 adults 40 years or older who were given a diagnosis of cutaneous melanoma in 1999-2000. Cases were matched by age and sex to 373 patients with colon cancer given diagnoses during the same period. All research subjects were white. Both groups completed a questionnaire regarding demographic and clinical information and submitted a toenail clipping for determining arsenic content via graphite furnace atomic absorption spectrophotometry.

Results.—Compared with research subjects with the lowest toenail arsenic content (lowest quartile, ≤0.020 µg/g), those with the highest toenail arsenic content (highest quartile, ≥0.084 µg/g) had double the risk of cutaneous melanoma (odds ratio, 2.1; *P* for trend, .001). This relationship was modified by a self-reported prior history of skin cancer. At the highest quartile of toenail arsenic content, the odds ratios for cutaneous melanoma were 1.7 among patients with no prior skin cancer diagnosis and 6.6 among patients who reported a prior skin cancer.

Conclusion.—In this sample of white Iowans, higher arsenic concentrations in toenail clippings were significantly associated with an elevated risk of cutaneous melanoma, particularly when a prior history of skin cancer was present. This possible link between environmental arsenic exposure and cutaneous melanoma warrants further study.

▶ This article is an interesting epidemiologic exploration. Arsenic is a known human carcinogen and has been associated with the development of nonmelanoma skin cancer. This investigation demonstrates an increased risk of melanoma in patients with high toenail arsenic concentrations. For this reader, it generated more questions than answers. Further investigation is needed before a true causal relationship can be established.

J. Cook, MD

Three-Point Checklist of Dermoscopy: A New Screening Method for Early Detection of Melanoma

Soyer HP, Argenziano G, Zalaudek I, et al (Univ of Graz, Austria; Second Univ of Naples, Italy; Univ Tor Vergata of Rome, et al)
Dermatology 208:27-31, 2004 17–9

Introduction.—The removal of all lesions that clinically or dermoscopically are suggestive of melanoma is warranted. However, excision of benign lesions should be minimized. Recent reports indicate that dermoscopy performed by experienced users is more accurate than clinical examination in the diagnosis of melanoma. The diagnostic performance of nonexperts using a new 3-point checklist based on a simplified dermoscopic pattern analysis was retrospectively examined to verify the reproducibility and validity of the new method.

Methods.—Clinical and dermoscopic images of 231 clinically equivocal and histopathologically verified pigmented skin lesions were evaluated by 6 non-experts and 1 expert in dermoscopy. Each lesion was evaluated by non-experts using the 3 dermoscopic criteria (asymmetry, atypical network, and blue-white structures) that compose the 3-point method. Additionally, all examiners made an overall diagnosis by use of standard pattern analysis of dermoscopy.

Results.—Asymmetry, atypical network, and blue-white structures were reproducible, with a kappa value that ranged between 0.52 and 0.55. The 3-point checklist diagnosis had similar reproducibility (kappa = 0.53) compared with overall diagnosis using the standard pattern analysis of dermoscopy.

When assigning an overall diagnosis, the expert had 89.6% sensitivity for malignant lesions (tested on 68 melanomas and 9 pigmented basal cell carcinomas) versus 69.7% sensitivity for the nonexperts. The sensitivity of the nonexperts using the 3-point checklist was 96.3%. The specificity of the expert using overall diagnosis was 94.2% versus 82.8% and 32.8% for nonexperts using overall diagnosis and the 3-point checklist.

Conclusion.—The 3-point checklist is both a valid and a reproducible dermoscopic algorithm that has high sensitivity for the diagnosis of melanoma when used by nonexperts. It may be used as a screening procedure for early identification of melanoma.

▶ Melanoma remains primarily a surgical disease; thus, early diagnosis is essential. Dermoscopy in the hands of experienced clinicians can increase the diagnostic sensitivity for melanoma by 35% compared to clinical examination alone. However, in the hands of the inexperienced, it is of little benefit. In this study, the authors used a simplified approach to dermoscopy by selecting what appear to be the 3 most important features which help distinguish benign from malignant pigmented skin lesions.

Using these 3 features, they then gave a "crash course" to novices, and then examined their ability to differentiate between benign and malignant pigmented skin lesions. The 3 dermoscopic criteria utilized were (1) asymmetry of color and dermoscopic structures, (2) an atypical pigment network with irregular holes and thick lines, and (3) the presence of blue or white colors. Using this 3-point checklist, the novices achieved a sensitivity of diagnosis of 96.3%; however, the specificity was only 32.8%. If the dermoscopic features were combined with the clinical impression, the specificity increased to 82.8%, although the sensitivity fell to 69.7%.

An expert dermoscopist had a sensitivity of 89.6% and a specificity of 94.2% when using combined dermoscopic and clinical criteria. Although specificity needed improvement, the authors correctly conclude that the experiment was a success from the standpoint of teaching novices to effectively use dermoscopy to recognize malignant pigmented skin lesions.

P. G. Lang, Jr, MD

Melanoma Computer-Aided Diagnosis: Reliability and Feasibility Study

Burroni M, Corona R, Dell'Eva G, et al (Univ of Siena, Italy; Istituto Dermopatico dell'Immacolata, Rome; Italian Cancer League, Siena, Italy)
Clin Cancer Res 10:1881-1886, 2004   17–10

Introduction.—The differential diagnosis of melanoma from melanocytic nevi is frequently not straightforward. There is growing interest in the auto-mated analysis of digitized images obtained by epiluminescence microscopy techniques in helping clinicians differentiate early melanoma from benign skin lesions. Diagnostic accuracy provided by various statistical classifiers was examined with the use of a large set of pigmented skin lesions (melano-mas and nevi) obtained by 4 digitized analyzers (DB-Mips) located in 2 dif-ferent dermatologic units in Rome and Siena, Italy.

Methods.—The DB-Mips System is composed of a 3CCD PAL video cam-era with 750 lines of image resolution and a 60-decibel signal noise ratio. The camera, operating in the visible spectrum, is attached to a patented hand-help optic system that provides dermoscopic images with a magnifica-tion ranging from x6 to x40, allowing a horizontal field view of 40 to 6 mm. Images from 391 melanomas and 449 melanocytic nevi were evaluated.

A linear classifier was created by using the method of receiver operating characteristic curves to determine a threshold value for a fixed sensitivity of 95%. A K-nearest-neighbor classifier, a nonparametric method of pattern recognition, was constructed by using all available image features and trained for a sensitivity of 98% on a large exemplar set of lesions.

Results.—For all parameters, a clearly elucidated difference between melanomas and nevi was seen. For an additional check on the feature se-lection procedure, a logistic regression model encompassing all of the se-lected features was run to evaluate each feature with melanoma, after ad-justing for the others. All except 2 geometric parameters (fractality of the border and variance of the contour symmetry) were independently linked with melanoma.

There were 3 linear classifiers (2 of which were trained on separate sets derived from the Rome and Siena centers). All 3 classifiers were indepen-dently tested on the Rome and Siena sets of lesions. One classifier with a fixed sensitivity of 95% achieved a specificity of 83% with use of the Rome test set.

Similar findings were achieved with the second classifier, constructed on the Siena training set, which yielded a sensitivity of 93% and a specificity of 81% on the set of lesions from the Rome center. The performance of the K-nearest-neighbor classifier on the same set of lesions had a fixed sensitivity of 98%. A specificity of 79% was achieved on all sets of histologically diag-nosed benign lesions, compared to that achieved by the linear classifiers.

Conclusion.—Computer-aided differentiation of melanomas from benign pigmented lesions obtained with DB-Mips is both feasible and reliable. The same equipment used in different units produced similar diagnostic accuracy. It remains to be determined whether this could improve early diagnosis of melanoma or decrease the incidence of unnecessary surgery.

▶ Attempts continue to develop diagnostic aids for the early detection of melanoma. These include dermoscopy, epiluminescence microscopy, and digital image analysis (DIA). This study examined the usefulness of DIA. The authors found that the analyzer used had a diagnostic sensitivity of 98% and a specificity of 79%. Although they cannot replace the clinician or the pathologist, diagnostic tools such as DIA can be used as an adjunct in the selection of pigmented skin lesions for biopsy.

P. G. Lang, Jr, MD

Digital Epiluminescence Microscopy Monitoring of High-Risk Patients
Robinson JK, Nickoloff BJ (Loyola Univ, Maywood, Ill)
Arch Dermatol 140:49-56, 2004   17–11

Introduction.—Experienced dermatologists diagnose melanomas with the unaided eye. Epiluminescence microscopy (ELM) improves the diagnostic accuracy of early cases and assists in selecting pigmented lesions that necessitate biopsy. Cutaneous photographs are used to monitor patients with new lesions and changes in atypical nevi. Digital ELM (DELM) archives images of nevi and helps surveillance of atypical nevi by providing 30-fold magnification of pigmented structural components. Reported was an experience with multiple atypical nevi monitored annually for 4 years with DELM using defined criteria of change to determine the need for biopsy.

Methods.—Between January 1, 1998, and December 31, 2000, baseline DELM was performed in 100 patients, followed by annual imaging of atypical nevi. Pigmentary changes or an increased DELM diameter of 1 mm or greater was an indication for excisional biopsy. The patient age range was 18 to 65 years (mean age, 38.4 years; 72% female). A minimum of 2 images were available for each lesion. The change in DELM was verified histopathologically. Patient confidence in and comfort with dermatologic surveillance and skin self-examination performance was evaluated.

Results.—A total of 1532 melanocytic skin lesions had a minimum of 3 sequentially recorded images and 1950 had 2 images by DELM. At annual follow-up examinations, 215 new nevi larger than 3 mm in diameter were added to total images and had only 1 recorded image. During the 4-year duration of the study, 3697 nevi had stored images.

The median follow-up period was 36.2 months (range, 12-48 months). During annual follow-up examination with DELM, 5.5% of lesions changed. Of 193 excisional biopsy specimens, 4 were melanoma in situ, 169 were dysplastic nevi, and 20 were common nevi. The confidence in and comfort with surveillance and skin self-examination were enhanced with the use of DELM.

Conclusion.—Criteria used to identify marked DELM changes were an increase in DELM diameter of 1 mm or greater and pigmentary changes, including radial streaming, focal enlargement, peripheral black dots, and "clumping" within the irregular pigment network. The use of DELM was beneficial in boosting confidence in and comfort with the performance of more extensive skin self-examination.

▶ Digital ELM (DELM) can be used to monitor patients with numerous atypical nevi who are at increased risk for developing melanoma. This report reflects the experience of 1 physician who has utilized this diagnostic aid. Over a 4-year period, images of 3482 lesions were recorded. Of these, 5.5% showed a significant change in size or pigmentation and were subsequently subjected to biopsy. Of these, only 2% were melanomas, the majority (88%) being dysplastic nevi. Thus, although DELM allowed the early diagnosis of a few melanomas, unfortunately it did not allow one to distinguish melanoma from dysplastic nevi undergoing change with enough certainty to obviate the need for a biopsy.

P. G. Lang, Jr, MD

Presentation, Histopathologic Findings, and Clinical Outcomes in 7 Cases of Melanoma In Situ of the Nail Unit
High WA, Quirey RA, Guillén DR, et al (Univ of Texas, Dallas)
Arch Dermatol 140:1102-1106, 2004   17–12

Introduction.—Melanoma of the nail unit is both rare and associated with a poorer prognosis than melanoma at other sites. Early diagnosis is difficult because pigmentation may be absent or attributed to a traumatic cause. Tissue-sparing Mohs micrographic surgery has the potential benefit of avoiding amputation in cases of thin melanoma of the nail unit. Patients with melanoma in situ (MIS) of the nail unit were reviewed for presentation, histopathologic findings, and clinical outcome.

Methods.—Over a 5-year period, 7 of 166 patients treated by a single Mohs micrographic surgeon had biopsy-proven MIS of the nail unit. Patients were 5 women and 2 men who ranged in age from 34 to 87 years. Fingernails were affected in 5 patients (3 index fingers) and toenails in 2 patients (the great toe in both). Duration of pigmentation ranged from 7 months to 6 years. The primary indication for biopsy was melanonychia in all cases. Both biopsy and surgical specimens were reviewed.

Results.—Pigmentation of the proximal nail fold (Hutchinson sign) was positive in 3 cases. Biopsy specimen photomicrographs revealed asymmetry, atypia, and limited pagetoid spread. No patient had lymphadenopathy or signs of systemic disease at the time of excision, and histopathologically tumor-free margins were obtained in all cases. Four tumors were cleared in a single stage, 2 required 2 stages, and 1 required 3 stages. Three patients underwent partial distal interphalangeal amputation. With a mean follow-up period of 24 months, 1 patient had a recurrence of pigmentation at the operative site 5 months after surgery. Another biopsy revealed atypical melanocytic hyperplasia, and the patient elected to have a partial amputation. No other recurrences or metastatic disease have occurred.

Conclusion.—A diagnosis of MIS of the nail unit should be considered in white patients with longitudinal melanonychia. Because Hutchinson sign may be absent, the threshold for biopsy should be low. Mohs surgery should be explored as a tissue- and digit-sparing procedure.

▶ Traditionally, patients with a subungual melanoma or squamous cell carcinoma have been managed by amputation of the digit. However, the advent of Mohs surgery has offered such patients another option that allows preservation of the digit. There have been a number of reports demonstrating the efficacy of Mohs surgery for such tumors. This report confirms the usefulness of this technique for managing melanomas of the nail unit. However, several observations should be made. First, 3 patients underwent partial amputation after Mohs surgery. This was unfortunate since the purpose of Mohs surgery is to preserve the digit. These 3 patients not only underwent partial amputation but also had to suffer through additional painful surgery before this. Unfortunately, one cannot always predict the amount of subclinical tumor spread, and thus after tracing out the tumor the simplest way to manage the defect may be partial amputation. Although the details of the Mohs surgery are not given, based on the example shown it would appear that these authors customarily resect the entire nail bed, matrix, and lateral nail folds as a unit. Although not exactly tissue conserving, this approach does obviate several potential problems: (1) leaving a remnant of a nail that is nonfunctional and not cosmetically pleasing, and (2) attempting to trace out tumor in a nail bed that has been partially denuded by avulsion of the nail plate.

P. G. Lang, Jr, MD

Amelanotic/Hypomelanotic Melanoma: Clinical and Dermoscopic Features

Pizzichetta MA, Talamini R, Stanganelli I, et al (Centro di Riferimento Oncologico, Aviano, Italy; Ravenna-Niguarda Hosp, Milano, Italy; IDI, Rome; et al)
Br J Dermatol 150:1117-1124, 2004   17–13

Background.—Amelanotic malignant melanoma is a subtype of cutaneous melanoma that presents with little or no pigment at visual inspection. This type of melanoma is most likely to occur in sun-exposed skin, particularly in elderly persons with photodamage. Dermoscopy is a noninvasive technique introduced to increase the accuracy of diagnosis of pigmented skin lesions and to improve the sensitivity and specificity of melanoma diagnosis. Whether dermoscopy is also useful for the diagnosis of amelanotic/hypomelanotic melanoma (AHM) was determined.

Methods.—A retrospective clinical study was conducted of 151 AHM skin lesions from 151 patients with a mean age of 47 ± 17.5 years. The lesions included 55 AHM nonmelanocytic lesions (AHNML), 52 AHM benign melanocytic lesions (AHBML), and 44 AHM lesions. Of the AHM lesions, 10 (23%) were nonpigmented, truly amelanotic melanomas. The 44 AHM lesions were grouped as thin melanomas (TnM) (≤1 mm; 29 cases) and thick melanomas (TkM) (>1 mm; 15 cases) according to the Breslow index. Five clinical features and 10 dermoscopic criteria were evaluated to achieve clinical and dermoscopic diagnoses.

Results.—The most frequent and significant clinical features for TnM and TkM were asymmetry and ulceration (with ulceration significant only for TkM) compared with AHBML. The most relevant dermoscopic criteria for TnM compared with AHBML were the presence of irregular dots/globules, regression structures, irregular pigmentation, and blue-whitish veil. TkM differed significantly from AHBML in the frequency of occurrence in irregular pigmentation, irregular dots/ globules, regression structures, blue-whitish veil, and hypopigmentation. Linear irregular vessels and a combination of dotted and linear irregular vessels associated with TnM and TkM were not observed in these cases of AHBML and were only rarely observed in AHNML (3.6% and 1.8%, respectively). Sensitivity and specificity were higher for the dermoscopic diagnosis than for the clinical diagnosis (89% and 96% vs 65% and 88%, respectively).

Conclusions.—Dermoscopy is a useful technique for pigmented melanoma and hypomelanotic melanoma. Vascular patterns alone may not be adequate for the diagnosis of "true" amelanotic melanoma. An approach that combines dermoscopy with clinical findings should aid in the detection of "true" amelanotic melanoma.

▶ In the hands of experienced clinicians, dermoscopy can improve the ability to diagnose melanoma. Dermoscopic criteria assessed during the examination include not only pigmentary features but also vascular features of the lesion. In this study of AHM, the authors found that if sufficient pigment was present, dermoscopy was useful for making the correct diagnosis. However, if pigment was totally absent, one had to rely heavily on the history and clinical features to make the correct diagnosis. Although amelanotic melanomas have characteristic vascular patterns, unfortunately these are seen with other nonpigmented lesions such as basal cell carcinoma, and this criterion alone cannot be used to diagnose melanoma.

P. G. Lang, Jr, MD

Cutaneous Melanoma in a Multiethnic Population: Is This a Different Disease?

Hemmings DE, Johnson DS, Tominaga GT, et al (Univ of Hawaii at Manoa, Honolulu)

Arch Surg 139:968-973, 2004   17–14

Background.—Cutaneous melanoma is most typically found in persons with blue/green eyes, who have blond or red hair and fair to light complexions, and those who are sun sensitive and tan poorly. Cutaneous melanoma is relatively unusual in nonwhite persons, and the effects of educational programs to improve outcomes is unknown, particularly in an increasingly ethnically diverse population. The experience with the management of cutaneous melanoma in nonwhite patients in a multiethnic population was reviewed.

Methods.—The study group was composed of 357 consecutive patients with melanoma seen at a tertiary care, university-affiliated community medical center in a multiethnic setting. The main outcome measures were ethnicity, age, sex, primary tumor site, tumor thickness, nodal status, stage at diagnosis, and survival.

Results.—The patients included 208 men and 149 women ranging in age from 15 to 93 years (mean, 58 years). The primary site was unknown in 22 patients. Of the 357 patients, 67 (18.7%) were nonwhite. No statistically significant difference was observed in the age or sex distribution of the white and nonwhite populations. The nonwhite patients at initial diagnosis had thicker tumors, more frequently had ulcerated primary tumors and positive nodes, and were at a more advanced stage than the white patients. There was a significant difference in the anatomic distribution between the 2 populations, with a high incidence of melanoma on the sole and subungual locations and significantly less frequent occurrence on the head and neck, trunk, and extremities in the nonwhite populations compared with the white population. The overall survival rate of the nonwhite patients was significantly worse than that of the white patients; however, no difference in outcome was present when survival was stratified by stage.

Conclusions.—In a multiethnic population, cutaneous melanoma in nonwhite persons is unusual but not rare. The diagnoses are distinctly different at initial examination, which suggests a potential biologic component. However, the stage-for-stage outcomes are similar between white and nonwhite persons, which suggests a need for early diagnostic interventions in nonwhite patients with unusual pigmented lesions.

Association Between Female Breast Cancer and Cutaneous Melanoma
Goggins W, Gao W, Tsao H (Univ of Hong Kong; Jinan Univ, Guangzhou, China; Massachusetts Gen Hosp, Boston)
Int J Cancer 111:792-794, 2004   17–15

Background.—Findings from epidemiologic studies have suggested a link between cutaneous melanoma (CM) and breast cancer (BC). In addition, carriers of mutations in *BRCA2*, the breast cancer predisposition gene, appear to have an increased risk of melanoma, whereas carriers of mutations in the melanoma susceptibility gene, *CDKN2A*, show a higher than expected risk of breast cancer. Thus, pathways involved in the development of CM and BC may overlap, and survivors of one form of cancer may be prone to the development of the other. The hypothesis that survivors of BC have an increased risk of CM, and vice versa, was tested.

Methods.—Female patients with BC registered in the 1973-1999 Surveillance, Epidemiology, and End Result (SEER) database were monitored for development of a subsequent CM, and female patients with CM were monitored for the development of a subsequent BC. The expected number of cases was then compared with the observed number of cases by using standardized incidence ratios.

Results.—Overall, a modest but statistically significant increased risk of CM was present among female survivors of BC and vice versa. Young patients with BC were found to have a 46% elevated risk of a subsequent CM. Women who were treated with radiation therapy had a 42% increased risk of CM. The risks of BC among female survivors of CM and CM among survivors of BC were also increased, although to a lesser extent (11% and 16% overall, respectively). A mutual association was found between female BC and CM.

Conclusions.—The suggestion of the observed elevated risk for CM, particularly among younger patients with BC, is that the genetic observations from high-risk groups may also be at work, although at a much lower level, in the general BC population.

▶ Studies on familial melanoma, especially those associated with a mutation in *CDKN2A*, have suggested that there may be an increased risk for BC in these cohorts. Likewise, BC patients with a mutation in *BRCA2* have been reported to be at increased risk for development of CM. In this study, the investigators found that BC patients were at increased risk for developing CM, especially if they had received radiation therapy, and vice versa. These findings are in contrast to another article addressed by this reviewer (Abstract 17–16), which suggested the possibility of a genetic link between the 2 diseases but could not document a strong enough association to justify routine screening for BC. Goggins et al could not explain the influence of radiation therapy on the development of CM.

P. G. Lang, Jr, MD

Heterogeneity of Risk for Melanoma and Pancreatic and Digestive Malignancies: A Melanoma Case-Control Study
Rutter JL, Bromley CM, Goldstein AM, et al (Natl Cancer Inst, Bethesda, Md; BioStat Solutions LCC, Damascus, Md; Univ of Pennsylvania, Philadelphia; et al)
Cancer 101:2809-2816, 2004   17–16

Introduction.—Two genes, *CDKN2A* and *CDK4*, are implicated in the etiology of melanoma, but the reported incidence of *CDKN2A* mutations in patients with melanoma is extremely low. Evidence for heterogeneity of risk for melanoma and other malignancies believed to cluster in melanoma-prone families was examined in a case-control study.

Methods.—Without regard to family history, eligible patients were newly diagnosed with invasive cutaneous melanoma between January 1, 1991, and December 31, 1992. A control group, matched for age, race, sex, and geographic distribution, was recruited from 12 clinics that focused on other illnesses. All participants were interviewed about melanoma risk factors and cancer status of first-degree relatives. Full-body skin examinations were also performed. A family's melanoma risk was based on the observed deviation from the expected incidence of melanoma.

Results.—The 737 cases and 1021 controls were similar in sex, age, and number of family members reported. First-degree relatives with melanoma were reported by 8% of patients with melanoma versus 4% of control subjects. Three of 10 control subjects and 6 of 22 cases with a previous diagnosis of melanoma had a family history of melanoma. The overall estimated relative risk conferred by a family history of melanoma was 1.7 (with adjustment for dysplastic nevi, age, sex, and study site). Risk of melanoma was not significantly increased by family histories of pancreatic, brain, breast, gastrointestinal, or lymphoproliferative disease. Significant evidence was present of familial heterogeneity for melanomas, but not for pancreatic or gastrointestinal malignancies, among case families. Screening for *CDKN2A* germline mutations in 133 melanoma case probands identified 2 mutations in *CDKN2A* associated with melanoma risk. Families with high and low heterogeneity scores did not differ in rates of mutation detection.

Conclusion.—Melanoma was the major cancer clustering in families of these patients with melanoma, and the occurrence of other cancers previously reported to cluster in melanoma families was rare. Because few *CDKN2A* mutations were found in families considered to be at increased risk, other susceptibility genes may be involved in the cause of melanoma. Widespread testing for *CDKN2A* in the general population does not appear to be warranted.

▶ Two genes, *CDKN2A* and *CDK4*, have been implicated in the etiology of melanoma. Mutations in *CDKN2A* have been found in approximately 20% of melanoma-prone families, whereas mutations in *CDK4* have been detected in only 3 melanoma-prone families. The incidence of mutations in *CDKN2A* in large population-based studies in patients with melanoma is, however, extremely low (0.2%). In certain melanoma-prone families an increased incidence of other malignancies has been reported (pancreatic, digestive tract, breast, brain, soft tissue sarcomas, and lymphoproliferative malignancies). Mutations in *CDKN2A* have been observed in some of these families. A question that arises when evaluating a patient with melanoma or a melanoma-prone family is whether it is worthwhile screening for associated malignancies and for mutations in *CDKN2A*. Based on the findings of these authors, routine screening for associated malignancies is not indicated, and the incidence of mutations in *CDKN2A* is so low, even in melanoma-prone families, that screening for these mutations is not worthwhile.

P. G. Lang, Jr, MD

Surgical Margins for Lentigo Maligna and Lentigo Maligna Melanoma: The Technique of Mapped Serial Excision
Huilgol SC, Selva D, Chen C, et al (Univ of Adelaide, Australia; Wakefield Clinic, Adelaide, Australia)
Arch Dermatol 140:1087-1092, 2004   17–17

Introduction.—Lentigo maligna (LM), a form of melanoma in situ, can progress to lentigo maligna melanoma (LMM), a subtype of invasive melanoma. Surgical excision is preferred for both LM and LMM, but the clinical margins of these lesions are often poorly defined. Consecutive patients with head and neck LM or LMM were studied prospectively to assess the margins required for excision by the technique of mapped serial excision (MSE).

Methods.—The single-center study included patients who underwent MSE between March 1, 1993, and October 31, 2002. All had histologically confirmed LM or LMM larger than 1 cm. The tumor borders were marked, and a 5-mm margin was added. Patients received local anesthetic, and excision to the middle-to-deep subcutaneous fat level was performed. Further 5-mm excisions continued to be made, if necessary, until histopathologic assessment confirmed clear margins. Patients were monitored for new lesions at the site or for changes in pigmentation or the appearance of the scar.

Results.—A total of 161 LMs or LMMs in 155 patients were treated in the study period. Thirty-seven LMs (30%) required more than 5-mm margins. Among LMMs less than 1 mm in Breslow thickness, 4 (12%) required more than 10-mm margins for complete excision. All additional 5-mm levels for both LM and LMM were for marginal in situ disease. The preoperative clinical lesion size was not significantly related to the number of 5-mm levels needed for a complete histologic excision. Forty-six (29%) of the 161 cases (34 of LM and 12 of LMM) had recurred before MSE. None of these were previously treated by MSE; surgical excision had been used in 32 cases, cryotherapy had been used in 12, and argon or carbon dioxide laser therapy had been used in 2. Recurrent LM was more likely than primary LM to require more than 1 level for a complete clear-margin excision. Of the 155 cases with follow-up (mean, 38 months' duration), 4 cases that were initially primary LM recurred at intervals of 12, 31, 39, and 40 months after MSE.

Conclusion.—Current recommendations of 5-mm margins for in situ melanoma and 10-mm margins for invasive melanoma less than 1 mm in Breslow thickness are often insufficient for head and neck LM and LMM. Complete excision is the treatment of choice, and MSE appears to be effective in achieving a high cure rate.

▶ The National Institutes of Health recommendation of 5-mm margins for the resection of lentigo maligna is, in many circumstances, inadequate. My experience dealing with these difficult lesions on sun-damaged skin echoes that of Zitelli et al.[1-3] When lentigo maligna is resected with the use of the Mohs technique and surgical margins are determined, it has been found that subclinical extension is frequently present. Moreover, determination of a true positive margin may be problematic given that melanocyte hyperplasia is common in significantly actinically damaged skin. This study failed to find any association between the diameter of the lesion and the margins required for excision. My experience, like that of Zitelli et al, suggests that larger diameter melanomas, especially on the head, neck, hands, and feet, require larger surgical margins to achieve a clinical cure. The treating physician should be very respectful of lentigo maligna in anatomically challenging areas such as those mentioned above. The utilization of Mohs micrographic surgery and its method of horizontal tissue mapping allows for a more complete examination of the true surgical margins. The use of Mohs surgery for melanoma requires an experienced Mohs surgeon and a technically proficient laboratory.

J. Cook, MD

References

1. Zitelli JA, Brown CD, Hanusa BH: Mohs micrographic surgery for the treatment of primary cutaneous melanoma. *J Am Acad Dermatol* 37:236-245, 1997.
2. Zitelli JA, Moy RL, Abell E: The reliability of frozen sections in the evaluation of surgical margins for melanoma. *J Am Acad Dermatol* 24:290-294, 1991.
3. Zitelli JA, Brown CD, Hanusa BH: Surgical margins for excision of primary cutaneous melanoma. *J Am Acad Dermatol* 37:422-429, 1997.

Management of Lentigo Maligna and Lentigo Maligna Melanoma With Staged Excision: A 5-Year Follow-up
Bulb JL, Berg D, Slee A, et al (Univ of Washington, Seattle)
Arch Dermatol 140:552-558, 2004   17–18

Introduction.—The number of cases of lentigo maligna (LM) and LM melanoma (LMM) increases with age, and the incidence of these lesions is highest in geographic areas with greater sun exposure. Because cryosurgery, radiotherapy, and topical agents have high recurrence rates, complete surgical excision is considered the treatment of choice. Outcome after staged excision with permanent sectioning for LM was assessed in a retrospective follow-up of 62 lesions.

Methods.—Fifty-nine patients underwent treatment at the study institution between January 1, 1990, and December 31, 2001. Fifty-five lesions were LMs and 7 were LMMs. The surgical technique included vertical excision with initial 2- to 3-mm margins examined by rush permanent sections, with histologic findings guiding further excision. Medical records were reviewed and follow-up was obtained by direct examination, contact with the referring physician, or telephone interview with the patient or nearest relative. Biopsy was performed if clinical recurrence was suspected.

Results.—With a mean follow-up time of 57 months, 95% of patients were free of recurrence. Two local recurrences were of previously excised LM and 1 was of an LMM. Three lesions initially read as LM were found to be invasive LMM at the time of definitive excision. Thirty-two of 62 lesions required 2 or more stages and 1 required more than 4 stages. The average excision margin was 5.5 mm, which reflected subclinical tumor spread. In the 3 patients who had local recurrence, as well as those without recurrence, no signs of metastasis were present. One patient had died in 1996 after metastatic melanoma developed from a different primary tumor.

Conclusion.—A staged, margin-control surgical technique for the treatment of LM and LMM achieved a 95% cure rate during an average follow-up time of 57 months. Many such techniques use initial excision margins equal to or greater than the 5-mm recommended standard excision margin, but the technique described here is able to attain similar margin control with a smaller defect size.

▶ The difficulty in prescribing appropriate care for patients with LM and LMM is well known. Based on this reviewer's experience and that in the published literature, 5 mm margins are grossly inadequate for the successful extirpation of melanoma in situ arising on sun-damaged skin, particularly on the head, neck, hands, or feet. For this reason, the Mohs technique has been used for the management of these melanomas. The published success of the Mohs technique equals or surpasses that of conventional surgical resection.

The debate over the use of rush permanent sections or frozen sections with or without immunohistochemistry during Mohs surgery for melanoma continues. This report addressed a modified technique of radial-oriented vertical sections in these patients. The follow-up data showed disease-free and survival rates comparable to Mohs surgery or other techniques. For this reason, one may certainly argue "there is more than one way to skin a cat." The arrival of imiquimod and its anecdotal published success in the treatment of melanoma in situ on sun-damaged skin further clouds the issue. Alternative techniques, such as dermabrasion, cryotherapy, and chemical peels, are not recommended because of their high failure rates.

J. Cook, MD

A Pilot Study of Treatment of Lentigo Maligna With 5% Imiquimod Cream

Fleming CJ, Bryden AM, Evans A, et al (Ninewells Hosp, Dundee, Scotland)
Br J Dermatol 151:485-488, 2004   17–19

Introduction.—Lentigo maligna (LM), 90% of which occurs on the head and neck, is often challenging to treat. Surgical excision is frequently unsatisfactory and the benefit of Mohs surgery is uncertain. New methods of treatment should be considered. Imiquimod is an immune response modifying agent that induces a cell-mediated T-helper 1 type cytokine profile, particularly interferon-α, interferon-γ, and interleukin 12. The histologic and clinical responses of surgically resectable LM after treatment with 5% imiquimod cream were examined in 6 patients with LM.

Methods.—The patients ranged in age from 42 to 79 years. Five LM lesions were on the face and 1 was on the forearm. Imiquimod 5% cream was applied once daily to the visible tumor, with a 1-cm margin around the tumor, for 6 weeks. Standard surgical excision of the original area and a 5-mm margin, ascertained by reference to pretreatment photographs, was performed within 2 weeks of completion of treatment. Clinical and histologic responses were determined via consensus opinion of 3 dermatologists. Histologic grading scores ranged from 0 to 4+.

Results.—Complete or nearly complete clearance of pigmentation was observed with minimal residual histological evidence of LM in 4 patients; 1 patient demonstrated no clinical or histologic improvement; and 1 patient had almost no residual pigmentation clinically after treatment, yet had histopathologic changes that were as severe as those before treatment.

Conclusion.—Topical imiquimod is worth considering for treatment of LM when surgical excision is either impossible or inappropriate. Patients must be observed carefully when this treatment approach is used.

▶ The quest for nonsurgical management of LM continues, especially given the difficulty of microscopically identifying what constitutes a truly positive surgical margin. Imiquimod has recently gained interest in the treatment of such patients. This study was too small to conclude whether imiquimod is useful for treating LM. The 2 issues of concern are the lack of histologic response in 2 patients, including near clinical clearing in 1 patient with histologically persistent LM. It is clearly prudent to carefully follow such patients with biopsies following a prescribed topical imiquimod regimen. Other investigators have also described the development of LM melanoma in LM patients treated with imiquimod.[1] Clearly, largely prospective trials are needed to determine the efficacy of this topical medication for treating melanoma in situ on sun-damaged skin.

J. Cook, MD

Reference

1. Fisher G, Lang P: Treatment of melanoma in situ on sun-damaged skin with topical 5% imiquimod cream complicated by the development of invasive disease. *Arch Dermatol* 139:945-947, 2003.

A Retrospective Observational Study of Primary Cutaneous Malignant Melanoma Patients Treated With Excision Only Compared With Excision Biopsy Followed by Wider Local Excision

McKenna DB, Lee RJ, Prescott RJ, et al (Royal Infirmary of Edinburgh, Scotland; Univ of Edinburgh, Scotland)
Br J Dermatol 150:523-530, 2004
17–20

Background.—Current guidelines for the surgical management of primary cutaneous malignant melanoma call for the use of a 2-stage procedure in which an excisional biopsy of the suspected lesion with a narrow margin of normal skin is the first step. This first step permits confirmation of the diagnosis and allows the second stage of wider local excision to account for the Breslow thickness when surgical margins are planned. A previous article has shown superior survival rates with the use of excisional biopsy before wider local excision, whereas other studies have found either no advantage or impaired survival rates. The clinicopathologic features, surgical margins, and survival of patients from the Scottish Melanoma Group database whose tumors were removed by excision only (1-stage) were retrospectively compared with the features, margins, and survival of patients who underwent excisional biopsy followed by wider local excision (2-stage) surgery.

Methods.—A total of 1595 patients were identified over a 19-year interval from 1979 to 1997 with follow-up until the end of December 1999. Univariate and multivariate statistical methods were used to examine the overall survival rate, the disease-free survival rate, and the recurrence-free interval.

Results.—The 547 patients in the 1-stage excision group were statistically significantly older, had thicker melanomas, a higher proportion of lentigo maligna melanomas, head and neck melanomas, and ulcerated lesions compared with the 1048 patients in the 2-stage group. The margins of excision were significantly narrower in the 1-stage than in the 2-stage group. More than half (52%) of all 1-stage excisions were performed with margins less than 1 cm compared with 20% of the 2-stage group. The excision margin was more positively correlated with the Breslow thickness for the 2-stage than for the 1-stage group. Overall survival, disease-free survival, and recurrence-free survival rates were all statistically significantly better in the 2-stage than in the 1-stage excision group. After adjustment was made for prognostic factors (ie, age, sex, tumor thickness, site, histologic type, and ulceration), overall survival, disease-free survival, and recurrence-free survival rates were still significantly better in the 2-stage than in the 1-stage group.

Conclusions.—One-stage excisions were more common in patients with poorer prognostic features, and excision with margins narrower than those suggested by current guidelines was more likely. The patient survival rate was statistically significantly better with the 2-stage procedure, but the reasons for this improved survival rate were not clear.

▶ Current recommendations for the management of pigmented lesions suspected of being melanoma include conservative excision followed by re-excision of the lesion with currently recommended margins should the lesion prove to be a melanoma. In this study, the authors examined whether any difference in overall survival, disease-free survival, and recurrence-free survival rates occurred between patients who had an excisional biopsy before definitive treatment and those who had "definitive" excisions as their initial and only treatment. Survival rates (overall, disease free, and recurrence free) were found to be significantly better in patients having an initial excisional biopsy followed by definitive excision. No clear-cut explanation for this observation could be given; however, it should be noted that patients undergoing single-stage excisions had their tumors removed with narrower margins. Although this group also had higher risk lesions, this difference in survival was observed even after subjecting the data to multivariate analysis.

P. G. Lang, Jr, MD

A Comparison of Dermatologists', Surgeons' and General Practitioners' Surgical Management of Cutaneous Melanoma
McKenna DB, Marioni JC, Lee RJ, et al (Royal Infirmary of Edinburgh, Scotland; Univ of Edinburgh, Scotland)
Br J Dermatol 151:636-644, 2004   17–21

Introduction.—Patients in Scotland with suspected melanomas usually see their general practitioner (GP), who is likely to refer the patient to a dermatologist or a surgeon. Information obtained from the Scottish Melanoma Group database was used to compare the characteristics, management, and survival outcomes of patients with melanomas treated by GPs, dermatologists, general surgeons, or plastic surgeons.

Methods.—The study period extended from 1979 to 1997, and follow-up continued to the end of December 1999. Included were patients with primary invasive cutaneous malignant melanomas without metastasis at the time of surgery. A potentially confounding influence was avoided by the exclusion of patients who underwent an incisional biopsy before the excision and the exclusion of those with an amputation.

Results.—Information was available for 1536 patients: 663 (43%) treated initially by a dermatologist, 486 (32%) treated by a general surgeon, 257 (17%) treated by a plastic surgeon, and 130 (8%) treated by a GP. The percentage of patients treated by a dermatologist rose during the study period, from 18% in 1979-1984 to 51% in 1991-1997. A corresponding decrease occurred during these years in the percentage treated by general surgeons. Older patients were most often seen by general and plastic surgeons; a higher proportion of female patients were managed by dermatologists. The median tumor thickness, lesion diameter, and frequency of ulceration were all greater in patients treated by general surgeons. More patients treated by a dermatologist or GP underwent wider local excision after the initial excision. Compared with other specialists, general surgeons used wider excision margins. Patients treated by dermatologists had significantly better overall survival, disease-free survival, and recurrence-free survival rates than did those treated by general and plastic surgeons.

Conclusion.—Dermatologists in Scotland are now managing a greater proportion of patients with melanomas, and patients treated by dermatologists experience significantly better survival rates than do those treated by surgeons. Even after adjustment was made for poor prognostic features in the surgeon-group patients, this group still had the worst survival rate.

▶ Although this review is based on data from Scotland, it still has some relevance to the very different health care system in the United States. Dermatologists are becoming increasingly important in the management of patients with cutaneous melanomas. Previously published studies have documented that dermatologists offer the highest level of care for patients with cutaneous neoplasia, as evidenced by the appropriateness of biopsy use, treatment rendered, and clinical outcomes. This study shows that, after a correction was done for prognostic variables (eg, surgical colleagues saw patients with more aggressive melanomas), those patients cared for by dermatologists have statistically significantly improved better rates. The specialty of dermatology is becoming more surgically oriented, and we should (correctly) view ourselves as *the* experts in the treatment of skin cancer. The management of cutaneous melanoma has recently been reviewed.[1]

J. Cook, MD

Reference

1. Tsao H, Atkins MB, Sober AJ: Management of cutaneous melanoma. *N Engl J Med* 351:998-1012, 2004.

Excision Margins in High-Risk Malignant Melanoma
Thomas JM, for the United Kingdom Melanoma Study Group, the British Association of Plastic Surgeons, and the Scottish Cancer Therapy Network (Royal Marsden Hosp Natl Health Service Trust, London; et al)
N Engl J Med 350:757-766, 2004   17–22

Background.—The risk of death from cutaneous melanoma is determined primarily by tumor thickness, the presence or absence of tumor ulceration and microdeposits of melanoma in sentinel lymph nodes, the site of the tumor, and the sex of the patient. In the past, wide margins of excision were used to prevent lymphatic spread; in the last 10 years, these margins have become smaller because trials have suggested that narrower margins are safe. Inadequate excision margins increase the risk of local recurrence and in-transit metastases, and unnecessarily large margins are associated with greater morbidity and increased cost. The effect of width of excision margin on the outcome of patients with high-risk melanoma was investigated.

Methods.—From an enrollment of 900 patients with a melanoma at least 2-mm thick on the trunk or limbs (excluding the palms and soles), 453 were randomly assigned to undergo surgery with a 1-cm margin of excision, and 447 patients were assigned to surgery with a 3-cm margin of excision. The median follow-up time for these patients was 60 months. The main outcome measures were local recurrence, which was defined as recurrence within 2 cm of the scar or graft, and in-transit recurrence, which was defined as a recurrence from beyond the first 2 cm of the scar or graft to the regional nodes.

Results.—The patients who underwent surgery with a 1-cm margin of excision were at a significantly increased risk of locoregional recurrence. There were 168 cases of locoregional recurrence in the group with 1-cm margins of excision compared with 142 cases of locoregional recurrence in the group with 3-cm margins. A total of 128 deaths attributable to melanoma were recorded in the group with 1-cm margins compared with 105 in the group with 3-cm margins. Overall survival was similar in the 2 groups.

Conclusion.—In patients with melanoma with a poor prognosis (tumor thickness 2 mm or greater), a 1-cm margin of excision is associated with a significantly greater risk of regional recurrence than is a 3-cm margin, but with a similar overall survival rate.

▶ Multiple previously published prospective clinical trials from groups including the World Health Organization, Swedish melanoma, and Intergroup melanoma trials have demonstrated no difference in disease-free or overall survival in patients undergoing resection of intermediate-thickness melanomas with narrow versus wide surgical margins. A relative deficiency of higher risk (more invasive) melanomas in these clinical trials led to the initiation of the United Kingdom melanoma trial. In this prospective clinical trial, patients with melanomas measuring more than 2 mm in thickness were included. These patients were randomized to excisions with 1 cm or 3 cm margins.

This is the first prospective clinical trial showing increased locoregional recurrence with narrow versus wider margin excision of melanomas. However, one must interpret these data with a degree of skepticism. As noted, multiple clinical trials have demonstrated the efficacy of narrow margin resection for melanoma. This trial underwent statistical reconfiguration once undertaken because of a lower than anticipated frequency of disease recurrence. Moreover, although the narrow margin excision group showed an increase in locoregional recurrence, there were no differences in overall survival comparing narrow versus wide excision margins. Nevertheless, it is interesting to note that the increased locoregional recurrence rate in the narrow margin resection group was predominantly caused by an increase in nodal metastasis. There was no significant increase in local recurrence at or near the resection site of the melanoma.

Although this prospective trial somewhat clouds the picture of narrow margin resection for melanoma, the above qualifications must certainly be considered. It will be interesting to observe how these patients' data mature over the coming years. The physician may safely and effectively resect malignant melanoma with narrow margins based on the preponderance of previously generated clinical data. However, one must be aware of this clinical trial and its associated medicolegal ramifications.

J. Cook, MD

▶ Current recommendations for the margins of excision of primary invasive melanoma are as follows: (1) lesions less than 2 mm thick, 1 cm margin, and (2) lesions more than 2 mm thick, 2 cm margin. In this study, the authors examined the difference in locoregional recurrence (local recurrence, in-transit metastases, and regional nodal metastases) and survival in patients with primary melanoma more than 2 mm thick whose lesion was excised with a 1 cm versus a 3 cm margin. The authors found that narrower margins were associated with a higher incidence of locoregional recurrence but had no effect on survival. The authors explained this observation by postulating that in patients whose melanoma had been excised with a 3 cm margin and recurred, the tumor was probably more aggressive, resulting in a higher mortality rate.

Although this seems plausible, it is reasonable to question if the patients were truly randomly distributed, why would the 3 cm group have more aggressive tumors? If one examines Table 3 (see original article), it would appear that when locoregional recurrences are broken down by type there is no difference in recurrence rates between the 2 groups. Moreover, why would a patient who had not suffered a local recurrence be more likely to have nodal metastases develop?

Finally, satellite lesions are lumped with "true" local recurrences, a fact that can effect the conclusions of the study. Taking wide margins to encompass microscopic satellites is futile and, as noted in this study, has no effect on prognosis because microscopic satellites are associated with occult regional nodal metastases and systemic spread. In summary, although based on a large and well-intended study, this article fails to convince this reviewer that wide margins are associated with a lower local recurrence rate or a better prognosis.

P. G. Lang, Jr, MD

Geographic and Patient Variation in Receipt of Surveillance Procedures After Local Excision of Cutaneous Melanoma
Barzilai DA, Cooper KD, Neuhauser D, et al (Case Western Reserve Univ, Cleveland, Ohio)
J Invest Dermatol 122:246-255, 2004   17–23

Introduction.—Little is known concerning the variation in surveillance practices after the diagnosis of invasive melanoma. Geographic, patient, and tumor variation in the use of follow-up surveillance testing were examined in patients with local or regional stage melanoma.

Methods.—A cohort of Medicare beneficiaries aged 65 years or older who were diagnosed with invasive melanoma between 1992 and 1996 and lived in a Surveillance, Epidemiology, and End Results registry area were evaluated. Both outpatient and inpatient Medicare claims 3 months after diagnosis were assessed for up to 2 years for surveillance procedures of interest. The use of chest radiographs, chest CT scan, abdominal or pelvic CT scan, abdominal US, head CT scan, head MRI, laboratory testing, and skin examination were compared among patient groups and geographic regions.

Results.—Of 11,293 patients with a diagnosis of melanoma, 3389 were included in the analysis. The cohort was 57% male, 98% white, with 50% at least 75 years of age. Surveillance testing ranged from 13% for abdominal US to 80% for laboratory testing. Multivariate analysis controlling for potentially confounding factors revealed a significant variation in the use of chest radiographs, head CT, liver enzymes or lactic dehydrogenase, complete blood count, and the sensitive and specific measures of follow-up visits.

With some exceptions, there was no significant variation across regions in surveillance for chest CT, abdominal or pelvic CT, abdominal US, or head MRI. Follow-up skin examinations were conducted in 70% to 90% of the cohort. The use of most surveillance procedures was linked to younger age, male gender, regional stage tumors, and geographic area, with up to 2-fold differences seen ($P < .01$) across regions.

Conclusion.—Future trials are needed to ascertain the etiology and impact of the observed disparities in surveillance after local excision of cutaneous melanoma, along with the influence of surveillance procedures on morbidity and mortality.

▶ Although a number of studies have been published regarding the follow-up of patients with a history of melanoma, there appears to be no consensus of opinion as to the best method to accomplish this. In this study, the authors, as anticipated, found considerable variation in methodology, based on geographic location. Most commonly included in the follow-up visit was a skin exam, a complete blood count, a liver panel, and a chest x-ray. Younger patients, males, and those with more advanced disease and thicker lesions were more closely monitored.

P. G. Lang, Jr, MD

Thin Primary Cutaneous Malignant Melanoma: A Prognostic Tree for 10-Year Metastasis Is More Accurate Than American Joint Committee on Cancer Staging
Gimotty PA, Guerry D, Ming ME, et al (Univ of Pennsylvania, Philadelphia)
J Clin Oncol 22:3668-3676, 2004   17–24

Introduction.—Most patients diagnosed with primary cutaneous melanoma have thin (≤ 1.00 mm) invasive lesions that usually have a good prognosis. In some cases, however, regional metastases and disseminated disease develop and patients may die of their disease. A prospective cohort study of 884 patients with thin invasive melanoma was undertaken to examine potential prognostic factors, in addition to Clark level and ulceration, that might identify those at high risk and low risk for a metastatic event by 10 years after definitive surgical excision of the lesion.

Methods.—A total of 1114 patients seen between 1972 and 1991 were eligible for the study. All lesions were retrospectively reviewed by pathologists blinded to patients and clinical outcomes. Complete clinical and histologic data were available for 884 patients, 736 of whom were alive at the last follow-up examination. The first recurrences after surgery were classified as local, regional metastasis, disseminated disease, and mixed. Eleven factors were used to develop a prognostic tree for 10-year metastasis: age, sex, anatomic site, thickness, level, growth phase, mitotic rate (MR), regression, tumor-infiltrating lymphocytes (TILs), ulceration, and microscopic satellites.

Results.—The median age of the patient group was 45.6 years; 87% of lesions were superficial spreading melanomas. Within 10 years of definitive excision, 57 patients had metastatic disease and 40 had died from melanoma. Overall 10-year metastasis and melanoma-specific death rates were 6.5% and 4.5%, respectively. Four of 11 factors were significantly associated with 10-year metastasis in multivariate analysis: sex, growth rate, MR, and TIL. Odds of metastasis were 3.1-fold higher for men than for women, 42-fold higher for vertical growth phase (VGP) versus radial growth phase lesions, 7.7-fold higher for lesions with an MR greater than 0 versus an MR of 0, and 2.34-fold higher for lesions with brisk/nonbrisk TIL compared with those without TIL. The prognostic tree identified a high-risk group (in men with VGP lesions that had MRs <0, the 10-year metastasis rate was 31%), a moderate-risk group (in women with VGP lesions that had MRs >0, the rate was 13%), a low-risk group (in patients with VGP lesions that had an MR of 0, the rate was 4%), and a minimal-risk group (in patients with invasive lesions without VGP, the rate was 0.5%).

Conclusion.—Among patients with thin primary cutaneous melanoma, growth phase, MR, and sex are important prognostic factors that can identify subgroups at minimal to high risk for metastasis.

Prognostic Factors of Thin Cutaneous Melanoma: An Analysis of the Central Malignant Melanoma Registry of the German Dermatological Society

Leiter U, Buettner PG, Eigentler TK, et al (Eberhard-Karls-Univ, Tuebingen, Germany; James Cook Univ, Townsville, Australia)
J Clin Oncol 22:3660-3667, 2004   17–25

Introduction.—With early detection, more patients are being diagnosed with thin (≤1 mm) cutaneous melanoma (CM) than with more extensive lesions. Such thin tumors are classified on the basis of ulceration and level of invasion (T1a/1b). A need to identify additional prognostic factors prompted a follow-up study of 12,728 patients with thin incident primary invasive (Clark level ≥II) CM.

Methods.—The patients had follow-up data recorded between 1976 and 2000 by the German-based Central Malignant Melanoma Registry, which records approximately 35% to 50% of all patients in Germany with melanoma. After surgery, patients were scheduled for regular examinations every 3 to 6 months for 10 years. Data recorded included case history and tumor characteristics, body site of the primary CM, patient age, and histopathology reports.

Results.—The mean age at diagnosis was 50 and the mean tumor thickness was 0.58 mm; 41.4% of patients were men. The median follow-up time was 4.0 years, but 31.8% of patients were followed for 5 to 10 years. The overall 5-year survival rate was 98.8%; overall 10-year survival was 96.5%. Tumor thickness was the strongest significant survival factor. Compared with tumors 0.5 mm or less thick, tumors with a thickness between 0.76 and 1.0 mm had a relative risk of 3.9. Additional significant prognostic factors were sex, age, body site, and histopathologic subtype. Men with more than 0.75-mm tumor thickness had the worst prognosis. Acral lentiginous melanoma had a relative risk of 3.1 compared with other histologic subtypes, and risk was greater for head and neck and posterior trunk tumors that for tumors at all other sites. Ulceration, regression, and Clark level of invasion did not appear to have a significant effect on prognosis.

Conclusion.—Among patients with thin primary invasive CM, tumor thickness predominated as the strongest prognostic factor. Female patients had a better outcome, and age, body site, and histologic subtype also contributed to the estimate of prognosis.

▶ There are a bewildering number of published histologic and clinical variables that on multivariate analysis are claimed to be statistically significant for predicting survival in patients with primary CM. Breslow thickness and sentinel lymph node status are the only 2 variables that consistently strongly correlate with survival. Even ulceration, a major parameter in the new staging system for CM developed by the American Joint Committee on Cancer, has not always been shown to be a significant prognostic variable. Although the incidence of CM continues to increase, most newly diagnosed lesions are thin (<1.0 mm thick). Although most patients with thin lesions do well, some suffer recurrence and eventually die of their disease. Because the majority of patients with CM have thin lesions, it is important to identify which patients in this group are at significant risk for recurrence so that they may be targeted for interventional therapy (eg, sentinel lymph node biopsy, adjuvant therapy) in addition to primary excision. These 2 studies (Abstracts 17–24 and 17–25) address this issue but unfortunately do not examine all the same variables or yield exactly the same results. Interestingly, neither study demonstrated a significant correlation between prognosis and the presence of ulceration or the Clark level of invasion, 2 variables that in the American Joint Committee on Cancer staging system are considered prognostically significant for patients with thin lesions. Also noteworthy is the fact that a significant number of patients suffered a recurrence more than 10 years after initial diagnosis and treatment.

P. G. Lang, Jr, MD

Impact of Ulceration in Stages I to III Cutaneous Melanoma as Staged by the American Joint Committee on Cancer Staging System: An Analysis of the German Central Malignant Melanoma Registry

Eigentler TK, Buettner PG, Leiter U, et al (Eberhard-Karls-Univ of Tuebingen, Germany; James Cook Univ, Townsville, Australia)
J Clin Oncol 22:4376-4383, 2004   17–26

Background.—An updated staging system for cutaneous melanoma (CM) was proposed in 2001 by the American Joint Committee on Cancer melanoma group to replace the 1987 classification. In this updated staging system, ulceration of the primary melanoma was introduced as a new key parameter being represented in respective subcategories of the tumor classification. The prognostic significance of ulceration in relation to tumor thickness and clinical stages (stages I to III) of CM was evaluated.

Methods.—A review was conducted of data on 15,158 patients with incident invasive primary nonmetastatic CM and follow-up data recorded between 1976 and 2000 by the German Central Malignant Melanoma Registry. The review was conducted by using survival analysis to evaluate prognostic factors such as tumor thickness, level of invasion, body site, histologic subtype, ulceration, regression, age, and sex.

Results.—Comparisons of survival probabilities according to the Kaplan-Meier method between ulcerated and nonulcerated CM were not statistically significant for subgroups with tumor thickness 1 mm or less and more than 4.00 mm but were significant for tumor thickness of 1.01 to 2.00 mm and 2.01 mm to 4.00 mm. Multivariate analysis provided confirmation of these findings. For stage III CM, the impact of ulceration on overall survival was statistically significant in the bivariate Cox model but not in the multivariate Cox model.

Conclusions.—Ulceration appeared to have a negative effect on the prognosis of patients with stages T2 and T3 CM, but a potential influence for patients with stages T1 and T4 could not be established. Tumor thickness, but not ulceration, should be the most important parameter when factors of the primary CM are considered in the assessment of prognosis of stage III CM.

▶ In 2001, the American Joint Committee on Cancer (AJCC) proposed a new staging system for CM. The presence of ulceration of the primary lesion plays a prominent role in this new staging system, both for patients without evidence of metastatic disease as well as those with regional nodal disease. In this staging system, the presence of ulceration is associated with a worse prognosis for these 2 groups of patients. In analyzing data from The German Central Malignant Melanoma Registry, these investigators came up with findings that are not completely in keeping with the data on which the AJCC staging system is based. On the basis of their analysis, ulceration had an adverse impact on survival in patients with lesions 1- to 4-cm thick, but there was no effect on survival in patients with lesions less than 1-mm or more than 4-mm thick. The same was true of patients with regional nodal disease. In the latter instance, however, the thickness of the primary lesion did affect survival. On the basis of their findings, they suggest that the new AJCC staging system be revised. Obviously this is a significant finding that requires conformation and further scrutiny.

P. G. Lang, Jr, MD

Effect of Pregnancy on Survival in Women With Cutaneous Malignant Melanoma

Lens MB, Rosdahl I, Ahlbom A, et al (St James's Univ, Leeds, England; Univ of Linköping, Sweden; Karolinska Inst, Stockholm, Sweden)
J Clin Oncol 22:4369-4375, 2004   17–27

Introduction.—Melanoma may be the malignancy most frequently encountered during pregnancy, with an incidence of 2.8 to 5 cases per 100,000 pregnancies. Anecdotal reports suggest that the hormonal and immunological changes that occur during pregnancy have an adverse effect on melanoma prognosis. A population-based, retrospective cohort study compared overall survival of women diagnosed with melanoma during pregnancy with that of women of the same childbearing age diagnosed with melanoma while not pregnant.

Methods.—Swedish women in their reproductive years who were diagnosed with a first primary cutaneous melanoma between January 1958 and December 1999 were eligible for inclusion in the study. The main end point was overall survival. Potential confounders analyzed included age, Breslow tumor thickness, site of melanoma, and Clark level of invasion. In a secondary analysis, pregnancy status subsequent to the diagnosis of the primary melanoma was examined for long-term effects.

Results.—The cohort was composed of 185 women (3.3%) diagnosed with melanoma during pregnancy and 5348 (96.7%) diagnosed with melanoma while not pregnant. Melanoma diagnosis in pregnant women occurred during the first trimester in 31.4%, the second trimester in 28.1%, and the third trimester in 40.5%. The median follow-up time was 11.6 years and 11.4 years, respectively, for the pregnant and nonpregnant groups. The 2 groups did not differ significantly in mean tumor thickness, and most lesions in each group were superficial spreading melanoma with Clark level less than IV. At the end of the follow-up period, 4544 women were alive (85.0% of the pregnant group and 82.0% of the nonpregnant group, not a significant difference). Pregnancy status after the diagnosis of melanoma was not a significant predictor of survival in the multivariable analysis. The major single determinant of overall survival in both pregnant and nonpregnant groups was tumor thickness.

Conclusion.—Pregnancy status limits treatment options in melanoma, but this study showed no adverse effect of pregnancy on survival at the time of diagnosis with melanoma. Similarly, no evidence was found that pregnancy subsequent to diagnosis affects outcome. Thus, deferral of pregnancy is not necessary for women with a good-prognosis, thin tumor.

▶ Although controversial, recent studies have suggested that pregnancy has no adverse effect on survival in patients who have melanoma develop during pregnancy. Lens et al corroborate these findings and also demonstrate that pregnancy does not adversely effect survival in patients with a history of melanoma who subsequently become pregnant. In this study, although there was no difference in tumor thickness between pregnant and nonpregnant patients, third-trimester patients did have thicker tumors, suggesting perhaps a delay in diagnosis.

P. G. Lang, Jr, MD

Hormone Replacement Therapy After Surgery for Stage 1 or 2 Cutaneous Melanoma
MacKie RM, Bray CA (Public Health and Health Policy Univ of Glasgow, Scotland)
Br J Cancer 90:770-772, 2004   17–28

Background.—Because the average age of women diagnosed with invasive melanoma is the early 50s, many of these women may seek advice on the safety of hormone replacement therapy (HRT). The safety or hazards of HRT after surgery for primary melanoma were investigated.

Methods.—Two hundred six women born between 1935 and 1950 who had melanoma diagnosed between 1990 and 1995 were included in the study. Melanoma had been confirmed in every patient. Data after a minimum of 5 years of follow-up after primary melanoma surgery were analyzed to determine whether HRT adversely affected prognosis.

Findings.—Twenty-three women died of melanoma. One hundred twenty-three women received no HRT, and 83 received HRT for varying amounts of time. The no-HRT group included 22 deaths, and the HRT group had 1. After adjustment for known prognostic factors, HRT did not appear to affect prognosis adversely in the group of women who had had surgery for melanoma.

Conclusion.—HRT does not adversely affect outcomes after surgery for localized melanoma. Women who have had successfully treated stage 1 or 2 melanoma should be considered for HRT using the same parameters as women who have never had melanoma.

▶ Although controversy continues on the possible increased incidence of breast cancer in women receiving HRT, results of this prospective observational study showed that HRT had no adverse effect on outcome after surgery for localized melanoma. The apparent improvement in prognosis in HRT-treated patients may result from selection bias, ie, patients with thick, ulcerated tumors, which inherently would be associated with the worst prognosis, generally were less likely to receive HRT.

B. H. Thiers, MD

Reduced Apaf-1 Expression in Human Cutaneous Melanomas

Dai DL, Martinka M, Bush JA, et al (Univ of British Columbia, Vancouver)
Br J Cancer 91:1089-1095, 2004   17–29

Background.—The lifetime risk for melanoma is estimated to have increased 15-fold in the past 60 years. Patients with metastatic melanoma have a poor prognosis, because the disease is resistant to conventional chemotherapy. A key mechanism to the rapid growth of cancer cells in melanoma is thought to be their resistance to apoptosis, although the exact mechanism for failure in the apoptotic pathway is unclear. The tumor suppressor gene, p53, is only rarely mutated in melanoma, but Apaf-1 gene, a downstream effector of p53, recently was found to be inactivated in metastatic melanoma. Loss of heterozygosity of the Apaf-1 gene was reported in 40% of metastatic melanomas.

Methods.—To further investigate the role of Apaf-1 in melanoma progression, tissue microarray technology and immunohistochemistry were used to evaluate the Apaf-1 expression level in primary human melanoma at different stages. Tissue samples from 70 patients (38 men, 32 women; mean age, 58 years) had Apaf-1 staining available. The most common diagnosis was superficial spreading melanoma (32 cases), and 56 of the 70 melanomas were located in sun-protected sites. Sixteen nevi were also examined.

Results.—Expression of Apaf-1 was significantly reduced in melanoma cells compared with normal nevi, and the staining pattern differed significantly between the 2 types of lesions. No association was apparent between loss of Apaf-1 and tumor thickness, ulceration or subtype, patient gender or age, and 5-year survival. Results of an in vivo apoptosis assay indicated that overexpression of Apaf-1 can sensitize melanoma cells to chemotherapy.

Conclusion.—Acquired resistance to apoptosis allows cancer cells to survive, metastasize, and resist chemotherapy. Malignant melanoma is particularly resistant to chemotherapeutic agents. Because expression of Apaf-1 is significantly reduced in melanoma compared with normal nevi, reversion of the reduced Apaf-1 expression may represent a future therapeutic strategy for this deadly skin cancer.

▶ Apaf-1, a downstream target of p53, is inactivated in metastatic melanoma. Dai et al show that Apaf-1 expression is significantly reduced in melanoma cells compared with normal nevi, and loss of Apaf-1 is independent of tumor thickness, ulceration or subtype, gender, age, and 5-year survival. They also use an in vitro apoptosis assay to demonstrate that overexpression of Apaf-1 can sensitize melanoma cells to anticancer drug treatment. The data suggest that Apaf-1 expression is significantly reduced in melanoma and that methods to enhance Apaf-1 expression may provide a strategy for treatment of this highly chemoresistant tumor.

B. H. Thiers, MD

Effects of Angiogenesis Inhibitors on Vascular Network Formation by Human Endothelial and Melanoma Cells
van der Schaft DWJ, Seftor REB, Seftor EA, et al (Northwestern Univ, Chicago; Maastricht Univ, The Netherlands; Univ of Minnesota, Minneapolis)
J Natl Cancer Inst 96:1473-1477, 2004   17–30

Introduction.—Many new angiogenesis inhibitors have shown efficacy against tumor growth in animal models, but clinical studies have not duplicated these results. One explanation might be the heterogeneous composition and plasticity of cells of growing tumors. In a phenomenon referred to as vasculogenic mimicry, aggressive melanoma cells can express some genes typically expressed by endothelial cells and can form extracellular tubular networks. The effects of 3 angiogenesis inhibitors on vasculogenic mimicry were examined in human metastatic melanoma MUM-2B (uveal) and C8161 (cutaneous) cells and then compared with their effects in human microvascular endothelial cells (HMEC-1) and human umbilical vein endothelial cells (HUVECs).

Methods and Findings.—The angiogenic inhibitors were anginex, TNP-470, and endostatin. Compared with vehicle control, each inhibitor of angiogenesis markedly inhibited vascular cord and tube formation by HMEC-1 and HUVECs in vitro. Tubular network formation by MUM-2B and C8161 cells was relatively unaffected. Because the process of angiogenesis requires cell growth and migration as well as tube assembly, the effects of the 3 angiogenesis inhibitors on endothelial and melanoma cell growth over the course of 6 days was examined. Anginex and TNP-470 resulted in statistically significant inhibition of endothelial cell proliferation versus the control. In contrast, neither melanoma cell line showed statistically significant changes in their apoptotic indices, relative to control treatment, when treated with any of the 3 inhibitors. The finding that endothelial cells expressed higher messenger RNA and protein levels for 2 putative endostatin receptors (α_5 integrin and heparin sulfate proteoglycan 2) than did melanoma cells suggests that a mechanistic basis exists for the varying responses to angiogenic inhibitors seen in the 2 cell types.

▶ van der Schaft et al demonstrate that a "cookie cutter" approach to antiangiogenic therapy is likely to fail. Using a receptor-specific approach to design such drugs is more likely to yield positive clinical results.

B. H. Thiers, MD

Vascular Endothelial Growth Factor C mRNA Expression Correlates With Stage of Progression in Patients With Melanoma

Goydos JS, Gorski DH (MDNJ-Robert Wood Johnson Med School, New Brunswick, NJ)

Clin Cancer Res 9:5962-5967, 2003   17–31

Introduction.—Vascular endothelial growth factor (VEGF)-C is a pro-lymphangiogenic peptide implicated in many different tumor types, including melanoma. The orderly pattern of metastasis to the regional lymph nodes typically seen in patients with melanoma led investigators to hypothesize that VEGF-C expression is involved in disease progression. Human melanoma samples representing different stages of progression and both the vertical and horizontal growth phases of the same primary tumor were examined for VEGF-C mRNA levels.

Methods.—Melanoma samples from operative specimens had total RNA extracted and subjected to quantitative real-time polymerase chain reaction. Included in the samples were 15 primary melanomas, 6 local recurrences, 11 regional dermal metastases, 12 nodal metastases, and 10 distant metastases. Expression of the lymphatic endothelial marker LYVE-1 was measured as a surrogate for lymphatic density, and its expression was correlated with the previously obtained VEGF-C levels.

Results.—Levels of VEGF-C were significantly higher in vertical growth phase melanomas than in horizontal growth phase melanomas. The highest levels were expressed in nodal metastases, followed by dermal regional metastases. Relatively low levels of VEGF-C appeared in primary and local recurrences and also in negative lymph nodes and distant metastases. There was a strong correlation between VEGF-C and LYVE-1 mRNA levels for all stages of melanoma, especially for regional dermal metastases and nodal metastases.

Conclusion.—The findings suggest that the expression of VEGF-C increases significantly as a melanoma progresses from the horizontal to the vertical growth phase. This progression produces a concurrent, though far more variable, increase in LYVE-1 expression. Levels of VEGF-C and LYVE-1 may be used to identify tumors at high risk for nodal metastases, which may respond to antilymphangiogenic therapy.

▶ The clinical importance of VEGF-C as a facilitator of metastasis and the usefulness of antiangiogenic therapy in tumor control are areas of intense research. The data presented by Goydos et al suggest that high tumor levels of VEGF-C may aid in identifying melanomas with a high risk for nodal metastases. The authors also argue that the identification of different isoforms of VEGF-C may be a factor in determining whether a tumor spreads locally or to distant sites.

B. H. Thiers, MD

Diagnosing Melanoma Patients Entering American Joint Committee on Cancer Stage IV, C-Reactive Protein in Serum Is Superior to Lactate Dehydrogenase
Deichmann M, Kahle B, Moser K, et al (Univ of Heidelberg, Germany)
Br J Cancer 91:699-702, 2004   17–32

Introduction.—Lactate dehydrogenase (LDH) has prognostic value in melanoma and other tumors, including small cell and non–small cell lung cancer. It has recently been introduced into the new American Joint Committee on Cancer (AJCC) staging system for cutaneous melanoma. LDH may be useful in discriminating patients entering AJCC stage IV melanoma from those staying in AJCC stages I, II, or III. This study compared LDH with the acute phase protein, C-reactive protein (CRP), which has been observed to reflect the course of melanoma in earlier reports.

Methods.—Both LDH and CRP were prospectively measured in the serum of 91 consecutive patients with melanoma progressing into AJCC stage IV, and compared with 125 patients staying in AJCC stages I, II, or III.

Results.—Comparing distribution of the parameters by median values and quartiles by the Mann-Whitney test, LDH was not significantly elevated in patients entering AJCC stage IV melanoma ($P = .785$) versus CRP, which was significantly elevated ($P < .001$). Analyzing the sensitivity and specificity jointly by the areas under the receiver-operating characteristic curves (ROC-AUC), LDH did not discriminate between the defined groups of patients (AUC = 0.491; 95% confidence interval [CI], 0.410-0.581), compared with CRP, which did discriminate (AUC = 0.933; 95% CI, 0.900-0.966; $P < .001$). Logistic regression analysis was performed to calculate the ROC-AUC values upon the predictive probabilities and showed that LDH offered no additional information to CRP. With a cutoff point of 3.0 mg^{-1}, CRP provided a sensitivity of 0.769 and a specificity of 0.904 for diagnosing AJCC stage IV entry.

Conclusion.—For discriminating patients with melanoma entering AJCC stage IV from those staying in AJCC stages I, II, or III during follow-up, LDH is not useful, regardless of its proven prognostic value in patients who have AJCC stage IV disease. The unexpected finding was that CRP was the more favorable serum marker and contributed substantially to discriminating patients with melanoma entering AJCC stage IV from those staying in AJCC stages I, II, or III.

▶ In patients with melanoma, the usefulness of serial radiologic investigations or of serum markers of tumor progression remains controversial. Serum LDH levels have been included in the staging classification system of the AJCC. Interestingly, this study showed the inability of LDH levels to discriminate stage IV from stages I, II, and III melanoma patients. However, CRP (a nonspecific marker of inflammation) did offer the power of discrimination in patients with advanced melanoma compared to stages I, II, and III. Thus, this series suggests that CRP may more effectively identify patients with tumor progression.

J. Cook, MD

▶ Lactate dehydrogenase (LDH) has traditionally been used to assess the progression of disease in patients with melanoma. In this report, the authors present data to suggest that the nonspecific reactive protein, CRP, may be a better tool for doing this. In this study, CRP correlated better with progression to stage IV disease than did LDH. CRP production is stimulated by interleukin 6, whose possible source could include melanoma cells, surrounding fibroblasts and endothelial cells, T-cells, macrophages, and monocytes. Melanoma is not the only tumor associated with increased levels of CRP. Increases can be observed during the progression of any number of tumors, including renal cell carcinoma and colorectal carcinoma.

P. G. Lang, Jr, MD

Sentinel Node Biopsy Provides More Accurate Staging Than Elective Lymph Node Dissection in Patients With Cutaneous Melanoma
Doubrovsky A, de Wilt JHW, Scolyer RA, et al (Univ of Sydney, Australia; Royal Prince Alfred Hosp, Sydney, Australia; Daniel den Hoed Cancer Ctr, Rotterdam, The Netherlands)
Ann Surg Oncol 11:829-836, 2004   17–33

Background.—Elective lymph node dissection (ELND) has been performed widely in patients with melanoma who were considered at high risk for locoregional recurrence. However, most centers no longer consider ELND an appropriate treatment option because of the morbidity associated with this procedure. The sentinel node biopsy (SNB) procedure is an alternative to ELND. The SNB procedure has been shown to improve staging when compared with a historic group of patients treated with standard axillary lymphadenectomy. However, no overall survival benefit for the SNB procedure has been demonstrated. The nodal staging accuracy and duration of survival for SNB and ELND were compared.

Methods.—A retrospective cohort study was conducted of patients with American Joint Committee on Cancer stage II disease treated at a single center between 1983 and 2000 with either SNB (672 patients) or ELND (793 patients). Multivariate analyses were performed with the logistic regression model for nodal staging accuracy and Cox proportional hazards regression model for survival.

Results.—The patient factors that influenced nodal positivity included age, Breslow thickness, ulceration, head or neck primary, and operation type (SNB or ELND). SNB was superior to ELND in the detection of micrometastases, but survival was not influenced by operation type.

Conclusions.—More nodal micrometastases were identified with SNB than with ELND. However, SNB did not influence survival, although complete regional node dissection was performed in all patients who were SNB positive.

▶ This study confirms what has been stated previously: SNB is a more accurate way of staging melanoma patients than ELND. This is because (1) in the past, for ELNDs, lymphoscintigraphy was not usually performed; thus, in many instances, the wrong lymph nodes were removed. (2) Sentinel lymph nodes undergo a much more thorough pathologic examination than do the multiple nodes removed during ELND. In terms of survival, there was no difference between the SNB group and ELND group. Of note, the authors mention an observation-only control group, yet one does not seem to be included in the analysis of survival. This would have been a very important piece of information to assess whether SNB improves survival or is simply a staging tool.

P. G. Lang, Jr, MD

Failure to Remove True Sentinel Nodes Can Cause Failure of the Sentinel Node Biopsy Technique: Evidence From Antimony Concentrations in False-Negative Sentinel Nodes From Melanoma Patients
Scolyer RA, Thomspon JF, Li L-XL, et al (Royal Prince Alfred Hosp, Camperdown, Australia; Univ of Sydney, Australia)
Ann Surg Oncol 11:174S-178S, 2004   17–34

Background.—Sentinel node biopsy (SNB) has been shown to be highly accurate for the staging of cutaneous melanoma. In addition, the presence or absence of metastases in the sentinel node (SN) is the most important prognostic factor for patients with melanoma. Long-term follow up of SN-negative patients has shown a small but definite incidence of recurrence in the mapped and sampled nodal basin. These patients may be considered to have a false-negative (FN) result on SNB. A multidisciplinary approach is needed for assessment of SNs. "True" SNs should be removed and examined thoroughly. Antimony can be measured in tissue sections from archival paraffin blocks of SNs through inductively coupled plasma mass spectrometry (ICP-MS) to confirm that the removed nodes were true SNs.

Methods.—From March 1992 to June 2001, 1330 patients with a single primary cutaneous melanoma underwent SNB and were followed at the Sydney Melanoma Unit. From this population, 957 patients were included in the retrospective analysis. After histopathologic confirmation of the diagnosis of cutaneous melanoma in the primary lesion, lymphoscintigraphy was performed in all but 3 of the 957 patients. The SNs were biopsied within 24 hours of the isotope injection. All the patients were treated by wide excision of the primary site after SNB. A retrospective review was conducted of antimony concentrations in these 957 patients.

Results.—Among the 957 patients were 27 (2.8%) patients with an FN SNB result. Of these 27 patients, 25 recurred in the mapped and sampled nodal basin, and 2 patients had their original specimens reviewed for other reasons and were then found to be positive. The overall FN rate for the entire series was 13.3%. Archival paraffin blocks of the SNs were available for antimony concentration assay in 20 of 27 patients with a FN SN result. Of these, 5 had antimony concentrations of less than the concentration threshold and probably represented non-SNs. The antimony levels of SNs of all 7 nodes in whom melanoma cells were detected on pathologic review were greater than the concentration threshold, a finding that reconfirmed that each of these SNs was a "true" SN. After a median follow-up period of 21.5 months, 9 of the 27 patients with an FN SNB had died of disease and 2 were alive with disease.

Conclusion.—FN SNBs can occur because of histopathologic misdiagnosis or a failure to remove the true SN.

▶ Despite a negative SNB specimen, some patients will have melanoma recurrence in the same nodal basin. Greater scrutiny of the SLN with techniques such as immunohistochemistry and reverse transcription–polymerase chain reaction has revealed, in some instances, that the tumor was not detected by routine hematoxylin and eosin staining. However, this does not explain all cases of FN SNB. Another possibility could be that the incorrect node was sampled. It has now been demonstrated that antimony, which originates from one of the colloids used by some institutions for lymphoscintigraphy, can be detected in the SNs to confirm that the correct node has been sampled. The authors utilized this new technology in 20 patients with FN SNBs; 5 were found to have low concentrations of antimony, suggesting that the wrong lymph node had been removed. It should be noted that the overall FN rate for this series of 957 patients undergoing SNB was 2.8%.

P. G. Lang, Jr, MD

Is the Identification of In-transit Sentinel Lymph Nodes in Malignant Melanoma Patients Really Necessary?
Vidal-Sicart S, Pons F, Fuertes S, et al (Univ of Barcelona)
Eur J Nucl Med Mol Imaging 31:945-949, 2004   17–35

Background.—The metastatic spread of primary malignant melanoma is usually an orderly progression through the lymphatic system. The sentinel lymph node (SLN) is the first node in a nodal basin to receive the direct lymphatic flow from a malignant melanoma. However, lymphoscintigraphic studies have shown the presence of lymphatic nodes in some patients in the area between the primary melanoma and the regional basin. These nodes are called in-transit nodes or interval nodes and are also SLNs. The incidence and location of in-transit SLNs in patients with malignant melanoma and whether harvesting is necessary were determined.

Methods.—The study group was composed of 600 consecutive patients (279 men and 321 women) with a mean age of 52.1 years with malignant melanoma and who were referred to the nuclear medicine department. The primary tumors were located in the head and neck region in 75 patients, on the trunk in 239 patients, on the arm in 91 patients, on the leg in 188 patients, and on the genitalia in 7 patients. Lymphoscintigraphy was performed on the day before surgery after intradermal injection of 74 to 111 MBq of technetium 99m nanocolloid in 4 doses around the primary melanoma or the biopsy scar.

Results.—Dynamic and static images revealed SLNs in 599 of the 600 patients. The SLN was intraoperatively identified with patent blue dye and a handheld gamma probe. Lymphoscintigraphy revealed in-transit SLNs in 59 (9.8%) of 599 patients. All these in-transit SLNs were harvested during surgery; the SLNs most difficult to identify and excise were those in the popliteal and epitrochlear regions. Metastatic deposits were identified in 10 (16.9%) of these in-transit SLNs.

Conclusions.—Lymphoscintigraphy has a key role in the identification of in-transit SLNs. The incidence of these nodes is relatively low in patients with malignant melanoma; however, these SLNs contain metastatic deposits in a significant number of cases. Thus, identification of in-transit SLNs is vital in these patients.

▶ This study demonstrates the importance of identifying and harvesting in-transit or interval SLNs in patients with cutaneous melanoma. In this series of patients, 9.8% had interval SLNs; when these were harvested, 16.9% contained metastatic disease. In patients with positive internal SLNs, 50% also had metastases to regional nodes. In patients with negative SLNs, only 1 had involvement of regional nodes. Other studies have demonstrated interval SLNs were most commonly associated with truncal lesions. As the authors state, if these SLNs are overlooked, they may be a source of recurrent disease, not only when they are the only SLN involved but also in patients who have a positive SLN in the nodal basin and undergo a complete lymphadenectomy. It should be noted that only 78% of these nodes stained with the blue dye.

P. G. Lang, Jr, MD

Indications for Lymphatic Mapping and Sentinel Lymphadenectomy in Patients With Thin Melanoma (Breslow Thickness ≤1.0 mm)
Stitzenberg KB, Groben PA, Stern SL, et al (Univ of North Carolina, Chapel Hill; CancerVax Corp, Carlsbad, Calif; Evanston Northwestern Healthcare, Ill)
Ann Surg Oncol 11:900-906, 2004   17–36

Introduction.—The prognosis is good (5-year survival rate > 90%) in patients with thin (Breslow thickness ≤ 1.0 mm) melanoma. However, the added benefit of lymphatic mapping and sentinel lymphadenectomy (LM/SL) in these patients is debatable. It is possible that LM/SL with a focused evaluation of the sentinel node (SN) could identify a significant number of metastases in patients with thin melanoma and that particular clinical or histopathologic factors might act as predictors of SN tumor involvement. These possibilities were investigated in a prospective 6-year study.

Methods.—Between January 1998 and January 2004, every patient with a primary melanoma of Breslow thickness 0.75 mm or greater and no evidence of nodal or distant metastases on clinical examination was offered LM/SL; a total of 349 underwent LM/SL and were prospectively entered into an institutional review board-approved database. The LM/SL procedures were performed with a combined radiotracer and blue dye technique. The SNs were serially sectioned and every section was examined by a dermopathologist at multiple levels, using hematoxylin and eosin and immunohistochemical stains.

Results.—A total of 146 (42%) patients had a melanoma with a Breslow thickness 1.0 mm or less. Six (4%) of these patients had a tumor-involved SN. Multivariate analysis revealed that none of the clinical or histopathologic factors evaluated were significantly linked with SN tumor involvement in patients with thin melanoma. All patients with a tumor-involved SN underwent completion lymphadenectomy; none had non-SN tumor involvement.

Conclusion.—The prevalence of SN tumor involvement in patients with thin melanoma is considerable. It was not possible to identify predictors of SN tumor involvement for patients with thin melanoma, but efforts to identify predictors of SN tumor involvement need to continue. Until better predictors are identified, it is recommended that LM/SL be offered to patients with thin melanomas with clinical or histopathologic characteristics historically linked with an increased risk of recurrence or death.

▶ Unfortunately, the survival rate for patients with thin melanomas (Breslow depth < 1.0 mm) is not 100%. Certain risk factors have been associated with a worse prognosis in these patients; these include ulceration, young age, high mitotic rate, regression, Clark level IV or V, male sex, and location on the trunk. Using this information, certain investigators have advocated sentinel lymph node biopsy (SLNB) in subsets of these patients (eg, patients with Clark level IV or V lesions), but it is not clear what variables are more likely to predict SLN involvement. In this series, 4% of patients with thin melanomas had positive SLNBs, but none of these had involvement of non-SLNs. There was no correlation between SLN involvement and any clinical or histological variable(s). What are the therapeutic implications of this article? If the incidence of a positive SLNB is only 4%, is the procedure justifiable without evidence that it significantly alters prognosis? Also, is a complete node dissection necessary in patients with a thin melanoma and a positive SLNB?

P. G. Lang, Jr, MD

Sentinel Lymph Node Biopsy in Patients With Cutaneous Melanoma: Outcome After 3-Year Follow-up
Mozzillo N, Caracò C, Chiofalo MG, et al (Natl Cancer Inst, Naples, Italy)
Eur J Surg Oncol 30:440-443, 2004   17–37

Background.—The management of patients with cutaneous melanoma without lymph node metastases at diagnosis continues to be controversial. Sentinel node biopsy may identify patients with nodal micrometastases as candidates for lymph node dissection. The 3-year disease-free survival and overall survival rates for all patients who underwent sentinel node biopsy at one cancer institute in Naples, Italy, were analyzed.

Methods.—A total of 265 sentinel node biopsies have been performed at one institution in 242 patients since 1996. All patients had melanomas with a Breslow thickness greater than 1 mm or Clark IV-V, previously excised with a margin of less than 1 cm. Most were treated within 3 months of their primary diagnosis. All patients were studied by clinical evaluation, chest radiograph, and liver ultrasound to exclude nodal or distant metastases. Patients with a tumor less than 1.9 mm deep received wide excision of the primary lesion with a margin of 1 cm. Patients with a Breslow thickness greater than 2 mm received an excision with a 2-cm margin. Data from the sentinel node biopsy specimens were reviewed to determine the effect of the treatment on the disease-free survival rate, and the overall survival rate was used to stratify the patients by nodal status and tumor ulceration.

Results.—The statistical analysis showed a 3-year survival advantage for patients with negative sentinel nodes compared with patients with positive sentinel nodes. The 3-year survival rates were 88.4% and 72.9%, respectively.

Conclusions.—Sentinel node biopsy was shown to provide accurate staging of nodal status in the absence of clinical evidence of metastases in patients with melanoma. Longer follow-up and the final results from a multicenter selective lymphadenectomy trial are needed to clarify the role of this procedure.

▶ This article confirms previous reports documenting the value of sentinel lymph node biopsy (SLNB) in patients with melanoma; however, it presents no new information. As noted by others, the 3 most important prognostic factors in patients with primary melanoma are tumor thickness, the presence or absence of tumor ulceration, and sentinel lymph node status. The presence of tumor ulceration confers a worse prognosis, even for patients with positive SLNB results. The false-negative rate for SLNBs was approximately 5% in this series of patients.

P. G. Lang, Jr, MD

Mitotic Rate and Younger Age Are Predictors of Sentinel Lymph Node Positivity: Lessons Learned From the Generation of a Probabilistic Model

Sondak VK, Taylor JMG, Sabel MS, et al (Univ of Michigan Health System, Ann Arbor)
Ann Surg Oncol 11:247-258, 2004   17–38

Background.—The concept of lymphatic mapping and sentinel lymph node biopsy has been one of the most significant advances in the management of primary cutaneous melanoma. This technique has allowed surgeons to identify patients with subclinical nodal involvement who may benefit from a lymphadenectomy and, possibly, adjuvant therapy. Several factors in the selection of patients who require sentinel lymph node biopsy have been variably and, in some cases, discordantly reported to be predictive of sentinel lymph node metastasis. The factors that most strongly influence the probability of finding positive sentinel lymph nodes in patients with cutaneous melanoma were evaluated.

Methods.—A group of 419 patients who underwent sentinel lymph node biopsy for melanoma were reviewed from a prospectively collected melanoma database. A stepwise variable selection method was used to fit a multivariate logistic model that, in turn, was used to derive a probabilistic model for the occurrence of a positive sentinel lymph node. The accuracy of each model was evaluated with receiver operator characteristic curves.

Results.—Univariate analysis showed that the number of mitoses per square millimeter, increasing Breslow depth, decreasing age, ulceration, and a melanoma on the trunk showed a significant relationship to a positive sentinel lymph node. Multivariate analysis showed that once age, mitotic rate, and Breslow thickness were included, no other factor, including ulceration, was significantly associated with a positive sentinel lymph node. Thus, younger patients with tumors less than 1 mm may yet have a substantial risk of having a positive sentinel lymph node, particularly if the mitotic rate is high.

Conclusions.—In addition to Breslow depth, the number of mitoses per square millimeter and younger age were identified as factors that are independent predictors of a positive sentinel lymph node. The model presented in this study may identify patients with thin melanoma who are at sufficient risk of metastases to justify a sentinel lymph node biopsy.

▶ This study is based on multivariate analysis and a complex statistical model to assess the predictability of a positive sentinel lymph node. As identified by the model, the 3 most important variables were Breslow thickness, decreasing age, and a high mitotic rate. One observation, a lack of effect of ulceration, is in contrast to the findings of most other studies and was difficult for the authors to explain. In their experience, a high mitotic rate in a young person is associated with an increased risk of nodal metastases and is one of the criteria that they use when considering sentinel lymph node biopsy in patients with lesions less than 1 mm thick.

P. G. Lang, Jr, MD

Standard Immunostains for Melanoma in Sentinel Lymph Node Specimens: Which Ones Are Most Useful?

Karimipour DJ, Lowe L, Su L, et al (Univ of Michigan, Ann Arbor)
J Am Acad Dermatol 50:759-764, 2004   17–39

Introduction.—Sentinel lymph node (SLN) biopsy is being used with increasing frequency in melanoma. Pathologic assessment of SLNs using immunohistochemistry enhances diagnostic accuracy. There is no universally accepted standard protocol for pathologic processing of SLNs. The experience with 3 commonly used immunostains (S-100, HMB-45, and Melan-A) for examining SLNs for metastatic melanoma was evaluated to determine whether the SLN protocol could be improved and streamlined.

Methods.—Ninety-nine positive SLNs from 72 patients were retrospectively examined for the presence of microscopic metastatic melanoma using hematoxylin and eosin (H&E), S-100, HMB-45, and Melan-A stained sections. The sensitivities for each of the immunohistochemical stains was calculated.

Results.—There were no discordant findings among the 3 dermopathologists who read the slides during the course of clinical care. Ninety-seven of the 99 positive SLNs had available H&E-stained sections, of which 20 (21%) were negative and required immunohistochemistry to make the diagnosis of metastatic melanoma. Sixty-three SLNs had S-100 staining performed, of which 97% (61/63) were positive. Fifty-nine had HMB-45–stained sections, of which 75% (44/99) were positive. Fifty-three SLNs were stained for Melan-A, of which 96% (51/53) were positive.

The sensitivities of S-100, HMB-45, and Melan-A in SLNs were 97%, 75%, and 96%, respectively. Of 52 positive SLNs in which all 3 immunostains were performed, 39 (75%) were positive for all 3 immunostains and 13 (25%) demonstrated inconsistent results (9 were positive for both Melan-A and S-100, 2 were positive for S-100 only, and 2 were positive for Melan-A only).

Conclusion.—The lower sensitivity of HMB-45 prompted development of a modified protocol in which combinations of H&E, S-100, and Melan-A without HMB-45 are used. If the H&E sections are negative or equivocal for metastatic melanoma, the sections undergo immunohistochemistry staining with S-100 protein and Melan-A.

▶ Previous studies have demonstrated that immunostains should be performed on SLN biopsy specimens from patients with high-risk melanoma to maximize the detection of occult disease. However, the protocol for pathologic examination of SLNs has not been standardized and varies from institution to institution.

In this study, the authors found that the use of immunostains increased their detection of melanoma by 21%. Of the 3 immunostains, S-100, HMB-45, and Melan-A/Mart-1, HMB-45 was the least sensitive for detecting melanoma deposits and probably need not be used routinely. However, HMB-45 might be useful to distinguish benign nevi from melanoma cells, in which case HMB-45 would be negative, but S-100 and Melan-A would be positive.

P. G. Lang, Jr, MD

Serial Follow-up and the Prognostic Significance of Reverse Transcriptase-Polymerase Chain Reaction–Staged Sentinel Lymph Nodes From Melanoma Patients
Kammula US, Ghossein R, Bhattacharya S, et al (Mem Sloan-Kettering Cancer Ctr, New York)
J Clin Oncol 22:3989-3996, 2004   17–40

Introduction.—Sentinel lymph node (SLN) histologic status is the most significant predictor of survival in patients with melanoma who have no clinical evidence of nodal metastasis, yet histologic examination with hematoxylin and eosin (H&E) staining or immunohistochemical techniques (IHC) is of limited sensitivity in detecting micrometastatic deposits. Reverse transcriptase-polymerase chain reaction (RT-PCR) allows more precise detection of occult disease with an apparently strong negative predictive value. The role of a single-marker RT-PCR assay for tyrosinase mRNA in the detection of melanoma SLN metastases was determined in 112 patients with extended follow-up.

Methods.—Patients with stage I and II primary cutaneous melanoma and clinically negative lymph nodes were enrolled and evaluated between October 1996 and November 1999. According to a standard protocol, preoperative lymphoscintigraphy was followed by wide local excision of the primary melanoma with selective lymphadenectomy. The SLNs were bivalved, with half of each specimen evaluated by histologic methods and half by nested RT-PCR for tyrosinase.

Results.—The study included 60 men and 52 women (median age, 52 years) with a median tumor thickness of 2.2 mm. Conventional H&E analysis was performed in 60 (54%) patients, whereas step sectioning, H&E, and IHC were performed in 52 (46%). Fifteen patients (13%) had histologically positive SLNs that were also positive by RT-PCR (HISTO+/PCR+). In 39 patients (35%), SLNs were negative by both histology and RT-PCR (HISTO−/PCR−). Fifty-eight (52%) patients who were histologically negative were upstaged with a positive RT-PCR result (HISTO−/PCR+). Rates of recurrence were statistically different among these 3 groups at a median follow-up of 42 months (53%, 0%, and 14%, respectively), but after a median follow-up time of 67 months, the differences in recurrence rates between HISTO−/PCR+ (24%) and HISTO−/PCR− (15%) were not of statistical significance. The median times-to-relapse in these groups were 31 months and 41 months, respectively.

Discussion.—The HISTO−/PCR− group had a defined long-term failure rate that was not different from the HISTO−/PCR+ group, with the exception of time-to-recurrence. To provide clinically relevant information regarding staging and outcome in patients with occult melanoma metastases, approximately 5 years of median follow-up time will be needed.

▶ Prior studies have demonstrated that sentinel lymph nodes (SLNS) that are negative by routine histology and immunostaining may harbor melanoma cells that are only detectable by tyrosinase RT-PCR. These patients appear to have a prognosis that is intermediate between patients who are HISTO+/PCR+ and those who are HISTO−/PCR− However, follow-ups have been relatively short in reported patients. In this study, the authors followed patients who were HISTO−/PCR+ or Histo−/PCR− for a median of 67 months. The recurrence rates were similar, although the latter group tended to relapse 10 months later than the former group. These late recurrences in the HISTO−/PCR− group, however, were more commonly systemic recurrences as opposed to nodal recurrences, suggesting hematogenous dissemination. Why this was the case is not clear.

P. G. Lang, Jr, MD

The Staging of Malignant Melanoma and the Florida Melanoma Trial
Reintgen DS, Jakub JW, Pendas S, et al (Lakeland Regional Cancer Ctr, Fla)
Ann Surg Oncol 11:186S-191S, 2004   17–41

Background.—Lymphatic mapping and sentinel lymph node (SLN) biopsy have provided a less-morbid procedure for nodal staging in patients with solid tumors. In the American Joint Committee on Cancer melanoma database, the 5-year survival rate of patients with primary tumors 1.0 mm or thicker was 65% when nodes were staged negative with clinical examination, 75% when nodes removed during elective lymph node dissection (ELND) were negative, and 90% when patients were staged to be node negative with the SLN procedure. The Florida Melanoma Trial is a multi-institution trial that will enroll more than 3200 patients with melanoma over a 5-year period. The purpose of the FMT is to determine whether a complete lymph node dissection (CLND) after a positive SLN biopsy contributes to disease control and survival.

Methods.—Patients with clinical stage I or II melanoma were recruited from 1992 to 2002 for inclusion in the study. All the patients underwent preoperative lymphoscintigraphy to determine the actual lymphatic basin(s) at risk for metastases and the approximate number and location of SLNs in the basin. The patients then underwent intraoperative lymphatic mapping and SLN biopsy under general anesthesia. The SLN examination included histologic examination and tissue culture or reverse transcription–polymerase chain reaction (RT-PCR).

Results.—Of the 326 patients who underwent SLN biopsy from 1992 to 2002, 69% were male. Patients had a mean age of 57 years. The mean thickness of the primary cutaneous melanoma was 2.18 mm. Nearly all the patients (94%) had Clark level III and IV melanoma, and ulceration was present in 64% of the specimens. Routine hematoxylin and eosin (H&E) staining showed that 64 patients (19%) had metastatic melanoma in 1 or more SLNs. In 16 of these patients the metastatic cells were initially found with S-100 immunohistochemical (IHC) staining and confirmed to be malignant with H&E stain after metastatic cells had not been detected by the initial H&E screening. These cases would have been inaccurately staged with ELND specimens. Correlation of the RT-PCR assay of the SLN with clinical outcome showed that patients whose SLNs were histologically positive and PCR positive had a recurrence rate of 42% at 3 years, whereas patients whose SLNs were negative in both assays had a recurrence rate at 3 years of 6.6%. Patients whose SLNs were histologically negative but PCR positive had an intermediate prognosis, with 22% recurring at 3 years. RT-PCR positivity of the regional nodes or SLNs was found to correlate with tumor thickness at diagnosis, a prognostic factor related to survival. Patients with relatively thin melanomas (0.76 to 1.5 mm) had an RT-PCR positive-node rate of 33%, whereas 80% of the patients with thick melanomas had tyrosinase mRNA in the regional node.

Conclusion.—The lymphatic mapping procedure is the most accurate method for determining tumor status of the regional lymph nodes.

▶ This article summarizes the experience of the Florida Melanoma Trial as it relates to lymphatic mapping and SLN biopsy. Of particular interest is the authors' experience with RT-PCR analysis of SLNs. Patients positive by light microscopy and RT-PCR had a recurrence rate at 3 years of 42%, whereas those patients negative by both investigations had a recurrence rate of 6.6%. Those positive by RT-PCR only had a recurrence rate of 22%. On the basis of this significant recurrence rate, the authors plan to design trials for patients positive only by RT-PCR to assess whether treatments can be devised to affect recurrence rate and survival. It should be noted that these authors' results for this group of patients positive by RT-PCR only are in contrast to those of Kammula et al (Abstract 17–40), who did not note a higher incidence of relapse in a similar group of patients. However, their RT-PCR positive patients did relapse 10 months earlier.

P. G. Lang, Jr, MD

Sentinel Lymphonodectomy and S-Classification: A Successful Strategy for Better Prediction and Improvement of Outcome of Melanoma
Starz H, Siedlecki K, Balda B-R (Klinikum Augsburg, Germany)
Ann Surg Oncol 11:162S-168S, 2004   17–42

Introduction.—Sentinel lymphonodectomy (SLNE) has been incorporated into primary melanoma treatment at many centers, yet some continue to follow the practice of performing lymph node dissections only when a nodal macrometastasis becomes clinically evident. Outcome of melanoma was compared for patients at the study institution treated before and after (since 1995) SLNE was used routinely. The predictive value of SLNE was also investigated.

Methods.—The outcomes of an SLNE cohort of 324 patients were compared with those of a pre-SLNE cohort of 274 consecutive patients with the same distribution of clinical stages. The 2 cohorts were similar in sex, age, and site of the primary melanoma. Immediately after SLNE, SLNs were fixed and prepared for hematoxylin and eosin staining and immunohistochemical analysis with anti-S100 and HMB45. When completion lymph node dissection (CLND) was performed, the entire CLND specimen was fixed in formalin and cut into thin tissue slices to permit detection of even small lymph nodes. Performance of CLND was strongly recommended (and refused by only 3 patients) in all 39 cases with SIII metastases, defined as a depth of invasion more than 1 mm below the capsular level. Patients were followed for metastases for at least 10 years.

Results.—Both SLN tumor status and S-classification were strongly associated with thickness of the primary melanoma. The rate of SIII metastases was less than 1% when thickness was 1 mm or less, but reached 22% with primary melanomas greater than 4 mm. The risk of nonsentinel node metastases was 11% to 13% with SI and SII metastases versus 53% with SIII metastases. Both survival without distant metastases and overall survival were significantly better in the SLNE cohort than in the pre-SLNE cohort. Regional nodal metastases developed in 20.8% of patients in the pre-SLNE cohort (median follow-up, 95 months), but in only 3.1% of those in the SLNE cohort (median follow-up, 45.5 months). In both cohorts, 79% of patients never showed evidence of regional nodal involvement. These subgroups were similar in overall survival and frequency of distant metastases.

Conclusion.—Most regional lymph node metastases can be detected in microstages by SLNE and by thorough histological and immunohistochemical evaluation of SLNs. In addition to being a highly sensitive staging tool, SLNE allows early elimination of a major source of systemic metastasis.

The Microanatomic Location of Metastatic Melanoma in Sentinel Lymph Nodes Predicts Nonsentinel Lymph Node Involvement

Dewar DJ, Newell B, Green MA, et al (St George's Hosp, London; Royal Surrey County Hosp, Guildford, England)

J Clin Oncol 22:3345-3349, 2004   17–43

Introduction.—Sentinel node (SN) status is the strongest prognostic criterion for melanoma and is used to determine subsequent therapy. Patients with a positive SN usually undergo completion lymphadenectomy (CLND) of the involved basin, but only 20% may have involvement beyond the SN. A method for categorizing SN metastases that is based on physiologic microanatomy was used to predict nonsentinel node (NSN) involvement, so that only selected patients would have to undergo CLND.

Methods.—Patients eligible for the study had clinical stage I or II malignant melanoma and a primary tumor Breslow thickness greater than 1.0 mm. Also included were those with a Breslow thickness less than 1.0 mm if the lesion was Clark's level III or more, showed evidence of regression, or was in the vertical growth phase. SNs were examined by conventional histologic and immunohistochemical analyses. The metastasis deposit within each node was classified as subcapsular, combined subcapsular and parenchymal, parenchymal, multifocal, or extensive. The rate of NSN involvement was calculated for each SN subtype.

Results.—SN and corresponding CLND specimens were available for 146 patients (146 lymph node basins). The mean patient age was 49.9 years, with men comprising 55.2% of the patients. No relationship was found between patient age and sex or site of the CLND and either microanatomical location of the SN metastasis or NSN involvement. SNs were classified as subcapsular in 28% of patients, combined in 37%, parenchymal in 11%, multifocal in 13%, and extensive in 13%. No NSNs were positive in the subcapsular group; rates of positivity in the 4 remaining subgroups were 11.1%, 18.8%, 36.8%, and 42.1%, respectively. The overall rate of NSN involvement was 22.2%. Breslow thickness was not significantly correlated with NSN involvement.

Conclusion.—The probability of NSN involvement is extremely low for patients in whom SN metastases are confined to a subcapsular site. In such patients, CLND may not be necessary. The microanatomical location of metastases should be noted routinely in histopathologic reports of positive SNs.

Factors Predictive of Tumor-Positive Nonsentinel Lymph Nodes After Tumor-Positive Sentinel Lymph Node Dissection for Melanoma

Lee JH, Essner R, Torisu-Itakura H, et al (John Wayne Cancer Inst, Santa Monica, Calif)

J Clin Oncol 22:3677-3684, 2004   17–44

Introduction.—The mortality rate for malignant melanoma correlates with thickness of the primary lesion, presence of ulceration, and number of regional lymph node (LN) metastases. Controversy exists over the performance of elective lymph node dissection (ELND) versus reserving the procedure for only those with clinical evidence of LN metastasis. Records of patients who underwent lymphatic mapping and sentinel lymphadenectomy (LM/SL) and were found to have a tumor-positive sentinel node (SN) were reviewed to identify clinicopathologic factors that might correlate with non-SN (NSN) tumor positivity.

Methods.—The study cohort included 191 patients who underwent LM/SL between 1990 and 2002. If the SN contained metastatic melanoma by either hematoxylin and eosin (H&E) staining or immunohistochemistry (IHC), the patient subsequently underwent completion lymph node dissection (CLND) of the involved nodal basin(s). The NSNs were evaluated by H&E staining alone.

Results.—Four of the 191 patients had tumor-positive NSNs identified at the time of LM/SL and 46 (24%) had tumor-positive NSNs found at the time of CLND. One of 3 patients found to have tumor-positive SNs only by IHC had tumor-positive NSNs. In a multivariate model, Breslow thickness and SN metastasis were significantly associated with patients having tumor-positive NSNs. Factors not predictive of tumor-positive NSN included sex, histology, ulceration, mitotic index, and SN basin locations. Risk stratification by the number of predictive factors (0, 1, or 2) yielded a low-risk group (0 factors) with a 12.3% risk of finding tumor-positive NSN. The risk increased to 30.9% in the intermediate group (1 factor) and to 41.9% in the high-risk group (2 factors).

Conclusion.—Factors predictive of NSN metastasis are similar to the prognostic factors for survival in patients with melanoma. The Breslow thickness and SN tumor burden correlate with risk of NSN metastasis, suggesting an orderly progression of locoregional spread of melanoma from the primary site to its draining lymph node basin. Patients most likely to benefit from CLND are those with thicker primaries ($\geq$3 mm) and higher SN tumor burden ($\geq$2 mm in diameter).

Micromorphometric Features of Positive Sentinel Lymph Nodes Predict Involvement of Nonsentinel Nodes in Patients With Melanoma

Scolyer RA, Li L-XL, McCarthy SW, et al (Royal Prince Alfred Hosp, Camperdown, Australia; Univ of Sydney, Australia; Westmead Hosp, Australia)
Am J Clin Pathol 122:532-539, 2004   17–45

Introduction.—The development of sentinel lymph node biopsy (SLN) as a staging procedure has allowed completion lymph node dissections (CLNDs) to be performed only in selected patients with melanoma, sparing most a major surgical procedure. Further lymph node involvement in CLND specimens is identified in fewer than one third of cases. Micromorphometric features of positive SLNs from patients with melanoma were examined for

TABLE 2.—Features of Positive SLNs in Patients With or Without Positive Non-SLNs in Corresponding CLND Specimens

Feature	Positive Non-SLNs (n = 24)	Negative Non-SLNs (n = 116)
No. of positive SLNs		
Median (mean)	1 (1.3)	1 (1.2)
Range	1-4	1-4
Deposit number		
Median (mean)	4 (4.8)	3 (4.6)
Range	1-11	1-11
Tumor penetrative depth (mm)		
Median (mean)	1.6 (2.4)	1.0 (1.7)
Range	0.1-7.5	0.0-12.0
Deposit diameter (mm)		
Median (mean)	1.1 (3.3)	1.0 (2.1)
Range	0.1-25.0	0.0-17.0
Deposit size (mm^2)		
Median (mean)	0.4 (22.9)	0.4 (8.2)
Range	0.0-300.0	0.0-153.0
Area of deposits (%)		
Median (mean)	2.0 (14.2)	2.0 (9.6)
Range	1.0-70.0	1.0-90.0

Abbreviations: CLND, Completion lymph node dissection; *SLN,* sentinel lymph node.
(Courtesy of Scolyer RA, Li L-XL, McCarthy SW, et al: Micromorphometric features of positive sentinel lymph nodes predict involvement of nonsentinel nodes in patients with melanoma. *Am J Clin Pathol* 122:532-539, 2004. Copyright 2004 by the American Society of Clinical Pathologists. Reprinted with permission.)

TABLE 3.—Correlation of Pathologic Features of SLNs With Detection of Melanoma
Metastases in Non-SLNs in CLND Specimens

Pathologic Feature	Patients With Positive CLND	Patients With Negative CLND	P
No. of positive SLNs			>.05
>1 (n = 30)	6 (20)	24 (80)	
1 (n = 110)	18 (16.4)	92 (83.6)	
Deposit number			>.05
>4 (n = 70)	13 (19)	57 (81)	
≤4 (n = 70)	11 (16)	59 (84)	
Tumor penetrative depth			<.05
>2 mm (n = 43)	12 (28)	31 (72)	
≤2 mm (n = 97)	12 (12)	85 (88)	
Tumor penetrative depth stratified at 1 mm†			>.05
>1 mm (n = 69)	13 (19)	56 (81)	
≤1 mm (n = 71)	11 (15)	60 (85)	
Deposit diameter			>.05
>4 mm (n = 25)	8 (32)	17 (68)	
≤4 mm (n = 115)	16 (13.9)	99 (86.1)	
Deposit size			<.01
>10 mm² (n = 20)	8 (40)	12 (60)	
≤10 mm² (n = 120)	16 (13.3)	104 (86.7)	
Area involved with deposits			>.05
>10% (n = 33)	8 (24)	25 (76)	
≤10% (n = 107)	16 (15.0)	91 (85.0)	
Subcapsular deposit			>.05
Present (n = 113)	18 (15.9)	95 (84.1)	
Absent (n = 27)	6 (22)	21 (78)	
Intraparenchymal deposit			>.05
Present (n = 73)	12 (16)	61 (84)	
Absent (n = 67)	12 (18)	55 (82)	
Effacement of nodal architecture			<.05
Present (n = 15)	6 (40)	9 (60)	
Absent (n = 125)	18 (14.4)	107 (85.6)	
Well-spread melanoma cells within the node			>.05
Present (n = 9)	3 (33)	6 (67)	
Absent (n = 131)	21 (16.0)	110 (84.0)	
Perinodal lymphatic involvement			<.01
Present (n = 4)	3 (75)	1 (25)	
Absent (n = 136)	21 (15.4)	115 (84.6)	
Extracapsular spread			>.05
Present (n = 6)	1 (17)	5 (83)	
Absent (n = 134)	23 (17.2)	111 (82.8)	

*Data are given as number (percentage).
†For comparison with the study by Starz et al.
Abbreviations: CLND, Completion lymph node dissection; SLN, sentinel lymph node.
(Courtesy of Scolyer RA, Li L-XL, McCarthy SW, et al: Micromorphometric features of positive sentinel lymph nodes predict involvement of nonsentinel nodes in patients with melanoma. Am J Clin Pathol 122:532-539, 2004. Copyright 2004 by the American Society of Clinical Pathologists. Reprinted with permission.)

their ability to predict which patients will demonstrate further involvement in their CLND specimens.

Methods.—Archival pathology slides and tissue blocks were retrieved for 986 patients with a single primary cutaneous melanoma who underwent successful SLN biopsy between March 1992 and February 2001. Metastatic melanoma cells were identified in at least 1 SLN in 175 patients, all but 8 of whom underwent subsequent CLND. All slides and specimens were available for review in 140 cases. Two independent observers assessed micromorphometric features of each positive SLN. Features included number of positive SLNs, number of metastatic foci, maximum diameter and size of the largest metastasis, percentage of nodal area involved, and tumor penetrative depth of metastasis.

Results.—Of the 140 patients with positive SLNs, 24 (17.1%) had further nodal involvement. The median and mean Breslow thickness (2.8 and 3.2 mm, respectively) of the primary melanomas of these 24 patients were similar to findings in the 116 patients with negative CLND specimens (2.5 and 3.4 mm, respectively), and the 2 groups were similar in other quantitative features of positive SLNs (Table 2). Micromorphometric features of SLNs that correlated significantly with the presence of metastases in CLND specimens were a tumor penetrative depth of more than 2 mm (Table 3), the presence of melanoma cells in perinodal lymphatic vessels, and the effacement of nodal architecture by metastatic melanoma cells.

Conclusion.—Patients with a negative SLN are spared an invasive CLND procedure, but not all patients with a positive SLN have further metastatic disease in non-SLNs. Thickness of the melanomas did not correlate with the presence or absence of non-SLN metastases in CLND specimens, but some morphometric features of melanoma deposits in SLNs did predict a likelihood of further nodal involvement.

Prediction of Metastatic Melanoma in Nonsentinel Nodes and Clinical Outcome Based on the Primary Melanoma and the Sentinel Node
Cochran AJ, Wen D-R, Huang R-R, et al (Univ of California, Los Angeles; John Wayne Cancer Inst, Santa Monica, Calif)
Mod Pathol 17:747-755, 2004   17–46

Introduction.—All patients who have a sentinel node (SN) positive for melanoma undergo completion lymphadenectomy, but in approximately two thirds of cases, only the SN contains metastatic tumor. A need exists for techniques that can identify patients who, despite a tumor-positive SN, have a low probability of metastatic tumor. Certain characteristics of the primary melanoma and the SN were assessed for their ability to predict the likelihood of tumor in nonsentinel lymph nodes (NSLNs).

Methods.—The study included 90 patients who had metastatic melanoma in at least 1 SN in sections stained by hematoxylin and eosin or on immunohistochemical analysis, using antibodies to S-100 protein and HMB-45. All NSLNs excised at complete lymph node dissection (CLND) were similarly examined for melanoma. Primary tumor thickness, the amount of tumor in the SN, and the area and density of interdigitating dendritic cells in the SN were assessed and correlated with the presence of melanoma in the NSLN. These parameters were also related to tumor recurrence and death from disease and were compared for their predictive abilities.

Results.—In univariate analysis, all examined parameters were significantly correlated with NSLN tumor status. The mean relative area of the SN occupied by tumor was 4.3% for patients who had no tumor in the NSLN, versus 30.46% for those with tumor present in the NSLN. The mean density of S-100$^+$ interdigitating dendritic cells in the SN of patients with tumor-free NSLN was twice that in the SN of patients with melanoma in the NSLN (69.34/ mm^2 versus 35.65/mm^2, respectively). In multivariate analysis, tumor burden in the SN and Breslow thickness of the primary melanoma were significant predictors of NSLN tumor status. A tree-based modeling technique was based on these findings. The combination of tumor burden, Breslow thickness, and dendritic cell density were also significantly correlated with tumor recurrence and death from melanoma.

Conclusion.—Data from this and other studies suggest that it is possible to identify patients with a positive SN who are unlikely to have metastatic tumor in NSLNs. The additions of the relative tumor area in the SN and the dendritic cell density to the Breslow thickness provide strong predictive information.

▶ One third or less of patients with a positive sentinel lymph node biopsy (SLNB) for melanoma who subsequently undergo a CLND will have involvement of nonsentinel lymph nodes (NSLNs). Thus, many patients appear to undergo unnecessary node dissection with its accompanying expense, risks and morbidity. Moreover, it remains to be proven whether a CLND improves survival rates in patients with a positive SLNB specimen. Unfortunately, attempts at predicting which patients will have NSLN involvement have been largely unsuccessful. Starz et al (Abstract 17–42) were the first to suggest that the area of the SLN occupied by tumor might correlate well with prognosis and predict which patients would have NSLN involvement. Subsequently, they simplified their classification by evaluating the depth of penetration of the tumor into the SLN. However, other investigators have been slow to adopt this approach to evaluating positive SLNs, possibly because of the cumbersome task of measuring the area occupied by tumor. The studies reviewed here (Abstracts 17–43 to 17–46) carry the concept of Starz et al regarding SLN staging 1 step further, and take into account not only the depth of penetration of the tumor and the number of adjacent tissue sections involved but also other variables, including the number of S100$^+$ interdigitating dendritic cells present, involvement of paranodal lymphatics, effacement of the nodal architecture, the maximum diameter of the tumor deposits, and the location of the tumor deposits (subcapsular vs other). Although there is no complete uniformity in these studies, it is obvious that staging of the SLNB specimen adds potentially valuable therapeutic and prognostic information. However, as is often the case, things are not black and white; that is, there are trends but there are no absolutes regarding how many variables should be assessed and their correlation with positivity or negativity of the NSLNs. Thus, a decision to perform a CLND in a patient with a positive SLNB specimen should be based on the probability that the patient would have involvement of the NSLNs. In this context, staging of the SLN may allow one to predict which patients are more likely to benefit from a CLND.

P. G. Lang, Jr, MD

Is Completion Lymphadenectomy After a Positive Sentinel Lymph Node Biopsy for Cutaneous Melanoma Always Necessary?
Elias N, Tanabe KK, Sober AJ, et al (Harvard Med School, Boston)
Arch Surg 139:400-405, 2004   17–47

Introduction.—Regional lymph node metastasis is the most important prognostic factor in patients with primary cutaneous melanoma. Completion lymph node dissection (CLND) is recommended when metastatic disease is identified at sentinel lymph node (SLN) biopsy, but only 15% to 20% of patients with a positive SLN biopsy are found to have further metastatic disease in the CLND specimen. A retrospective review tested the hypothesis that patients with negative lymph nodes included in the SLN specimen have low risk of metastases in the residual draining basin and may not require CLND.

Methods.—The 506 consecutive patients included in the review underwent SLN biopsy for staging between January 1, 1997, and May 31, 2003. All had a primary tumor thickness more than 1 mm or invasiveness to Clark level IV or greater and were free of clinical evidence of metastasis. In most patients the primary melanoma site was widely excised during SLN mapping. The number of nodes procured from each basin during SLN biopsy ranged from 1 to 10 (mean, 3.20); the number of positive nodes identified in the SLN specimen ranged from 1 to 3 (mean, 1.19).

Results.—Eighty (17.2%) of the 87 patients with metastatic melanoma at SLN biopsy underwent CLND, and 12 (15%) had further metastases. Primary tumor characteristics did not differ between patients with negative and positive CLND findings. In 28 cases, all SLNs contained metastatic melanoma; 7 of these patients (25%) had additional nodes with metastatic melanoma in the CLND specimen. Fifty-two of 80 patients had 1 or more SLNs without metastatic melanoma, and 5 of these patients had additional metastases in the CLND specimen.

Conclusion.—Most patients with positive SLNs and negative nodes at the initial biopsy were found to have no evidence of metastatic melanoma at CLND, but 10% did have further metastases. The subgroup of patients with positive SLNs and negative nodes in the SLN biopsy are at low risk for further metastasis, but CLND cannot be safely omitted in such cases. Thus, CLND remains the uniform recommendation for all patients with positive SLNs.

▶ In patients undergoing SLN biopsy for melanomas more than 1 mm thick, 15% to 20% will have positive findings. When this group of patients subsequently undergoes CLND, only 15% to 20% will be found to have involvement of the remaining nodes. Therefore, at least theoretically, 80% to 85% are subjected to an unnecessary procedure associated with significant morbidity, and it would be ideal to identify which patients with a positive SLNB require a CLND. In this study, the authors found that if there was a single positive SLN or if only some of the SLNs were positive, the patient was less likely to have involvement of non-SLNs (10%) as opposed to the patient with multiple positive SLNs (25%). Although there was a subset of patients with a positive SLNB who were less apt to have involvement of non-SLNs, the incidence of positive non-SLNs was significant enough that a CLND was still deemed advisable. In addition, the authors suggest that because non-SLNs are not as rigorously examined as SLNs, the true incidence of involvement of non-SLNs could actually be higher than 10%.

P. G. Lang, Jr, MD

Role of Sentinel Lymph Node Biopsy in Patients With Thick (>4 mm) Primary Melanoma

Jacobs IA, Chang CK, Salti GI (Univ of Illinois, Chicago)
Am Surg 70:59-62, 2004   17–48

Background.—Patients with thick melanomas (>4 mm) have been shown to have a high risk (60% to 70%) of regional nodal micrometastatic disease and a high risk (70%) of occult systemic disease at initial presentation. It is thought that the risk of distant microscopic metastases is so high in these patients that it may negate any potentially curative benefit of a regional operation; thus, these patients have not been considered candidates for elective lymph node dissection. Instead, they have been targeted for adjuvant therapy. This therapy may benefit patients who subsequently have nodal metastases, but data supporting its use in patients with thick melanomas are limited and controversial. Lymphatic mapping and sentinel lymphadenectomy have become routine components of the treatment of primary melanoma, and their role in the management of thick lesions (>4 mm) is evolving. The influence of sentinel lymph node (SLN) histologic variables on the survival of patients with thick melanomas was evaluated.

Methods.—A computerized patient database was accessed to obtain records on patients with thick melanomas. Survival curves were constructed with the Kaplan-Meier method, and a Cox regression analysis was used to establish statistical significance. A total of 266 SLN biopsy procedures were performed on 259 patients with malignant melanomas between 1997 and 2002, and both radioisotope and blue dye were used.

Results.—Thick melanomas were found in 45 patients (17%), of whom 20 patients (44%) had at least 1 positive SLN. The mean disease-free survival duration of patients with SLN-positive nodes was 44 months compared with 53 months in patients with SLN-negative nodes. Increasing Breslow thickness was associated with a decrease in disease-free survival duration, but no other histologic variables, such as Clark level, mitotic rate, or ulceration, affected disease-free survival.

Conclusion.—The status of the SLN seems to be predictive of disease-free survival in patients with thick melanomas.

Sentinel Lymph Node Biopsy Does Not Change Melanoma-Specific Survival Among Patients With Breslow Thickness Greater Than Four Millimeters
Caracò C, Celentano E, Lastoria S, et al (Natl Cancer Inst, Naples, Italy)
Ann Surg Oncol 11:198S-202S, 2004   17–49

Background.—The management of cutaneous melanomas has changed in the past decade with the introduction of the sentinel lymph node concept. Sentinel lymph node biopsy can provide accurate identification of patients with nodal micrometastases who are eligible for complete lymph node dissection. In the present study, data from 359 sentinel lymph node biopsy procedures at the National Cancer Institute in Naples, Italy were analyzed to determine 3-year disease-free survival and overall survival rates, particularly in patients with thick melanomas (>4 mm thick), who have a worse prognosis related to the early appearance of distant metastasis.

Methods.—Data from 359 sentinel lymph node biopsy procedures performed over a period of 5 years were reviewed to determine the effect of the treatment on disease-free survival and overall survival after stratification of patients for nodal status, tumor ulceration, and Breslow thickness. All patients had undergone excision of their primary melanomas with a margin less than 1 cm within 3 months before sentinel lymph node biopsy. Patients who had undergone wide excision (>3 cm) of the primary melanoma or reconstruction with a cutaneous rotation flap were excluded.

Results.—Statistical analysis showed a better 3-year survival rate for patients with negative sentinel nodes than for patients with positive sentinel nodes (88.4% and 72.9%, respectively). Tumor ulceration continued to have prognostic significance despite lymph node status, indicated by a higher risk of development of distant metastases. Survival curves associated with thicker melanomas did not demonstrate significant differences between patients with negative sentinel nodes and patients with positive sentinel nodes.

Conclusions.—Sentinel lymph node biopsy can provide accurate staging of nodal status in patients with melanomas who have no clinical evidence of metastases. However, the role of sentinel lymph node biopsy should be clarified by longer follow-up and the final results from ongoing trials.

▶ Both these studies (Abstracts 17–48 and 17–49) address the utility of sentinel lymph node biopsy (SLNB) in patients with melanomas that are more than 4 mm thick and demonstrate a better 3-year overall survival rate for patients with negative SLNB specimens. This difference in survival is even greater if the primary tumor is not ulcerated. These findings are in keeping with prior studies that support a role for SLNB in patients with tumors more than 4 mm thick. Of note, however, is the observation of Caracò et al (Abstract 17–49) that no difference in disease-free survival was seen for patients with negative versus positive SLNB specimens.

P. G. Lang, Jr, MD

Sentinel Lymph Node Dissection and Lymphatic Mapping for Local Subcutaneous Recurrence in Melanoma Treatment: Longer-term Follow-up Results
Coventry BJ, Chatterton B, Whitehead F, et al (Univ of Adelaide, North Terrace, South Australia; Royal Adelaide Hosp, North Terrace, South Australia; Inst of Med and Veterinary Sciences, West Terrace, Adelaide, South Australia)
Ann Surg Oncol 11:203S-207S, 2004   17–50

Background.—Lymphatic mapping and sentinel lymph node dissection (LM/SLND) for the surgical staging of primary cutaneous melanoma can identify patients who are likely to benefit from a complete regional lymphadenectomy. However, the role of this approach in patients with recurrent (secondary) melanoma has not been well explored. The current authors have used the LM/SLND technique since 1993 for primary melanoma and breast cancer treatment and as part of the international Multicenter Selective Lymphadenectomy Trial and other clinical trials. In recent years, this group has used peritumoral injection techniques, similar to those used for breast cancer, for subcutaneous recurrent melanoma deposits and have identified a sentinel node in the majority of cases. It was hypothesized that LM/SLND can be used to map sentinel nodes from solitary, subcutaneous, locally recurrent melanoma deposits and that theses techniques may aid in the identification of regional lymph node basin metastases. Follow-up data are presented from the preliminary clinical experience with this technique in the treatment of local subcutaneous melanoma recurrence.

Methods.—The 12 patients (median age, 60.5 years; range, 19-78 years) in the study had a solitary subcutaneous or cutaneous melanoma recurrence after previous wide local excision as the sole treatment for their primary melanoma. The methods used for LM/SLND were similar to those used in the Multicenter Selective Lymphadenectomy Trial. Patients were followed with clinical examinations every 3 months for 2 years, every 6 months for 2 years, and yearly thereafter and by interim examinations as required. CT scans of the head, chest, abdomen, and pelvis were performed before enrollment and at 6-month intervals unless otherwise indicated clinically.

Results.—The melanoma recurrence was located on an extremity in 8 patients, on the trunk in 2 patients, and on the head in 2 patients. All instances of recurrence were less than 5 cm from the initial primary melanoma resection site. Wider local excision and primary closure or skin grafting was performed in all cases after LM/SLND. The experience in these patients indicated the potential usefulness of this technique in the management of locally recurrent melanoma at subcutaneous sites. Mapping was also used to localize the sentinel node draining a subcutaneous local recurrence after previous LM/SLND.

Conclusion.—The application of LM/SLND may be extended beyond primary melanoma management as more is learned about the technical issues and appropriate selection of patients.

▶ LM/SLND is a well-established technique for staging and managing patients with primary melanomas; however, data is limited regarding the usefulness of this technique in patients with a local recurrence. In this article, the authors discuss their observations in 12 patients with locally recurrent melanomas who underwent LM/SLND. Unfortunately, no definitive conclusions could be drawn. Although sentinel node(s) could be identified, the significance of a negative SLND result was not clear because some of these patients experienced systemic dissemination or in-transit metastases.

P. G. Lang, Jr, MD

Desmoplastic and Neurotropic Melanoma: Analysis of 33 Patients With Lymphatic Mapping and Sentinel Lymph Node Biopsy
Su LD, Fullen DR, Lowe L, et al (Univ of Michigan, Ann Arbor)
Cancer 105:598-604, 2004   17–51

Background.—Desmoplastic and neurotropic malignant melanoma (DNMM) occasionally metastasizes to regional lymph nodes and extranodal sites. In patients with DNMM without clinical evidence of regional lymph node involvement, the general consensus is that combined lymphatic mapping and sentinel lymph node biopsy (SLNB) is the most appropriate strategy for obtaining staging information. However, articles in the literature thus far have suggested that the use of SLNB may not be reliable for DNMM. The utility of SLNB for the management of patients with DNMM was determined.

Methods.—A total of 33 patients (25 men, 8 women; median age, 61 years; range, 31-86 years) with DNMM who were seen during a 5-year period at one institution were included in the study. All patients underwent lymphatic mapping and SLNB. Clinical and histologic data were reviewed.

Results.—More than half (52%) of the tumors were on the head and neck region, and 24% were associated with lentigo maligna. Four of 33 patients (12%) without clinical evidence of metastatic disease who underwent SLNB had at least 1 positive sentinel lymph node. No additional positive lymph nodes were identified on subsequent therapeutic regional lymphadenectomy in any of these 4 patients.

Conclusions.—In this study, SLNB detected subclinical metastases of DNMM to regional lymph nodes. SLNB at the time of resection can provide useful information for guiding early treatment and, in combination with lymphadenectomy in patients with positive findings, may limit the spread of tumors and prevent a recurrence at the draining lymph node basin.

▶ Several prior studies have suggested that SLNB may not be reliable for staging patients with DNMM. In this retrospective study, the authors found that SLNB was very reliable and worthwhile for staging patients' tumors. Although these tumors were quite thick (mean thickness, 4 mm), SLNB showed positive findings in only 12% of patients. This observation is in keeping with anecdotal reports that thick DNMMs are less apt to metastasize than are other melanomas of comparable thickness.

P. G. Lang, Jr, MD

Selective Lymphadenectomy in Sentinel Node-Positive Patients May Increase the Risk of Local/In-transit Recurrence in Malignant Melanoma
Thomas JM, Clark MA (Royal Marsden Hosp, London)
Eur J Surg Oncol 30:686-691, 2004   17–52

Introduction.—Sentinel lymph node biopsy (SLNB) is performed in patients with melanoma to identify microscopic nodal metastases and to assess the need for formal lymph node dissection (selective lymphadenectomy [SL]). Yet there is no evidence at present that SL in sentinel node (SN)-positive patients offers a survival advantage, and some reports suggest that SL adversely affects the pattern of spread and recurrence of melanoma. A literature overview of SLNB with or without SL sought to quantify the risks of this practice.

Methods.—Investigators sought to identify all publications providing details of the site(s) of first recurrence of melanoma, with specific reference to the incidence of local/in-transit recurrence. Findings were compared to the incidence of such recurrence after wide local excision (WLE) alone.

Results.—The natural incidence of local/in-transit recurrence after WLE alone, as reported from 3 large randomized clinical trials, ranged from 2.5% to 6.3%, and, as reported previously, the natural incidence of local/in-transit recurrence increased with tumor thickness. Trials reporting patients who underwent SLNB found 68 (5.7%) local/in-transit recurrences in 1199 SN-negative patients and 43 (20.9%) in 206 SN-positive patients who underwent SL. Given the natural incidence of local/in-transit recurrences, patients undergoing SLNB with or without subsequent SL are at significantly increased risk for development of local/in-transit recurrence.

Conclusion.—The incidence of local/in-transit recurrence after SL in patients who are SN-positive may be 4 times greater than the expected incidence when the procedure is not performed. Until further evidence is gathered from a randomized controlled trial, the SLNB procedure should be viewed as experimental. Potential alternatives to SLNB include risk analysis of other prognostic factors and a more detailed investigation of the original WLE specimen.

High Incidence of In-transit Metastases After Sentinel Node Biopsy in Patients With Melanoma
Estourgie SH, Nieweg OE, Kroon BBR (Netherlands Cancer Inst, Amsterdam)
Br J Surg 91:1370-1371, 2004   17–53

Introduction.—The performance of sentinel lymph node biopsy (SLNB) in patients with clinically localized melanoma may disturb the lymph flow, causing entrapment of tumor cells and leading to in-transit metastases. Such metastases are usually multiple, tend to recur, and are difficult to treat. The incidence of in-transit metastases in 61 patients who had sentinel lymph node dissection because of a tumor-positive sentinel node (SN) was compared with that in 60 patients who had palpable nodal metastases dissected.

Methods.—All patients had a clinically localized melanoma with a Breslow thickness of at least 1 mm (or thinner lesions with a Clark level of IV or V). Excluded were patients with head or neck melanoma. Patients with a tumor-positive SN were studied prospectively; those with palpable metastases were evaluated retrospectively.

Results.—The 2 groups were similar overall in patient and tumor characteristics, but mean Breslow thickness was greater in the positive SN group (3.8 mm) than in the palpable lymph node group (2.9 mm). In addition, more patients in the positive SN group had ulceration (48% vs 22%). In-transit metastases were seen during follow-up in 23% of patients with a positive SN versus 8% with palpable lymph nodes. Only lymph node status had a significant effect on the development of in-transit metastases.

Discussion.—The risk of in-transit metastasis is significantly higher in patients undergoing lymph node dissection because of a non-palpable tumor-positive SN than in patients with more advanced disease undergoing dissection of palpable nodal metastases. Thus, the findings do not support the routine practice of SLNB in the management of melanoma.

▶ Until now, the major criticism of sentinel lymph node biopsy (SLNB) and subsequent complete lymph node dissection (CLND) has been that there is no evidence that it improves survival, and there are associated risks and complications. Now another potential drawback to SLNB and CLND has been suggested, namely, an increased incidence of in-transit metastases. In-transit metastases are difficult to manage and are associated with a poorer prognosis. Thus, if this were a true complication of SLNB and CLND, it would suggest that the procedure may lead to additional problems in management that negate any potential benefit. The authors of these 2 articles (Abstracts 17–52 and 17–53) theorize that in SLNB-positive patients, a CLND, in the absence of clinical disease, could lead to the trapping of melanoma cells en route to the nodal basin, within the afferent lymphatics, which later could manifest as in-transit metastases. Obviously this is an important issue that needs to be addressed with some urgency because of the large number of SLNBs and CLNDs that are being performed on a daily basis.

P. G. Lang, Jr, MD

Sentinel-Lymph-Node Biopsy (SLNB) for Melanoma Is Not Complication-Free

Wasserberg N, Tulchinsky H, Schachter J, et al (Tel Aviv Univ, Israel)

Eur J Surg Oncol 30:851-856, 2004   17–54

Introduction.—Lymph node dissection is linked with substantial morbidity, whereas sentinel lymph node biopsy (SLNB) is regarded as relatively complication-free. The long-term incidence and severity of SLNB-related complications in patients with malignant melanoma (MM) were evaluated to determine possible risk factors.

Methods.—Data from a computerized database of all patients with MM who underwent SLNB between 1994 and 2002 were analyzed, and procedure-associated complications were documented.

Results.—The data included 250 patients (127 males, 123 females) with primary MM who underwent SLNB. Their ages ranged from 17 to 84 years (median, 56.5 years). A total of 309 lymphatic basins in the 250 patients were analyzed for SLNB; complications as a result of surgery occurred in 62 (20%) of the 309 (Table 2). Sensory morbidity was significantly linked with axillary SLNB ($P = .04$) and was more prevalent among younger patients. The use of blue dye alone or combined with a handheld gamma probe had no statistically important influence on the sentinel node identification rate. There were 6 (2.3%) false-negatives and an overall false-negative rate of 18%. A positive sentinel node was significantly linked with shortened overall survival ($P = .04$).

Conclusion.—Wound complications are more common than are usually reported. Sensory morbidity was most common in the axilla. Neck SLNB was correlated with the highest incidence of identification failure. Patient age, basin location, and number of excised nodes may act as prognostic factors of morbidity.

▶ The SLNB is often treated as a benign procedure and, indeed, in this reviewer's experience, this would appear to be the case. However, this article demonstrates that significant complications may occur, including thrombosis and cerebrovascular events. With respect to wound complications (infection and

TABLE 2.—Complications by Sentinel Node Location

Complication	Axilla (N = 164)	Groin (N = 110)	Basin Neck (N = 35)	Total (N = 309)
Wound	16	25	1	42
Sensory	12	1	1	14
Edema	—	3	—	3
Other[a]	—	2	1	3
Total	28	31	3	62
Identification failure	8	1	8	17
False-negative	1	4	1	6

[a]Other: urinary tract infection, deep vein thrombosis, cerebrovascular accident.
(Courtesy of Wasserberg N, Tulchinsky H, Schachter J, et al: Sentinel-lymph-node biopsy (SLNB) for melanoma is not complication-free. *Eur J Surg Oncol* 30:851-856, 2004.)

seroma formation), these are more likely to occur with SLNBs of the groin, whereas sensory deficits and impaired mobility are more likely to follow SLNBs of the axilla, especially when more than 2 SLNs are removed. Transient lymphedema, sometimes requiring compression hose, has been reported after SLNBs of the groin. Although the complications reported in this article were usually transient and reversible, it does demonstrate that the procedure is associated with a significant complication rate and should be undertaken with care.

P. G. Lang, Jr, MD

Routine Imaging of Asymptomatic Melanoma Patients With Metastasis to Sentinel Lymph Nodes Rarely Identifies Systemic Disease

Miranda EP, Gertner M, Wall J, et al (Univ of California, San Francisco)
Arch Surg 139:831-837, 2004   17–55

Introduction.—Selective sentinel lymphadenectomy (SSL) has been established as the definitive staging procedure for regional draining lymph node basins in patients with malignant melanoma, but completion (radical) lymph node dissection might not be performed when there is evidence of distant metastatic disease. Most publications on the appropriate radiographic studies for detecting stage IV disease in patients with melanoma appeared in the "pre-sentinel lymph node (pre-SLN)" era. A retrospective analysis of patients who underwent SSL for primary melanoma was done to determine whether CT of the chest, abdomen, pelvis, and brain reveals systemic metastasis at the time of SSL.

Methods.—Eligible patients were those who had undergone SSL and chest radiography at a single tertiary care referral center between April 1994 and February 2003 and had pathologic evidence of metastasis to at least 1 SLN. Data from their medical records were examined, and patient demographics, characteristics of the primary tumor, and findings from imaging studies were analyzed.

Results.—Of 1183 patients, 185 (15.6%) met the entry criteria. The mean age of the group was 50.1 years; 67% were men. The Breslow thickness of the melanoma ranged from 0.8 to 14.5 mm. None of the patients had positive findings on initial chest radiography. At follow-up, 26% were found to have died. Results of 86% of imaging studies (chest radiographs, CT, and MRI) were negative for systemic disease, 14% were indeterminate; only 1 case (0.5%) was positive. Additional studies, ranging from repeated imaging to invasive procedures including thoracotomy and brain biopsy, confirmed the indeterminate results to be negative. The single patient with detectable systemic disease at the time of imaging also had symptoms of systemic disease. In this patient, 2 of 5 SLNs had been positive for macrometastatic disease but whole-body positron emission tomography (PET) and brain MRI were negative. Two months after SSL, dyspnea developed, and chest radiography showed evidence of metastatic disease.

Conclusion.—At the time of SSL in asymptomatic patients with melanoma, CT scans of the chest, abdomen, pelvis, and brain rarely demonstrate systemic metastasis. Thus, routine imaging of such patients at the time of SSL is not indicated. Chest radiography, however, is useful as an adjunctive test for preoperative risk stratification for morbidity directly related to operative procedures.

▶ A number of studies have demonstrated that in asymptomatic patients with primary melanoma, the yield from radiographic imaging studies, such as CT scan and MRI, is low and fraught with a significant number of false-positive results. This can lead to the performance of what is often unnecessary and expensive additional tests, including biopsies. This study takes these findings 1-step further; that is, what is the yield with imaging studies in patients with a positive sentinel lymph node biopsy (SLNB) who are asymptomatic and have no suspicious clinical findings suggesting systemic spread of disease? PET scans were not included in this analysis, probably because the numbers would have been too small. However, the authors found that the yield of true-positives for CT scan and MRI was extremely low but the incidence of false-positives was significant. Thus, they concluded that routine imaging of all patients with a positive SLNB is neither indicated nor cost effective. Although there are those who would argue that the same is true for chest radiographs, the authors suggest that the chest radiograph can be justified on the basis of the fact that (1) it is relatively inexpensive; (2) it occasionally is positive (which helps with staging); and (3) it can be justified because it is useful for the preoperative assessment of a patient undergoing general anesthesia. Unfortunately, despite the findings of this study and others, it has been this reviewer's experience that physicians, when dealing with high-risk melanoma patients, continue to order imaging studies that are not only expensive but usually negative. These tests are associated with a significant number of false-positive findings that, in turn, lead to more testing. I hope in time this will change.

P. G. Lang, Jr, MD

Is ¹⁸F-FDG PET More Accurate Than Standard Diagnostic Procedures in the Detection of Suspected Recurrent Melanoma?
Fuster D, Chiang S, Johnson G, et al (Univ of Pennsylvania, Philadelphia)
J Nucl Med 45:1323-1327, 2004   17–56

Introduction.—In asymptomatic patients who have been successfully treated for stage I or II melanoma, extensive staging workups are of limited value and may lead to unnecessary invasive procedures. Selective imaging studies are warranted, however, in patients with stage III or IV disease because of their risk of systemic recurrence. The accuracy of ¹⁸F-fluorodeoxyglucose positron emission tomography (¹⁸-FDG PET) in diagnosing recurrent melanoma was retrospectively investigated in patients with recurrence suspected by clinical examination or blood markers.

Methods.—Patients were 73 women and 83 men with a mean age of 53 years. Ninety-eight patients were stage I or II and 58 were stage III or IV. Results of PET were compared with those of clinical procedures (CP), including plain radiography, bone scanning, body CT, brain MRI, and ultrasound (US). The PET scans were assessed by 2 reporters without knowledge of CP results.

Results.—Eighty-six of 184 scans showed the patient to be disease free for at least 1 year after the scan; 98 scans revealed proven sites of active disease (146 lesions) that were confirmed by histologic examination or follow-up. Distant metastases were noted in 51 scans and locoregional involvement in 47. The overall accuracy for PET was 81%, compared with 52% for other methods. In 36% of patients PET led to a change in clinical management. Curative resection of 14 locoregional recurrences and 10 distant metastases was performed, and 12 patients received systemic therapy instead of inadequate surgery. CT had a better sensitivity than PET in the assessment of lung disease, but PET was more accurate in detecting skin lesions, malignant lymph nodes, and metastases to the abdomen, liver, and bone.

Conclusion.—Whole-body PET proved to be a useful tool in the diagnosis of recurrent melanoma, particularly in its ability to detect locoregional disease and distant metastases at all sites except the lung. The sensitivity of chest CT was higher (93%) than that of PET (57%), but PET was more specific (92%) than CT (70%) in showing solitary lung lesions.

▶ Previous studies have demonstrated that extensive staging workups in asymptomatic patients with stage I and II melanoma are unlikely to detect occult disease and may result in false-positive findings that lead to more extensive and expensive testing. In this study of patients with stage I to IV disease who were suspected of having a recurrence on the basis of clinical examination or laboratory testing, the authors found that ^{18}F-FDG PET was overall more sensitive and specific for detecting recurrent disease than was CT. Although CT was more sensitive for detecting subclinical lesions of the lung, false-positives were more common, suggesting that a combination of CT and PET might be best for evaluating patients for occult pulmonary disease. For suspicious brain lesions PET offered no advantage over MRI. Not only was PET more efficient at detecting occult disease, but the findings altered the course of treatment in a significant number of patients (36%). It obviated the need for further invasive procedures, which were based on false-positive findings by CT and allowed potential curative surgery in patients with locoregional disease or a single distant metastasis. It also saved some patients from undergoing surgery when it was found they had unresectable disease or were not suitable surgical candidates. This study, like others, confirms that FDG PET is more sensitive than CT in assessing melanoma patients for recurrent disease. It should be noted that, especially for stage I and II patients, PET was not performed in asymptomatic patients who had no clinical or laboratory evidence of recurrence.

P. G. Lang, Jr, MD

Adjuvant Interferon in High-Risk Melanoma: The AIM HIGH Study— United Kingdom Coordinating Committee on Cancer Research Randomized Study of Adjuvant Low-Dose Extended-Duration Interferon Alfa-2a in High-Risk Resected Malignant Melanoma

Hancock BW, Wheatley K, Harris S, et al (Weston Park Hosp, Sheffield, England; Univ of Birmingham, England; Selly Oak Hosp, Birmingham, England; et al)
J Clin Oncol 22:53-61, 2004   17–57

Introduction.—Phase I and II trials addressing metastatic melanoma have reported a response rate of about 15% with interferon alfa. Low-dose extended duration interferon-α was evaluated as adjuvant therapy in patients with completely resected high-risk melanoma in a randomized controlled trial.

Methods.—The effect of interferon alfa-2a (3 megaunits, 3 times weekly for 2 years or until recurrence) on overall survival (OS) and recurrence-free survival (RFS) was compared with that of no further treatment for patients with radically resected stage IIB and stage III cutaneous malignant melanoma. Between October 3, 1995, and December 22, 2000, a total of 674 patients with completely resected high-risk melanoma were enrolled. Of these, 338 were allocated to treatment with interferon alfa-2a and 336 to observation alone.

Results.—The median follow-up period was 3.1 years (range, 0-6.8 years). OS was 44% and RFS was 32% at 5 years. No significant differences were observed in OS or RFS between the interferon-treated and control arms (odds ratio, 0.94; 95% confidence interval, 0.75-1,18; $P = .6$; and odds ratio, 0.91; 95% confidence interval, 0.75-1.10; $P = .3$, respectively). Male gender ($P = .003$) and regional lymph node involvement ($P = .0009$) but not age ($P = .70$) were statistically adverse factors for OS.

Subgroup analysis by disease stage, age, and gender did not demonstrate any significant differences between the interferon-treated and control groups in either OS or RFS. Interferon-associated toxicities were modest. Grade 3 (grade 4 in 1 patient) fatigue or mood disturbance occurred in 7% and 4%, respectively. Fifty (15%) patients withdrew from interferon treatment because of toxicity.

Conclusion.—Extended-duration low-dose interferon does not appear to provide any benefit over observation alone in the initial treatment of completely resected high-risk malignant melanoma.

▶ The use of interferon as adjuvant therapy for patients with high-risk melanoma remains controversial. Conflicting results have been reported with high-dose interferon, which is often poorly tolerated. Studies have suggested that low-dose interferon is better tolerated but offers no clinical benefit.

This study examined the potential benefit of low-dose interferon alfa-2a (3 million units 3 times weekly) given for 2 years or until disease recurrence. Overall, there was no benefit on OS or RFS. However, in patients less than 50 years old, interferon did appear to prolong RFS but had no effect on OS. There was no difference in OS or RFS based on sex or stage of disease at time of treatment.

Although toxicity necessitating withdrawal from the study was noted in approximately 15% of patients, this regimen was much better tolerated than high-dose interferon. Being a male and having lymph node involvement had an adverse effect on OS, but age had no effect. In conclusion, based on this study and numerous others, it appears dubious that interferon alfa conveys any benefit to patients with high-risk melanoma.

P. G. Lang, Jr, MD

Ten-Year Experience of Carbon Dioxide Laser Ablation as Treatment for Cutaneous Recurrence of Malignant Melanoma
Gibson SC, Byrne DS, McKay AJ (Gartnavel Gen Hosp, Glasgow, Scotland)
Br J Surg 91:893-895, 2004   17–58

Introduction.—Cutaneous recurrence of malignant melanoma is historically linked with a poor prognosis because it indicates systemic disease. Surgical excision is useful when the number of lesions is limited. For more widespread lesions, carbon dioxide laser ablation, immunotherapy (including bacille Calmette-Guérin [BCG] vaccine, melanoma vaccine, and immunomodulators), cryotherapy, radiotherapy, and chemotherapy have been used. The 10-year experience with the use of carbon dioxide laser ablation was reviewed to ascertain the initial efficacy of the treatment, the time to recurrence, number of treatments needed, and the length of time for which palliation was achieved.

Methods.—The study included 42 patients (33 women and 9 men; ages 49-94 years; mean age, 73 years) who were treated between September 1992 and September 2002 for lower-limb recurrence of malignant melanoma. The lesion size varied between 0.5 and 6.0 cm in diameter; the number of lesions ranged from 1 to 60 (median, 14). The lesions were either too numerous or too large for surgical excision; isolated limb perfusion was either unsuccessful or was unsuitable. Twenty patients had undergone prior excision with or without grafting on more than 1 occasion, 29 had at least 1 isolated limb perfusion procedure, and 12 had undergone a regional lymph node dissection; 8 patients had more advanced disease with both local and regional recurrence. None had undergone radiotherapy or chemotherapy.

Results.—A total of 105 treatments were performed (mean, 2.5). The time to recurrence ranged from 1.2 to 72 months (median, 5.2). Twenty-three patients were still alive; The time from first laser ablation ranged from 0.5 to 10.0 years (median, 5.4). Nineteen patients had died after initial ablation at a period ranging from 0.1 to 5.3 years (median, 0.8 years). Ten of the 23 survivors were disease-free for more than 1 year. No limbs were amputated as a result of failure to control the disease.

Conclusion.—Laser ablation is both practical and useful in the palliative treatment of recurrent cutaneous malignant melanoma.

▶ The management of satellite lesions, in transit metastases, and distant cutaneous metastases in melanoma patients is a challenging problem. The physician does not want the patient to progress to the stage of a chronic nonhealing wound, yet cutaneous metastases are usually associated with systemic disease, and thus, mutilating or overly aggressive surgery is unlikely to alter the patient's prognosis. However, some patients have no other evidence of metastatic disease, or their body may be able to contain occult microscopic deposits of tumor for a prolonged period. Potential modalities for treatment include isolated limb perfusion, simple excision, cryosurgery, intralesional interferon or BCG, topical immunomodulators, and radiation therapy. Gibson et al report their experience with the carbon dioxide laser. Although their results are encouraging, this reviewer has a number of concerns with their reporting and methodology. First, no details are given regarding the parameters used nor their treatment protocol. Second, of all anatomical locations to select for treatment, what worse location (from the standpoint of wound healing and infection) could be chosen than the lower extremity? Moreover, even patients who had had previous node dissections were treated. It would appear that before this modality is used to treat cutaneous metastases in melanoma patients, one needs more information regarding the treatment protocol. The potential downside of treatment, a chronic nonhealing wound and a significant risk of infection, also must be considered.

P. G. Lang, Jr, MD

Contemporary Surgical Treatment of Advanced-Stage Melanoma
Essner R, Lee JH, Wanek LA, et al (Saint John's Health Ctr, Santa Monica, Calif)
Arch Surg 139:961-967, 2004   17–59

Background.—Cutaneous melanoma was at one time an uncommon malignancy, but it is rapidly becoming a major health concern in the United States. A total of 55,100 Americans are estimated to have had melanoma develop in 2004, with 7910 dying from the disease. The surgical treatment of patients with stage IV melanoma is controversial because the 5-year survival rate is approximately 5%. The outcome of patients with advanced-stage melanoma treated over a 29-year period at 1 institution in whom surgical resection was considered part of the curative intent was evaluated.

Methods.—A cohort analysis was conducted of 1574 successive patients who underwent surgical resection of metastatic melanoma at a tertiary cancer center over a 29-year period. The patients were followed on a routine basis with serial examinations and radiographic studies. The median follow-up time was 19 months, with a range of 1 to 382 months. The surgical technique used was based on the site of metastasis. The main outcome measure was a computer-assisted database with statistical analyses by log-rank tests and Cox regression models.

Results.—Of the 4426 patients with American Joint Committee on Cancer (AJCC) stage IV melanoma, 1574 patients (33%) underwent surgical resection. The majority of these patients (62%) were men, with a median age of 50 years. Of the primary melanomas, 46% arose on the trunk and 50% were Clark level IV or V, with a median thickness of 2.2 mm. A total of 697 patients (44%) had AJCC stage III melanoma (lymph node involvement) before the development of stage IV (metastases). The most common site for resection was the lung (42%), followed by the skin or lymph node (19%) and the alimentary tract (16%). Melanoma was present at a single site in 877 (56%) patients. The 5-year survival rate was significantly better for patients with a solitary melanoma than for those with 4 or more metastases. The survival rate was most favorable in patients with skin and lymph node metastases. On multivariate analysis, predictors of survival were early primary tumor stage (I vs II), an absence of intervening stage III metastases, solitary metastasis, and a long disease-free interval (>36 months) from AJCC stage I or II to stage IV.

Conclusions.—These findings provided evidence of the benefit of surgical resection for advanced-stage melanoma. Patients with limited sites and numbers of metastases should be considered for curative resection regardless of the disease location.

▶ In general, patients with stage IV melanoma are not considered surgical candidates. However, there have been reports of patients with a solitary metastasis who have long-term remission after resection of the metastatic lesion, and there are times when surgery is required for palliation (eg, intestinal obstruction). In this article, the authors report their experience over the past 29 years utilizing surgery to treat patients with stage IV disease. Unfortunately, they do not clearly delineate what criteria were used to select patients for surgery. However, their analysis of the group as a whole revealed that patients who benefited the most were those with 1 or 2 metastatic lesions, those who had a long remission (>36 months) before developing stage IV disease, and those who developed stage IV disease without a prior history of stage III disease. Patients with involvement of the skin or distal lymph nodes did the best, with a median survival of 35.1 months. The authors theorize that removing the metastatic lesion(s) allows the immune system to become more efficient in destroying or containing occult tumor deposits located elsewhere. Although there is no question that surgery can play a role in the management of patients with stage IV melanoma, strict criteria should be developed.

P. G. Lang, Jr, MD

Determinants of Outcome in Melanoma Patients With Cerebral Metastases

Fife KM, Colman MH, Stevens GN, et al (Univ of Sydney, New South Wales, Australia)
J Clin Oncol 22:1293-1300, 2004   17–60

Introduction.—Cerebral metastases are common in patients with melanoma; up to 10% of patients are ultimately diagnosed with them and 49% to 73% of patients who die as a result of melanoma have cerebral metastases on autopsy. The prognostic factors, effects of treatment, and survival were examined in patients with cerebral metastases from melanoma.

Findings.—All patients with melanoma who had cerebral metastases and were treated at a single institution between 1952 and 2000 were identified. Multivariate analyses were performed to determine prognostic factors for survival. Of 1137 patients with melanoma and cerebral metastases, 686 were treated between 1985 and 2000. Among those treated in the latter years, the median time from primary diagnosis to cerebral metastases was 3.1 years (range, 0-41 years). Of these, 646 (94%) died due to melanoma. Survival ranged between 0 to 17.2 years (median, 4.1 years) from the time of diagnosis of cerebral metastases. Treatment included surgery and postoperative radiotherapy in 158 patients, surgery alone in 47 patients, radiotherapy alone in 236 patients, and supportive care alone in 210 patients; median survival of the treatment groups was 8.9 months, 8.7 months, 3.4 months, and 2.1 months, respectively. Univariate analyses revealed that patients who underwent surgery with or without radiotherapy had significantly longer survival compared with those treated with supportive care or radiotherapy alone ($P < .001$). Patients who receive radiotherapy alone had significantly longer survival than those treated with supportive care alone ($P < .001$). Multivariate analyses showed that treatment received (surgical treatment; $P < .0001$) and the presence of concurrent metastases (no concurrent extracerebral metastases; $P < .0001$) were the most important determinants of survival; other factors were younger age ($P = .007$) and longer disease-free interval ($P = .036$).

Conclusion.—Appropriately selected patients with melanoma may benefit from aggressive treatment for intracerebral metastases.

▶ Brain metastasis from melanoma is not rare and may occur in up to 10% of patients. The overall prognosis is quite poor, as demonstrated in this study in which the survival rate was 6% and the median survival from the time the brain lesion was detected was 4 months. Improved survival was seen in younger patients and in those with no other evidence of metastases. Patients treated with surgery or surgery plus radiation did better than those treated by radiation alone or those who received only palliative therapy. The results are not entirely surprising as patients considered to be surgical candidates would be more likely to have a single cerebral metastasis and less likely to have extracerebral metastases. Patients undergoing surgery with or without radiation therapy had a median survival of 8.9 and 8.7 months, respectively.

P. G. Lang, Jr, MD

18 Lymphoproliferative Disorders

Lymphomatoid Papulosis in Children: A Retrospective Cohort Study of 35 Cases

Nijsten T, Curiel-Lewandrowski C, Kadin ME (Harvard Med School, Boston)

Arch Dermatol 140:306-312, 2004   18–1

Introduction.—Lymphomatoid papulosis (LyP) is a rare skin disease that can precede the development of malignant lymphoma in adult patients. Although LyP affects individuals at any age, only a few cases have been described in children. Thirty-five patients with childhood-onset LyP were evaluated for genetic and environmental risk factors, clinical characteristics, and the association between childhood onset of the disease and subsequent malignancies.

Methods.—Patients were identified through a retrospective registry established at Beth Israel Medical Center, Boston. Thirty-five of 48 patients were contacted in the spring of 2002. Participants were questioned about their personal and familial medical history, disease characteristics, treatment, and response to therapy.

Results.—The median age of the group at onset of LyP was 8.0 years, and the median age at the interview was 16.0 years. All patients but 1 (of Asian ancestry) were white; 19 were male, and 16 were female. The onset of LyP was at an earlier age in boys than in girls (median, 5.50 for boys vs 12.0 years for girls). During the follow-up period, a non-Hodgkin's lymphoma (NHL) developed in 3 patients (9%). Thus, the relative risk for NHL in patients with childhood-onset LyP was 226.2 (compared with the general population 44 years or younger in the United States). No other cancers occurred in the group. Papular lesions developed at some point in almost all patients, and about half reported at least 1 episode with 50 or more lesions. No relationship was noted between the number of lesions and the development of NHL. More than two thirds of patients had atopic dermatitis, seasonal allergies, and/or asthma at the time of the interview. Topical corticosteroids and antibiotics, the most common treatments, were less effective than phototherapy.

Conclusion.—The incidence of NHL in patients with childhood-onset LyP was 200 times more than expected. None of the patients in this series have been seriously ill or died of extracutaneous disease. No environmental or infectious precipitating factors for LyP in children were identified, and no clinical features predicted the development of malignancy.

▶ This study showed that the clinical presentation and course of LyP in children is similar to that in adults. Nine percent of 35 patients in this series developed NHL, and all apparently responded well to treatment. No clinical features were identified that could predict an increased risk of the malignancy. Children who develop LyP should be monitored throughout their life for the possible development of a lymphoproliferative disorder.

S. Raimer, MD

Outcome in 34 Patients With Juvenile-Onset Mycosis Fungoides: A Clinical, Immunophenotypic, and Molecular Study
Wain EM, Orchard GE, Whittaker SJ, et al (St Thomas' Hosp, London)
Cancer 98:2282-2290, 2003   18–2

Introduction.—The onset of mycosis fungoides (MF) before adulthood is rare, and few studies have examined the clinicopathologic, immunophenotypic, and prognostic factors of juvenile-onset MF. Thirty-four patients with MF, all of whom were diagnosed or showed signs of disease before age 16 years, were retrospectively reviewed for disease characteristics and outcome.

Methods.—Patients were identified through clinical and histologic databases of the study institution. Three authors reviewed all histology and immunohistochemistry slides and reached a consensus. T-cell receptor gene analysis was performed with skin biopsy samples and blood samples.

Results.—Cases of juvenile-onset MF accounted for approximately 4% of MF cases registered at the study center. Twenty-four (71%) of 37 patients were male, and 19 (56%) had been diagnosed by skin biopsy during childhood. The median age at onset of symptoms was 10 years; definitive diagnosis of MF was made at a median of 5 years after onset of symptoms. All patients had cutaneous patch or plaque-stage disease at diagnosis but no evidence of systemic disease. Stage 1A disease was present in 17 (50%) cases, stage 1B in 16 (47%), and stage IIA in 1. Six patients had associated lymphomatoid papulosis. A cytotoxic phenotype was noted in 38% of patients with juvenile-onset MF, including 71% of those with hypopigmented lesions. Twenty-eight patients had diagnostic histology, and 6 had compatible histology and a T-cell receptor clone in lesional skin. Treatments included emollients and topical steroids, psoralen and ultraviolet A irradiation, and local radiotherapy. During a median follow-up period of 6 years, 28 patients had no disease progression, but tumors developed in 2 patients and erythroderma in 3. One patient with tumors and lymph node involvement has been in remission after receiving an autologous peripheral blood stem cell transplant. The other patient with tumors died at age 53 years from a metastatic cutaneous Merkel cell carcinoma, possibly related to previous phototherapy or radiotherapy. One patient who did not respond to therapy died of MF at age 21 years.

Conclusion.—Overall disease-specific survival rates for juvenile-onset MF were 95% at 5 years and 93% at 10 years. Widespread cutaneous disease was associated with a less favorable outcome.

▶ This is the largest series reported to date of patients who developed MF before the age of 16 years. The most common clinical features were hypopigmented lesions (24%) and poikiloderma (26%); 18% of patients had associated lymphomatoid papulosis. Prognosis was good in this series, with disease-specific survival being 95% at 5 years and 93% at 10 years. Because widespread disease has a less favorable outcome, aggressive therapy with its resultant sequelae might be reserved for such patients or for those exhibiting uncomfortable symptoms or progression of disease.

S. Raimer, MD

Prognostic Value of Blood Eosinophilia in Primary Cutaneous T-Cell Lymphomas
Tancrède-Bohin E, Ionescu MA, de La Salmonière P, et al (Hôpital Saint-Louis, Paris)
Arch Dermatol 140:1057-1061, 2004   18–3

Background.—Primary cutaneous T-cell lymphomas include a variety of entities distinguished by clinical, histologic, and immunophenotypic features. These lymphomas are characterized by a proliferation of T lymphocytes in the skin. The prognostic value of initial characteristics, including blood eosinophilia, in patients with primary cutaneous T-cell lymphoma was investigated.

Methods.—One hundred four patients seen in 2 dermatology departments composed the retrospective cohort. Patients received their diagnoses between 1982 and 1998. The median follow-up period was 43 months. Sixty-nine patients had mycosis fungoides; 13, Sezary syndrome; and 22, nonepidermotropic cutaneous lymphoma. Variables recorded were age, sex, diagnosis by the European Organization for Research and Treatment of Cancer (EORTC) classification, type of skin involvement at diagnosis, initial absolute eosinophil count, lactate dehydrogenase value, date of disease progression, and cause and date of death or last contact date.

Findings.—The estimated rate of disease progression for 3 years was 19.5%, and of disease-specific death, it was 9.9%. In a univariate analysis, initial variables for disease progression with significant prognostic value were diagnosis according to EORTC classification, with a hazard ratio (HR) of 2.77; type of skin involvement, with an HR of 2.7; increased blood absolute eosinophil count, with an HR of 7.33; and increased serum level of lactate dehydrogenase, with an HR of 3.72.

Significant prognostic indicators for disease-specific death were diagnosis according to the EORTC classification (HR, 6.62) and increased blood absolute eosinophil count (HR, 10.57). Multivariate analysis indicated that only blood eosinophilia correlated with disease progression and disease-specific death.

Conclusion.—Blood eosinophilia at baseline was a prognostic indicator of poor outcome in patients with primary cutaneous T-cell lymphoma. Prospective, large-scale studies are needed to further investigate this result.

▶ The authors demonstrate that blood eosinophilia at baseline is a prognostic factor in patients with primary cutaneous T-cell lymphoma. This eosinophilia presumably results from secretion of cytokines from neoplastic type 2 T-helper (TH2) cells. Thus, the eosinophilia may be a sign that the TH2 response has overtaken the presumably antitumoral TH1 response. A prospective study that examines changes in blood eosinophilia with either successful treatment or disease progression would be interesting.

B. H. Thiers, MD

Topical Photodynamic Therapy for Patients With Therapy-Resistant Lesions of Cutaneous T-Cell Lymphoma
Coors EA, von den Driesch P (Univ of Erlangen-Nuremberg, Germany; Univ of Hamburg, Germany)
J Am Acad Dermatol 50:363-367, 2004   18–4

Background.—Despite multiple treatments including psoralen–ultraviolet A (PUVA), interferon-α, extracorporeal photopheresis, systemic chemotherapy, and total body electron beam irradiation, some patients with cutaneous T-cell lymphoma (CTCL) continue to have lesions. Photodynamic therapy (PDT) after topical application of a photosensitizing drug was used to treat 4 patients with recalcitrant CTCL. Results were described.

Case Report.—Man, 41, had disseminated large-cell anaplastic CD30+ T-cell lymphoma. Twelve months of PUVA and interferon-α2a therapy resulted in a complete response. But 3 years later, despite maintenance therapy with interferon-α, 2 new CD30+ lesions developed on the scalp. The patient refused PUVA, and thus PDT with 5-aminolevulinic acid (5-ALA) was instituted. The lesions were covered with a 20% 5-ALA ointment and protected from light for 6 hours. The area was then exposed to visible light from a PDT projector at 160 mW/cm² for 15 minutes, for a dosage of 144 J/cm².

The patient underwent another session of PDT within 4 weeks. There were no severe topical adverse events, and the patient did not require analgesia. Six weeks later, both tumors had completely resolved (Fig 2). The patient has remained in complete remission for 15 months with maintenance interferon-α2a therapy. The other 3 patients described (2 men and 1 woman, 54-65 years of age), 1 of whom had lesions on the forehead and eyelid, also had a complete response after 1 to 7 sessions with PDT using topical 5-ALA.

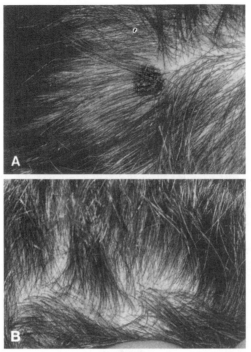

FIGURE 2.—Recidive lesion of CD30+ lymphoma on scalp before (**A**) and after (**B**) 2 treatments with photodynamic therapy. (Reprinted by permission of the publisher from Coors EA, von den Driesch P. Topical photodynamic therapy for patients with therapy-resistant lesions of cutaneous T-cell lymphoma. *J Am Acad Dermatol* 50:363-367, 2004. Copyright 2004 by Elsevier.)

Conclusion.—Application of a photosensitizer followed by PDT may be an option for patients with CTCL that does not respond to conventional treatment.

▶ PDT, when used for conditions as diverse as acne or CTCL, appears to be a useful modality for individual lesions. However, it cannot be expected to have any preventive effect against the development of new lesions. Thus, as the authors recommend, PDT can be used for patients with CTCL who have received more conventional approaches, such as topical mechlorethamine or phototherapy, but have residual treatment-resistant areas. An excellent review of the pathogenesis of CTCL has recently been published.[1]

B. H. Thiers, MD

Reference

1. Girardi M, Heald P, Wilson LD: The pathogenesis of mycosis fungoides. *N Engl J Med* 350:1978-1988, 2004.

Comparison of Selective Retinoic Acid Receptor– and Retinoic X Receptor–Mediated Efficacy, Tolerance, and Survival in Cutaneous T-Cell Lymphoma

Querfeld C, Rosen ST, Guitart J, et al (Northwestern Univ, Chicago)

J Am Acad Dermatol 51:25-32, 2004   18–5

Introduction.—The most common types of primary cutaneous T-cell lymphoma (CTCL), mycosis fungoides (MF) and Sézary syndrome, have responded in a limited manner to treatment with retinoids. The biologic effects of these compounds are triggered through specific receptor families, retinoic acid receptor (RAR) and retinoic X receptor (RXR). Patients with MF/SS who experienced disease relapse were studied retrospectively to compare the effects of the retinoic acid receptor (RAR) agonist, ATRA, and the retinoic X receptor (RXR) agonist, bexarotene.

Methods.—Thirty-three patients received ATRA between 1991 and 1999, and 19 patients received bexarotene between 2000 and 2003. Those given ATRA were participants in an institutional phase II trial in which treatment in responding patients was not permitted for more than 2 years. Patients were evaluated at baseline, weekly for the first 4 weeks, then monthly. The 2 groups were compared for response rates and duration, adverse effects, outcome, and survival.

Results.—The median follow-up time was 43 months for the ATRA group and 13.8 months for the bexarotene group. The 2 groups were similar in median age, number of patients with tumor stages IB to IVB, and response categories. In addition, ATRA and bexarotene groups did not differ statistically in response rates (12% vs 21%), response duration (20.5 vs 7.3 months), event-free survival time (4 vs 5 months), or median survival when corrected for length of follow-up. Fifteen patients in the ATRA cohort and 6 in the bexarotene-treated group have died of MF. Both treatments were tolerated well, but mild and moderate side effects were common. Hypertriglyceridemia developed in 15 patients treated with ATRA; hypothyroidism developed in 15 treated with bexarotene.

Conclusion.—No significant differences were observed in the modest response rates and survival times in patients with relapsed CTCL treated with ATRA, the RAR-selective retinoid, and bexarotene, the RXR-selective retinoid. Bexarotene was symptomatically better tolerated, but side effects of both therapies could be managed with medications. The optimal role of these retinoids may be as part of a combination treatment strategy.

▶ Much has been made of retinoic acid receptor-specificity in determining the clinical efficacy and toxicity of the various marketed retinoids. For example, it has been claimed that the RXR-specific retinoid, bexarotene, is especially well suited for the treatment of cutaneous T-cell lymphoma. In this study, Querfeld and colleagues found only modest objective responses with bexarotene and the RAR agonist, ATRA. They appropriately suggest that the best use for these agents in the treatment of cutaneous T-cell lymphoma may be in combination with other biologic immune response modifiers, phototherapy, or cytotoxic chemotherapy.[1]

B. H. Thiers, MD

Reference

1. Gorgun G, Foss F: Immunomodulatory effects of RXR rexinoids: Modulation of high-affinity IL-2R expression enhances susceptibility to denileukin diftitox. *Blood* 100:1399-1403, 2002.

Cutaneous T-Cell Lymphoma Treatment Using Bexarotene and PUVA: A Case Series
Singh F, Lebwohl MG (Mount Sinai School of Medicine, New York)
J Am Acad Dermatol 51:570-573, 2004   18–6

Background.—The most common form of cutaneous T-cell lymphoma (CTCL) is mycosis fungoides. This condition is often seen as chronic eczematous or psoriasiform patches and plaques that may resist a variety of single-agent treatments. The efficacy of combination therapy with bexarotene and psoralen plus ultraviolet A (PUVA) was determined in patients with CTCL recurring after monotherapy.

Methods and Outcomes.—The medical charts of 8 patients with CTCL were analyzed retrospectively. The patients had stage Ia to IIb disease that had not responded to a variety of single agents, including electron beam irradiation, interferon, PUVA, and topical steroids. Low-dose oral bexarotene and PUVA combination therapy was administered to all patients. All 8 patients showed an initial response to combination treatment. Five patients had a complete remission. The most common adverse event was pruritus.

Conclusion.—These anecdotal findings suggest that combination therapy with bexarotene and PUVA may be useful for patients with CTCL refractory to monotherapy. Prospective studies are needed to better define the role of this treatment approach for patients with refractory CTCL.

▶ The authors present anecdotal evidence to suggest that low-dose oral bexarotene in combination with PUVA may be effective in treating single-agent therapy–resistant CTCL. Whether its efficacy extends beyond combinations of acitretin with either ultraviolet A or ultraviolet B remains to be determined.

B. H. Thiers, MD

Pigmentary Characteristics, Sun Sensitivity and Non-Hodgkin Lymphoma

Hughes AM, Armstrong BK, Vajdic CM, et al (Univ of Sydney, Australia; Univ of New South Wales, Sydney; St Vincent's Hosp, Sydney; et al)
Int J Cancer 110:429-434, 2004   18–7

Introduction.—A study published in 1992 was the first to suggest a relationship between exposure to solar ultraviolet radiation (UVR) and a worldwide rising trend in the incidence of non-Hodgkin lymphoma (NHL). Evidence for such a relationship includes the immunosuppressive effects of UVR, a previously documented association between sun exposure and skin cancer, and the increased frequency of NHL among individuals with nonpigmented skin. A population-based case-control study conducted in Australia examined pigmentary characteristics, sun sensitivity, and other possible risk factors for NHL.

Methods.—Cases were drawn from patients notified to the New South Wales Central Cancer Registry with newly diagnosed NHL between January 1, 2000, and August 31, 2001. Eligible cases were aged 20 to 74 and had no history of transplantation or HIV infection. Pathology reports of cases were reviewed to confirm the diagnosis of NHL. Controls were randomly selected from electoral rolls in areas of the patients' residency and approximately matched the expected distribution of cases with respect to age and gender. Cases and controls completed a mailed questionnaire and a telephone interview designed to obtain data on ethnicity, skin color and tanning ability, smoking habit, skin cancer history, and socioeconomic status.

Results.—The risk of NHL was increased among individuals with hazel eyes (odds ratio [OR], 1.48), very fair skin (OR, 1.44), and poor ability to tan (OR, 1.70). Mild facial freckling as a child reduced the risk of NHL (OR, 0.77) relative to no or moderate to severe freckling. There was a slight, nonsignificant increase among individuals with a history of treatment for skin cancer, but smokers were not at increased risk of NHL. Previous radiation therapy and chemotherapy were associated with 1.5- to 2-fold increases in risk, although confidence intervals were wide.

Conclusion.—The hypothesis that sun sensitivity or sun exposure can increase the risk of NHL received only weak support in this study.

▶ The authors present rather tenuous data to suggest that sun sensitivity or sun exposure may increase the risk of NHL. Direct measurements of sun exposure would provide more convincing data.

B. H. Thiers, MD

Lymphoma-Specific Genetic Aberrations in Microvascular Endothelial Cells in B-Cell Lymphomas

Streubel B, Chott A, Huber D, et al (Med Univ of Vienna)
N Engl J Med 351:250-259, 2004   18–8

Background.—Most tumor growth relies on new blood vessel formation. Unlike genetically unstable tumor cells, endothelial cells of tumor vessels are thought to be normal diploid cells that do not mutate. However, this belief is contradicted by recent observations suggesting a genetic relationship between the lymphoma cells and the microvascular endothelial cells. B-cell lymphomas carrying specific chromosomal translocations were examined.

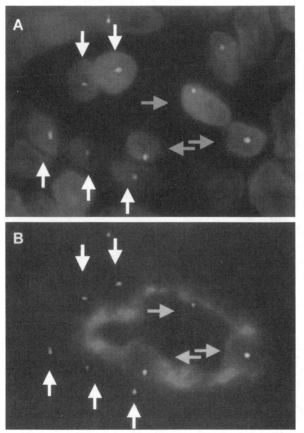

FIGURE 1.—Loss of the Y chromosome in lymphoma cells and tumor endothelial cells from a patient with posttransplantation lymphoma. In **Panel A,** fluorescence in situ hybridization analysis with probes for the centromeres of the X an Y chromosomes shows a single green signal for the X chromosome in the nuclei of both the tumor cells (*white arrows*) and the endothelial cells (*yellow arrows*). **Panel B** shows endothelial cells stained with CD31 antibody. (Reprinted by permission of *The New England Journal of Medicine* Streubel B, Chott A, Huber D, et al: Lymphoma-specific genetic aberrations in microvascular endothelial cells in B-cell lymphomas. *N Engl J Med* 351:250-259, 2004. Copyright 2004, Massachusetts Medical Society. All rights reserved.)

Methods and Findings.—In 27 B-cell lymphomas, endothelial cells were examined for cytogenetic changes known to be present in lymphoma cells. A combined immunohistochemical and fluorescence in situ hybridization assay was used. Lymphoma-specific chromosomal translocations were found in 15% to 85% (median, 37%) of microvascular endothelial cells in the B-cell lymphomas (Fig 1). Lymphoma and endothelial cells shared numerical chromosomal aberrations.

Conclusions.—A varying proportion of microvascular endothelial cells in lymphomas were demonstrated to have lymphoma-specific genetic aberrations. This suggests a close relationship between the 2 cell types.

▶ The authors report that microvascular endothelial cells within B-cell lymphomas express markers of the underlying neoplasm. Streubel et al found that cells lining the microvasculature possessed both endothelial-cell characteristics and the genetic aberrations of the surrounding B-cell lymphoma. The possible explanations underlying these findings were discussed in an editorial[1] that accompanied this article.

B. H. Thiers, MD

Reference

1. Fidler IJ, Ellis LM: Neoplastic angiogenesis: Not all blood vessels are created equal. *N Engl J Med* 351:215-216, 2004.

19 Thromboembolism and Other Lower Extremity Disorders

Combined Use of Rapid D-Dimer Testing and Estimation of Clinical Probability in the Diagnosis of Deep Vein Thrombosis: Systematic Review
Fancher TL, White RH, Kravitz RL (Univ of California at Davis, Sacramento; Center for Health Services Research in Primary Care, Sacramento, Calif)
BMJ 329:821-825, 2004   19–1

Background.—Two clinical probability tools are commonly used to determine the probability of venous thrombosis. The Wells tool uses a structured assessment of explicit historical and physical examination criteria (see Box) to stratify patients into different risk levels. The Perrier tool also stratifies patients, using semi-structured, implicit criteria. Both classify patients as having low, medium, or high risk.

The assessment of clinical probability can be used in combination with rapid D-dimer testing. A systematic review was done to evaluate the use of rapid D-dimer testing in conjunction with clinical probability assessment.

Box.—Wells Clinical Probability Tool

Wells explicit assessment
- Active cancer
- Paralysis, paresis or recent plaster, or immobilisation of lower limb
- Recently bedridden for more than three days or major surgery in the past four weeks or more
- Localised tenderness
- Entire leg swollen
- Calf swelling >3 cm compared with asymptomatic leg
- Pitting oedema
- Collateral superficial veins
- Alternative diagnosis as likely or greater than deep vein thrombosis

Each positive response is 1 point, except if an alternative diagnosis is as likely as or greater than DVT, where 2 points are deducted. 0 or fewer points: low probability; 1-2 points: moderate probability; 3 or more points: high probability.

(Courtesy of Fancher TL, White RH, Kravitz RL: Combined use of rapid D-dimer testing and estimation of clinical probability in the diagnosis of deep vein thrombosis: Systematic review. *BMJ* 329:821-825, 2004. With permission from the BMJ Publishing Group.)

Methods.—Twelve studies involving more than 5000 patients were identified for the review. All used rapid D-dimer testing and explicit criteria to classify consecutive outpatients as at low, intermediate, or high clinical probability of deep vein thrombosis (DVT) of the lower extremity. Two examiners independently abstracted data from the studies.

Findings.—With the less-sensitive SimpliRED D-dimer assay, the 3-month incidence of venous thromboembolism was 0.5% in the group with a low clinical probability of DVT and normal D-dimer levels. With a highly sensitive D-dimer assay, the 3-month incidence of venous thromboembolism was 0.4% in outpatients with low or moderate clinical probability of DVT and normal D-dimer results.

Conclusion.—A low clinical probability for DVT combined with a normal SimpliRED test result can safely exclude the diagnosis of acute venous thrombosis. Normal findings on a highly sensitive D-dimer test excludes DVT in patients categorized as having a low or moderate clinical probability of DVT.

Usefulness of Clinical Prediction Rules for the Diagnosis of Venous Thromboembolism: A Systematic Review

Tamariz LJ, Eng J, Segal JB, et al (Johns Hopkins Univ, Baltimore, Md)
Am J Med 117:676-684, 2004   19-2

Background.—Clinicians face important medical decisions when assessing patients with possible venous thromboembolism. The diagnostic accuracy of clinical prediction rules for deep vein thrombosis (DVT) and pulmonary embolism (PE) was investigated.

Methods.—In a search of the English language literature, 23 studies meeting eligibility were identified. All validated a clinical prediction rule prospectively against a reference standard and determined likelihood ratios, predictive values, and area under the receiver operating characteristic (ROC) curve for each rule.

Findings.—Seventeen studies assessed prediction rules for diagnosing DVT, and 6 assessed rules of PE. The most common DVT prediction rule evaluated was the Wells rule. This rule had median positive likelihood ratios of 6.62 for patients with a high pretest probability, 1 for a moderate pretest probability, and 0.22 for a low pretest probability. Area under the ROC curve was a median 0.82. Adding the D-dimer test to the prediction rule raised this median to 0.90.

The Wells prediction rule was also most often assessed for PE. Its median positive likelihood ratio was 6.75 for patients with high pretest probability, 1.82 for those with moderate pretest probability, and 0.13 for those with low pretest probability. The Wells prediction rule for PE yielded a median area under the ROC curve of 0.82.

Conclusion.—This literature review indicates that the Wells prediction rule is useful for identifying patients at low risk of a venous thromboembolism diagnosis. The overall performance of the prediction rule can be increased by adding a rapid latex D-dimer assay.

▶ Most ambulatory patients who present with symptoms suggesting DVT do not actually have the disease. Thus, ultrasound (US) testing is probably an overused modality in this patient population. Previous evidence has suggested that D-dimer testing and clinical probability assessment can safely reduce the need for US testing. Fancher et al (Abstract 19–1) show that a normal SimpliRED D-dimer test in patients at low risk can safely rule out DVT, and that a normal highly sensitive D-dimer test can safely rule out DVT in patients at low or moderate risk. Costly testing may be reduced even further by new stratification models.

B. H. Thiers, MD

D-Dimer for the Exclusion of Acute Venous Thrombosis and Pulmonary Embolism: A Systematic Review
Stein PD, Hull RD, Patel KC, et al (Saint Joseph Mercy-Oakland, Pontiac, Mich; Wayne State Univ, Detroit; Univ of Calgary, Alberta, Canada; et al)
Ann Intern Med 140:589-602, 2004   19–3

Background.—Many different D-dimer assays are available for diagnosing deep venous thrombosis (DVT) and pulmonary embolism (PE). The sensitivity, specificity, and likelihood ratios of these different D-dimer assays were reviewed.

Methods.—The authors searched the EMBASE and PubMed databases and relevant reference lists to identify trials in which a D-dimer assay was prospectively used to screen patients with suspected DVT or PE. At least 2 authors reviewed each study to determine its methodologic quality. Only high-quality studies were included in the primary analyses, whereas other, weaker studies were included in sensitivity analyses. The sensitivity, specificity, and negative and positive likelihood ratios for each specific D-dimer assay were compared.

Results.—The authors identified 108 studies meeting most of the inclusion criteria, including 31 studies deemed to be of high quality. For excluding DVT, sensitivity was highest with the enzyme-linked immunosorbent assay (ELISA) (96%) and quantitative rapid ELISA (96%). These 2 tests also had the best negative likelihood ratios (12% and 9%, respectively). Similarly, for excluding PE, ELISA and quantitative rapid ELISA had the best sensitivity (95% in both tests) and the best negative likelihood ratios (13% in both tests). Positive likelihood values with both tests were 1.5 to 1.77. Inclusion of the other, weaker studies did not substantially affect these results.

Conclusion.—The sensitivity of ELISA and quantitative rapid ELISA are sufficiently high and their negative likelihood ratios sufficiently low to allow the exclusion of DVT and PE with a high degree of certainty. These findings suggest that a negative result on quantitative rapid ELISA is as accurate in ruling out DVT and PE as a normal lung scan or a negative duplex ultrasonogram.

▶ Multiple D-dimer assays are available to aid in the exclusion of DVT and PE. Which test is superior is uncertain. Stein et al present data to suggest that negative ELISA results are strong evidence against the presence of either of these 2 conditions. Nevertheless, a patient with a negative D-dimer test who has findings consistent with DVT warrants further evaluation.[1]

B. H. Thiers, MD

Reference

1. Bates SM, Kearon C, Crowther M, et al: A diagnostic strategy involving a quantitative D-dimer assay reliably excludes deep venous thrombosis. *Ann Intern Med* 138:787-794, 2003.

Deep Vein Thrombosis and Pulmonary Embolism in Two Cohorts: The Longitudinal Investigation of Thromboembolism Etiology

Cushman M, Tsai AW, White RH, et al (Univ of Vermont, Burlington; Univ of Minnesota, Minneapolis; Univ of Washington, Seattle; et al)
Am J Med 117:19-25, 2004   19–4

Purpose.—To determine the incidence of deep vein thrombosis and pulmonary embolism in two cohorts representing regions of the United States.

Methods.—The sample comprised 21,680 participants of the Atherosclerosis Risk in Communities study and the Cardiovascular Health Study. Subjects were aged ≥45 years, resided in six communities, and were followed for 7.6 years. All hospitalizations were identified and thromboses were validated by chart review.

Results.—The age-standardized incidence of first-time venous thromboembolism was 1.92 per 1000 person-years. Rates were higher in men than women, and increased with age in both sexes. There was no antecedent trauma, surgery, immobilization, or diagnosis of cancer for 48% (175/366) of events. The 28-day case-fatality rate was 11% (29/265) after a first venous thromboembolism and 25% (17/67) for cancer-associated thrombosis. The recurrence rate 2 years after a first venous thromboembolism was 7.7% per year (95% confidence interval [CI]: 4.5% to 10.9% per year). Cancer was the only factor independently associated with 28-day fatality (relative risk [RR] = 5.2; 95% CI: 1.4 to 19.9) or recurrent thrombosis (RR = 9.2; 95% CI: 2.0 to 41.7).

Conclusion.—The incidence of venous thromboembolism in this cohort of middle- and older-aged subjects was similar to that observed in more geographically homogeneous samples. Half of cases were idiopathic. Short-term mortality and 2-year recurrence rates were appreciable, especially among subjects with cancer. Based on this study we estimate that 187,000 cases of first-time venous thromboembolism are diagnosed yearly in the United States among those aged 45 years or older.

▶ The authors demonstrate that approximately half of all cases of venous thromboembolism are idiopathic, with appreciable short-term mortality and 2-year recurrence rates, especially among patients with cancer. More study is required to define optimal prevention and management strategies for patients with a high risk of first and recurrent events.

B. H. Thiers, MD

The Risk of Recurrent Venous Thromboembolism in Men and Women
Kyrle PA, Minar E, Bialonczyk C, et al (Univ of Vienna; Wilhelminenspital, Vienna; Hanusch Krankenhaus, Vienna)
N Engl J Med 350:2558-2563, 2004   19–5

Background.—Whether a patient's sex is associated with the risk of recurrent venous thromboembolism is unknown.

Methods.—We studied 826 patients for an average of 36 months after a first episode of spontaneous venous thromboembolism and the withdrawal of oral anticoagulants. We excluded pregnant patients and patients with a deficiency of antithrombin, protein C, or protein S; the lupus anticoagulant; cancer; or a requirement for potentially long-term antithrombotic treatment. The end point was objective evidence of a recurrence of symptomatic venous thromboembolism.

Results.—Venous thromboembolism recurred in 74 of the 373 men, as compared with 28 of the 453 women (20 percent vs. 6 percent; relative risk of recurrence, 3.6; 95 percent confidence interval, 2.3 to 5.5; $P < 0.001$). The risk remained unchanged after adjustment for age, the duration of anticoagulation, and the presence or absence of a first symptomatic pulmonary embolism, factor V Leiden, factor II G20210A, or an elevated level of factor VIII or IX. At five years, the likelihood of recurrence was 30.7 percent among men, as compared with 8.5 percent among women ($P < 0.001$). The relative risk of recurrence was similar among women who had had their first thrombosis during oral-contraceptive use or hormone-replacement therapy and women in the same age group in whom the first event was idiopathic.

Conclusions.—The risk of recurrent venous thromboembolism is higher among men than women.

▶ Although the findings need to be confirmed, Kyrle et al present data to suggest that the risk of recurrent venous thromboembolism is higher among men than women. Future studies may examine the risks and benefits of prolonged anticoagulation in specific subgroups of patients with this disorder.[1]

B. H. Thiers, MD

Reference

1. Elliott CG, Rubin LJ: Mars or Venus: Is sex a risk factor for recurrent venous thromboembolism? *N Engl J Med* 350:2614-2616, 2004.

Elevated Plasma Factor VIII and D-Dimer Levels as Predictors of Poor Outcomes of Thrombosis in Children

Goldenberg NA, for the Mountain States Regional Thrombophilia Group (Univ of Colorado, Denver; Mountain States Regional Hemophilia and Thrombosis Ctr, Aurora, Colo)
N Engl J Med 351:1081-1088, 2004   19–6

Background.—Elevated levels of plasma factor VIII and D-dimer predict recurrent venous thromboembolism in adults. We sought to determine whether an elevation of factor VIII, D-dimer, or both at diagnosis and persistence of the laboratory abnormality after three to six months of anticoagulant therapy correlate with poor outcomes of thrombosis in children.

Methods.—We evaluated levels of factor VIII and D-dimer and additional components of an extensive laboratory thrombophilia (i.e., hypercoagulability) panel at the time of diagnosis in 144 children with a radiologically confirmed acute thrombotic event. All patients were treated initially with heparin and then with either warfarin or low-molecular-weight heparin for at least three to six months, according to the current standard of care. Patients were examined at follow-up visits 3, 6, and 12 months after diagnosis and then annually, at which times testing was repeated in children with previously abnormal factor VIII and D-dimer test results and a uniform evaluation for the post-thrombotic syndrome was performed.

Results.—Among 82 children for whom complete data were available regarding laboratory test results at diagnosis and thrombotic outcomes during follow-up, 67 percent had factor VIII levels above the cutoff value of 150 IU per deciliter, D-dimer levels above 500 ng per milliliter, or both at diagnosis, and at least one of the two laboratory values was persistently elevated in 43 percent of the 75 patients in whom testing was performed after three to six months of anticoagulant therapy. Fifty-one percent of the 82 patients had a poor outcome (i.e., a lack of thrombus resolution, recurrent thrombosis, or the post-thrombotic syndrome) during a median follow-up of 12 months (range, 3 months to 5 years). Elevated levels of factor VIII, D-dimer, or both at diagnosis were highly predictive of a poor outcome (odds ratio, 6.1; $P = 0.008$), as was the persistence of at least one laboratory abnormality at three to six months (odds ratio, 4.7; $P = 0.002$). The combination of a factor VIII level above 150 IU per deciliter and a D-dimer level above 500 ng per milliliter at diagnosis was 91 percent specific for a poor outcome, and after three to six months of standard anticoagulation, the combination was 88 percent specific.

Conclusions.—Elevated levels of plasma factor VIII, D-dimer, or both at diagnosis and a persistent elevation of at least one of these factors after standard-duration anticoagulant therapy predict a poor outcome in children with thrombosis.

▶ Lower concentrations of physiologic inhibitors of the coagulation system, along with more limited fibrinolytic capacity, are thought to account for the somewhat increased incidence of symptomatic venous and arterial thrombosis in neonates compared with older children. After the first year of life, the incidence of such vascular accidents decreases substantially, with a second peak during puberty and adolescence.[1] Little data document long-term outcomes in children with venous or arterial thrombosis. Goldenberg et al found that persistently elevated concentrations of factor VIII, D-dimer, or both, after a standard antithrombotic treatment regimen lasting for 3 to 6 months, was associated with a poor outcome, manifested as persistence of the thrombosis, occurrence of postthrombotic syndrome, or recurrence of thrombosis. These findings should stimulate further research into strategies to prevent thrombosis-related complications in children.

B. H. Thiers, MD

Reference

1. Nowak-Gottl U, and Kosch A: Factor VIII, D-Dimer, and thromboembolism in children. *N Engl J Med* 351:1051-1053, 2004.

Cost-Effectiveness of Testing for Hypercoagulability and Effects on Treatment Strategies in Patients With Deep Vein Thrombosis
Auerbach AD, Sanders GD, Hambleton J (Univ of California, San Francisco; Duke Univ, Durham, NC)
Am J Med 116:816-828, 2004   19–7

Purpose.—Among patients with deep vein thrombosis, hypercoagulable conditions impart a substantial risk of recurrent thrombosis. We sought to determine the cost-effectiveness of testing for these disorders, as well as which tests should be selected and how results should be used.

Methods.—Using a Markov state-transition model, strategies of testing or not testing for a hypercoagulable state followed by anticoagulation for 6 to 36 months were compared in a hypothetical cohort of patients with apparently idiopathic deep vein thrombosis who were followed for life. Strategies were compared based on lifetime costs, quality-adjusted life-years (QALYs), and marginal cost-effectiveness.

Results.—In the base case, testing followed by 24 months of anticoagulation in patients with a hypercoagulable condition was more cost-effective ($54,820; 23.76 QALYs) than usual care, which comprised 6 months of anticoagulation without testing ($55,260; 23.72 QALYs). All hypercoagulable conditions tested were common enough and associated with a sufficient risk of recurrence to justify inclusion in a test panel. Twenty-four months of initial anticoagulation was preferred (<$50,000/QALY) for most conditions, whereas lifetime anticoagulation was preferred for patients with antiphospholipid antibody syndrome ($2928/QALY) or homozygous factor V Leiden mutation ($3804/QALY). Models using newer evidence on recurrence suggested 18 to 36 months of anticoagulation without testing as the preferred approach.

Conclusion.—Testing for hypercoagulable disorders in patients with idiopathic deep vein thrombosis followed by 2 years of anticoagulation in affected patients is cost-effective. A simpler approach of treating all patients with prolonged anticoagulation without testing is justified if data confirm the persistent risk of recurrent thrombosis.

▶ Although the authors found that testing for hypercoagulable disorders in patients with idiopathic deep vein thrombosis followed by 2 years of anticoagulation is cost effective, a simplified approach of treating all at-risk patients with prolonged anticoagulant therapy (without testing) would be reasonable.

B. H. Thiers, MD

Withholding Anticoagulation After a Negative Result on Duplex Ultrasonography for Suspected Symptomatic Deep Venous Thrombosis
Stevens SM, Elliott CG, Chan KJ, et al (LDS Hosp, Salt Lake City, Utah)
Ann Intern Med 140:985-991, 2004   19–8

Background.—Compression ultrasound (US) is useful for detecting symptomatic proximal deep venous thrombosis (DVT) but not thrombi in the distal veins of the calf. Thus, a second examination is needed 5 to 7 days later to detect any distal clots that have propagated proximally. Comprehensive duplex US can image the deep veins from the inguinal ligament to the level of the malleolus during a single imaging session, but its utility in diagnosing DVT is unknown. This study examined whether comprehensive duplex US can safely and accurately rule out DVT in patients with a suspected initial episode of DVT of the leg.

Methods.—The research subjects were 445 nonpregnant patients with a suspected first episode of symptomatic DVT of the leg. All patients underwent comprehensive duplex US of the entire leg. Patients with positive results were given anticoagulants. Patients with negative results were not given anticoagulants, regardless of their signs or symptoms. Patients were followed for 3 months or more to determine new or progressive signs or symptoms of thromboembolism.

Results.—Of the 445 patients, 61 (13.7%) were shown to have DVT and were treated with anticoagulation; in one third of these cases (19, or 31.1%), DVT was present only in the deep veins of the calf. Among the 384 patients with negative US results, 9 (2.3%) were excluded from further analyses because they were given anticoagulation for reasons other than venous thromboembolism. Among the remaining 375 patients, only 3 (0.8%) had symptomatic DVT during the follow-up period.

Conclusion.—In nonpregnant patients with a suspected first episode of symptomatic DVT of the leg, negative results on comprehensive duplex US can safely rule out DVT and avoid the need for anticoagulation. Compared with simplified compression US, this approach is more convenient (it requires only 1 testing session) and reduces the risk for patients who might skip the second imaging session.

▶ When simplified compression US is performed to detect DVT, repeated testing is necessary 5 to 7 days later to detect proximal propagation from an unvisualized calf vein. In contrast, comprehensive duplex US examines deep veins from the inguinal ligament to the malleolus. In the current study, comprehensive duplex US was performed on consecutive patients with suspected symptomatic first episodes of DVT. Regardless of symptoms or clinical signs, anticoagulation was withheld if results were negative. The overall rate of symptomatic venous thrombosis was 0.8% at a 3-month follow-up. Thus, Stevens et al concluded that, given the low risk for false-negative results on comprehensive duplex US, repeated testing is not needed in the vast majority of patients with suspected first episodes of DVT. In an accompanying editorial, El Kheir and Büller[1] recommended studies to investigate the cost-effectiveness of a combined approach utilizing comprehensive duplex US in conjunction with pretest clinical probability or D-dimer testing, both of which were reviewed extensively in the 2004 YEAR BOOK OF DERMATOLOGY AND DERMATOLOGIC SURGERY.

B. H. Thiers, MD

Reference

1. El Kheir D, Büller H: One-time comprehensive ultrasonography to diagnose deep venous thrombosis: Is that the solution? *Ann Intern Med* 140:1052-1053, 2004.

Below-Knee Elastic Compression Stockings to Prevent the Post-Thrombotic Syndrome: A Randomized, Controlled Trial
Prandoni P, Lensing AWA, Prins MH, et al (Univ Hosp of Padua, Italy; Univ of Amsterdam; Academic Hosp, Maastricht, The Netherlands)
Ann Intern Med 141:249-256, 2004   19–9

Background.—Because only limited evidence suggests that elastic stockings prevent the post-thrombotic syndrome in patients with symptomatic deep venous thrombosis (DVT), these stockings are not widely used.

Objective.—To evaluate the efficacy of compression elastic stockings for prevention of the post-thrombotic syndrome in patients with proximal DVT.

Design.—Randomized, controlled clinical trial.

Setting.—University hospital.

Patients.—180 consecutive patients with a first episode of symptomatic proximal DVT who received conventional anticoagulant treatment.

Interventions.—Before discharge, patients were randomly assigned to wear or not wear below-knee compression elastic stockings (30 to 40 mm Hg at the ankle) for 2 years. Follow-up was performed for up to 5 years.

Measurements.—The presence and severity of the post-thrombotic syndrome were scored by using a standardized scale.

Results.—Post-thrombotic sequelae developed in 44 of 90 controls (severe in 10) and in 23 of 90 patients wearing elastic stockings (severe in 3). All but 1 event developed in the first 2 years. The cumulative incidence of the post-thrombotic syndrome in the control group versus the elastic stockings group was 40.0% (95% CI, 29.9% to 50.1%) versus 21.1% (CI, 12.7% to 29.5%) after 6 months, 46.7% (CI, 36.4% to 57.0%) versus 22.2% (CI, 13.8% to 30.7%) after 1 year, and 49.1% (CI, 38.7% to 59.4%) versus 24.5% (CI, 15.6% to 33.4%) after 2 years. After adjustment for baseline characteristics, the hazard ratio for the post-thrombotic syndrome in the elastic stockings group compared with controls was 0.49 (CI, 0.29 to 0.84; P = 0.011).

Limitations.—This study lacked a double-blind design.

Conclusions.—Post-thrombotic sequelae develop in almost half of patients with proximal DVT. Below-knee compression elastic stockings reduce this rate by approximately 50%.

▶ Although few studies have evaluated the effectiveness of elastic stockings to help prevent the postthrombotic syndrome, many physicians recommend them to their patients. Prandoni et al did, in fact, find that below-knee elastic compression stockings reduced postthrombotic sequelae in patients with proximal DVT. In an accompanying editorial, Ginsberg[1] recommends an initial conservative approach focused on lifestyle alteration, including frequent leg elevation, avoiding prolonged standing or sitting, and use of analgesics. Lightweight stockings (such as support hose) or full-strength stockings (30-40 mm Hg of pressure at the ankle) can be prescribed depending on the degree of associated edema. If the symptoms subside and the patient remains asymptomatic, he believes long-term stocking use can be avoided as long as the patient is carefully monitored for evidence of the postthrombotic syndrome.

B. H. Thiers, MD

Reference

1. Ginsberg JS: Routine stocking therapy after deep venous thrombosis: A clinical dilemma. *Ann Intern Med* 141:314-315, 2004.

Comparison of Surgery and Compression With Compression Alone in Chronic Venous Ulceration (ESCHAR Study): Randomised Controlled Trial

Barwell JR, Davies CE, Deacon J, et al (Cheltenham Gen Hosp, England; Gloucester Royal Hosp, England; Southmead Hosp, Bristol, England)

Lancet 363:1854-1859, 2004   19–10

Background.—Most patients with chronic venous ulceration of the leg respond to leg elevation, multilayer elastic compression bandaging, and supervised exercise. Still, about one fourth of these patients have a recurrence within a year. Saphenous vein ablation does not improve ulcer healing, but it does appear to reduce the incidence of recurrence. Whether compression plus surgery has a greater effect on ulcer healing or recurrence compared with compression alone was investigated.

Methods.—The research subjects were 500 patients (42% men; mean age, 73 years) with ulceration between the knee and malleoli for more than 4 weeks. All had isolated superficial venous reflux alone or mixed superficial and deep reflux (ie, <3 deep segments). Patients were randomly assigned to receive compression alone or compression plus surgery. Compression was delivered via multilayer bandages applied every week until lesions healed, then via class 2 below-knee elastic support stockings. Superficial venous surgery was performed based on the results of color duplex imaging. Patients were followed for 24 weeks to determine wound healing (ie, complete re-epithelialization) and for 12 months to determine recurrence (ie, epithelial breakdown).

Results.—Healing rates at 24 weeks were 65% in both groups. However, 12-month recurrence rates were significantly lower in the compression plus surgery group than in the compression alone group (12% vs 28%); the superior results in the combined treatment group were evident by 6 months. Few adverse events occurred, and most were minor. Adverse events related to surgery were wound infection (5 cases), deep vein thrombosis (1 case), hematoma (1 case), and phlebitis (1 case).

Conclusion.—Superficial venous surgery does not improve venous ulcer healing beyond that provided by multilayer elastic compression bandages. Surgery did, however, more than halve the rate of ulcer recurrence at 12 months. Subgroup analyses suggest surgery could benefit 85% of patients with chronic venous ulcers; thus, all patients should undergo venous duplex imaging to determine whether they are candidates for surgery.

▶ Barwell et al show that 85% of patients with chronic venous ulceration would benefit from surgery and suggest that all affected patients should undergo venous duplex imaging with this in mind. They believe that most patients (except the very elderly) should have long saphenous vein stripping to the knee in addition to a saphenofemoral junction disconnection. The latter procedure is necessary because, over a period of 5 years, recurrent reflux in the remaining long saphenous vein segment occurs in 15% of patients.[1]

The management of venous leg ulcers has recently been reviewed.[2]

B. H. Thiers, MD

Reference

1. Dwerryhouse S, Davies B, Harradine K, et al: Stripping the long saphenous vein in the treatment of reoperation for recurrent varicose veins: Five year results of a randomized trial. *J Vasc Surg* 29:589-592, 1999.
2. Simons DA, Dix FP, McCollum CN: Management of venous leg ulcers. *BMJ* 328:1358-1362, 2004.

Contact Sensitivity in Patients With Leg Ulcerations: A North American Study

Saap L, Fahim S, Arsenault E, et al (Boston Univ; Univ of Ottawa, Ont, Canada)
Arch Dermatol 140:1241-1246, 2004   19–11

Introduction.—Patch test results in patients with chronic leg ulcerations indicate a high incidence of multiple positive allergen sensitivities, particularly when the ulcer is of long duration. Various ointments and wound products, when applied for extended periods on a disrupted skin barrier, can lead to contact dermatitis of the leg and impair healing. A prospective study of patients with present or past leg ulcerations examined the prevalence of allergen sensitivity in North America versus Europe and proposed a standard battery of allergens for patch testing in North American patients.

Methods.—Fifty-four participants were recruited from wound healing centers located in Boston (22 patients) and Ottawa, Canada (32 patients). Excluded were patients receiving an oral prednisone dosage of 20 mg/d or greater or any oral immunosuppressive therapy. Patients completed a detailed questionnaire and underwent a physical examination and patch tests that included the North American Contact Dermatitis Group (NACDG) series and a supplemental leg ulcer series of 52 allergens.

Results.—Thirty-four patients (63%) were sensitive to 1 or more allergens; 6 (11%) had a single positive result, 28 (52%) had more than 1, and 11 (20%) had more than 5 positive results. The most common allergens from the NACDG series were balsam of Peru (30%), bacitracin (24%), and fragrance mix (20%). The most common allergens from the leg ulcer series were wood tar mix (20%) and control gel hydrocolloid (11%). Thirty-nine of 54 patients reported having dermatitis on the affected leg, and 22 (56%) of these patients had positive contact sensitivity to at least 1 allergen. There was a high cross-reactivity between positive allergic reactions to balsam of Peru and wood tar mix. No association was found between ulcer duration and number of allergen contact sensitivities. European studies showed similarly high frequencies of sensitization to balsam of Peru, fragrance mix, and hydrogel with propylene glycol, but different frequencies for many of the tested allergens.

Conclusion.—Because these North American patients with leg ulcers had a high incidence of positive allergen sensitivity, it is important to consider that contact allergy might impede healing. Products containing fragrances, propylene glycol, and other common allergens should be avoided.

▶ The authors show a high incidence of positive patch test results in patients with past and present leg ulcerations, and stress the importance of using a modified leg ulcer series along with standard patch test reagents in evaluating patients with leg ulcers and an associated dermatitis.

B. H. Thiers, MD

Ultrasound-Guided Injection of Polidocanol Microfoam in the Management of Venous Leg Ulcers

Cabrera J, Redondo P, Becerra A, et al (Vascular Surgery Clinic, Granada, Spain; Univ of Navarra, Pamplona, Spain)

Arch Dermatol 140:667-673, 2004   19–12

Introduction.—Venous leg ulceration is a common and severe complication of lower limb venous insufficiency. Compression therapy is associated with a protracted course of healing and many recurrences. Minimally invasive surgery (subfascial endoscopic perforating surgery) can only be performed in a subset of patients with leg ulcers. Several novel approaches to venous ulcers have been introduced, but none has become standard procedure because all are relatively expensive and require further evaluation. Reported is the first series of chronic venous leg ulcers treated with a novel procedure, ultrasound (US)-guided injection of polidocanol microfoam (UIPM). This minimally invasive technique is highly effective and able to achieve the selective and permanent disappearance of the sources and transmission routes of venous hypertension.

Methods.—Medical records, pretreatment and posttreatment color photographs, and echo Doppler examinations were retrospectively examined in 116 consecutive patients with venous leg ulceration. All patients were assessed at 6 months after therapy, 70% were assessed at 2 years, 25% at 3 years, and 14% at 4 or more years after treatment for complete (100%) ulcer healing, time to wound closure, and recurrence. The number of UIPM treatment sessions per patient was between 1 and 17 (mean, 3.6). Complete ulcer healing was defined as full reepithelialization of the wound with absence of drainage, and recurrence was defined as epithelial breakdown in the healed limb.

Results.—At 6-month follow-up, treatment with UIPM attained complete healing in 83% of patients (96/116). The median time to healing was 2.7 months. Seven patients never achieved cure and 1 was lost to follow-up. Ten patients experienced recurrent leg ulcers.

Conclusion.—The use of UIPM is highly effective in achieving stable ulcer healing with minimal invasion, even in elderly patients. Recurrent leg ulcers are easily treated with UIPM. This approach may become first-line treatment in the management of venous leg ulcers.

▶ Venous leg ulcers are thought to be the result of venous hypertension and are often difficult to heal. In this study, the authors used UIPM to sclerose incompetent tributary veins and incompetent perforators, thereby decreasing venous hypertension. Using this methodology, they were able to heal 83% of ulcers. A higher failure rate was seen in patients with long-standing leg ulcers and those with an incompetent deep venous system. The overall recurrence rate for the ulcers was 6.3%; however, the recurrence rate was higher for patients older than 65 years old, those with ulcers for longer than 72 months, those with ulcers larger than 6 cm², and those with deep venous incompetence.

P. G. Lang, Jr, MD

Efficacy of Sclerotherapy in Varicose Veins—A Prospective, Blinded, Placebo-controlled Study
Kahle B, Leng K (Univ of Heidelberg, Germany)
Dermatol Surg 30:723-728, 2004   19–13

Introduction.—Sclerotherapy is widely used in the treatment of varicose veins of the lower limbs. Currently, there are no placebo-controlled randomized trials to prove the efficacy of this technique. The efficacy of injection sclerotherapy for varicose veins for obliteration and hemodynamic improvement was examined with the use of duplex ultrasound (US) in a blinded placebo-controlled investigation.

Methods.—The mean age of 25 patients (18 women, 7 men) with primary varicose veins was 55.5 years. All patients had superficial varicose veins 3 to 6 mm in diameter; the saphenofemoral and saphenopopliteal junctions were competent. Fourteen patients were randomly assigned to treatment with injection sclerotherapy with 2% or 3% polidocanol (Aethoxysklerol) without preservatives and 11 patients received placebo injections (normal saline). External adhesive compression bandages were applied for 2 to 3 days, then knee-length compression stockings were used for 1 week after the procedure. At 1, 4, and 12 weeks after sclerotherapy, duplex US was performed. The quotient of venous flow volume by arterial volume flow was used to determine the venoarterial flow index. Patients and examiners were blinded to treatment assignment.

Results.—Compared with veins treated with normal saline, 76.8% of those treated with polidocanol were completely occluded ($P < .0001$). Eleven of 14 veins in the polidocanol group were completely occluded at 12-week follow-up, compared with none in the placebo group. In the placebo group, all 11 varicose veins were completely compressible at 4- and 12-week follow-up and spontaneous venous blood flow was documented before and within all duplex sonograms at 1, 4, and 12 weeks after treatment. In the polidocanol group, the venoarterial flow index dropped from 1.45 to 1.06 ($P = .05$); in the 11 occluded veins, the venoarterial flow index dropped from 1.5 to 0.98, a level seen in competent veins.

Conclusion.—Injection sclerotherapy with polidocanol is effective in obliterating varicose veins and improving venous hemodynamics.

▶ This study documents that sclerotherapy using polidocanol in conjunction with compression is effective for the obliteration of varicose veins. In patients with competent saphenofemoral and saphenopopliteal junctions, this procedure is associated with a concomitant improvement in venous hemodynamics.

P. G. Lang, Jr, MD

20 Miscellaneous Topics in Dermatologic Surgery and Cutaneous Oncology

Medical Malpractice and Cancer of the Skin
Lydiatt DD (Nebraska Med Ctr, Omaha)
Am J Surg 187:688-694, 2004   20–1

Introduction.—The growing costs of defensive medicine and malpractice premiums have led physicians to play a greater role in preventing litigation. Lawsuits involving cancer of the skin were analyzed with the use of a computerized legal database; a search was made for civil trials in the United States that involved malpractice in patients with a diagnosis of skin cancer.

Methods.—The WESTLAW database searches all federal and state cases from all 50 states. Included in the analysis were 99 cases from 30 states between 1986 and 2001. All cases had information available on the plaintiffs, defendants, medical evidence, verdict outcomes, and indemnity payments.

Results.—Important cancer cell types were represented equally in the suits: basal cell carcinoma, 25%; squamous cell carcinoma, 20%, and malignant melanoma, 24%. Sites of origin of the cancer were known in 78 suits: head and neck, 68%, extremity, 18%; trunk, 14%. The most common allegation was failure to diagnose (54%); of these, 48% alleged a biopsy should have been made and 20% alleged that a misdiagnosis occurred. In verdicts overall, 45% were for the defendant, 34% were for the plaintiff, and 20% of cases had a settlement. The mean plaintiff award was $969,000, which is a figure increased by the 8 awards for more than $1 million. The mean settlement award was $514,210. More and larger awards went to young patients and those with poor outcomes. The most common allegation against dermatologists and physicians in general practice was failure to diagnose. Allegations were highest for misdiagnoses by pathologists and for complications occurring while under care of surgeons. Evidence is lacking that a single uncomplicated trauma can cause skin cancer, but juries were found to have accepted trauma as constituting or contributing to negligence.

Conclusion.—Most litigation over skin cancer arose from cancers on the head and neck and were brought by patients with basal cell carcinoma of the face. In those for whom oncologic outcomes were known, 95% of plaintiffs were alive without evidence of disease. A misdiagnosis may be lessened by emphasizing a biopsy as the only definitive diagnostic test and by obtaining a second opinion.

▶ This analysis of litigation against physicians who treat cancer of the skin yields several interesting conclusions. For issues related to skin cancer, a failure to diagnose and a failure to order a biopsy are the most common reasons a physician would be sued. Given that a large number of skin cancers in the United States are treated by dermatologists, our diagnostic abilities should leave us reasonably well shielded from medical litigation. Dermatologists fared well compared with other specialty physicians in legal action eventuating in a trial. Surgeons, in contrast, fared much more poorly in the courtroom setting. This may be secondary to patient bias; that is, patients seen by dermatologists versus other specialty physicians may not be strictly comparable. The medical malpractice crisis continues in this country, and reviews such as this may educate the physician by providing insight into the current medicolegal climate.

J. Cook, MD

Glove Perforation in Outpatient Dermatologic Surgery
Dirschka T, Winter K, Kralj N, et al (Dermatologic Practice Ctr, Wuppertal, Germany; Univ Witten/Herdecke, Germany; Univ Wuppertal, Germany)
Dermatol Surg 30:1210-1213, 2004   20–2

Background.—Surgical gloves are an important barrier to infection via skin flora and bloodborne pathogens. The literature suggests that glove perforation rates for dermatologic surgeons operating on hospitalized patients only (up to 12%) are typically lower than those for surgeons in other specialties (eg, hip surgery, up to 83%). The glove perforation rate for outpatient dermatologic surgery was examined.

Methods.—Over a 2-month period, all 660 operating gloves used during outpatient dermatologic surgery were collected after surgery and were immediately tested. All gloves used were sterile, powder-free surgical latex gloves with an inner coating. Gloves were examined according to a standardized water leak test method, and perforations were examined with a microscope to determine their cause.

Results.—In all, 20 of the 660 gloves (3.0%) had perforations; in 15 of these cases (75%), the wearer had not noticed the perforation. Thirteen perforations (65%) were on the nondominant hand, and 7 (35%) were on the dominant hand. The most common site of perforation was the index finger of the nondominant hand (8 cases), and almost all perforations occurred at the fingertips or in the middle joints of the fingers. Microscopy indicated that all perforations were caused by needle sticks.

Conclusion.—The risk of glove perforations in outpatient dermatologic surgery is low. Nonetheless, the high number of outpatient dermatologic surgical procedures performed suggests that glove perforations could be a significant source of risk. This may be particularly relevant because most outpatient dermatologic surgeons do not recognize the glove perforation when it occurs.

▶ This study shows that, fortunately, glove perforations in the dermatologic surgical setting are relatively uncommon compared with more traditional operative settings. This most likely is due to the lower degree of complexity of our procedures versus that of other surgeons. Nevertheless, if one considers the large number of procedures a busy dermatologist does in an average operative day, a 3% glove perforation rate is certainly reason for concern. Dermatologic surgeons need to take every reasonable precaution to ensure their personal safety.

J. Cook, MD

Surgical Wound Infection as a Performance Indicator: Agreement of Common Definitions of Wound Infection in 4773 Patients
Wilson APR, Gibbons C, Reeves BC, et al (Univ College London Hosps; London School of Hygiene and Tropical Medicine; Medical School, Aberdeen, Scotland; et al)
BMJ 329:720-724, 2004   20–3

Introduction.—Surgical site infections are a significant burden to both patients and health services. The agreement between 4 common definitions of *surgical site infection* were compared: (1) the definition from the Centers for Disease Control (CDC), (2) the definition from the nosocomial infection national surveillance scheme (NINSS) modification of the CDC definition; (3) the presence of a purulent discharge; and (4) the definition from the ASEPSIS scoring method—all applied to the same series of surgical wounds. The percentages of infections based on the CDC definition and on the NINSS modification were examined to determine the potential effect of subjective CDC criteria and the variation between hospitals in data collection approaches.

Methods.—A total of 4773 surgical patients hospitalized for at least 2 nights was evaluated in a prospective observational investigation. The primary outcome measures were the number of wound infections based on the presence of purulent discharge alone, the number based on the CDC definition of wound infection, the number based on the NINSS version of the CDC definition, and the number based on the ASEPSIS scoring method.

Results.—A total of 5804 surgical wounds were evaluated during 5028 separate hospital admissions. The mean percentage of wounds categorized as infected differed markedly with different definitions: 19.2% (95% CI, 18.1%-20.4%) with the CDC definition, 14.6% (95% CI, 13.6%-15.6%)

with the NINSS version, 12.3% (95% CI, 11.4%-13.2%) with the purulent discharge only criterion, and 6.8% (95% CI, 6.1%-7.5%) using an ASEPSIS score greater than 20 as a benchmark. The agreement between definitions with regard to individual wounds was poor. Wounds with pus were automatically defined as infected with the use of the CDC, NINSS, and purulent discharge alone definitions; only 39% (283/714) of these had ASEPSIS scores greater than 20.

Conclusion.—Small changes made to the CDC definition or even in its interpretation, as with the NINSS version, produced important variations in the estimated percentage of wound infections. Many wounds were categorized differently using the varying criteria. A single definition used consistently would show changes in the percentage of wound infections over time at a single center and would provide a means of making comparisons between different centers.

▶ Although the percentage of surgical wounds classified as infected is a common performance indicator, some controversy exists as to what actually comprises a surgical infection. Clearly, the definition will affect the number of wounds classified as infected. Although comparing infection rates within a hospital with the use of a single definition may be helpful, infection rates cannot be used as a performance indicator to compare hospitals unless a single agreed-on definition is established.

B. H. Thiers, MD

Hand Hygiene Among Physicians: Performance, Beliefs, and Perceptions
Pittet D, Simon A, Hugonnet S, et al (Univ of Geneva Hosps)
Ann Intern Med 141:1-8, 2004   20–4

Introduction.—Hand hygiene promotion is a major challenge worldwide. Physician adherence to hand hygiene continues to be low in most hospitals. Risk factors for nonadherence were examined, along with beliefs and perceptions linked with hand hygiene among physicians.

Methods.—Hand hygiene practices during routine patient care were observed in 163 physicians participating in a cross-sectional survey in a large university hospital.

Methods.—Relevant risk factors were recorded. A self-reported questionnaire was used to measure beliefs and perceptions concerning hand hygiene. Logistic regression was used to identify variables independently correlated with adherence.

Results.—Adherence with hand hygiene recommendations was 57% and varied widely across medical specialties. Multivariate analysis revealed that adherence was correlated with the awareness of being observed, the belief of being a role model for other colleagues, a positive attitude toward hand hygiene after patient contact, and easy access to hand-rub solutions. Risk factors for nonadherence were a high workload, activities linked with a high risk for cross-transmission, and certain technical medical specialties, including surgery, anesthesiology, emergency medicine, and intensive care medicine.

Discussion/Conclusion.—The direct observation of physicians may have affected both adherence to hand hygiene and responses to the self-reported questionnaire. Physician adherence to hand hygiene is linked with work and system constraints, along with knowledge and cognitive factors. Physicians who work in technical specialty areas need to be targeted for improvement in hand hygiene. It may be useful to reinforce the idea that each individual can influence the behavior of colleagues.

▶ This study examined why physicians fail to practice good hand hygiene. The authors found that the overall adherence to hand hygiene guidelines was 57%. Busy workloads, performing activities with a high risk for cross-transmission, and work in technical specialties (such as surgery and anesthesiology) were associated with poor adherence. Easily accessible hand-rub solutions were associated with higher adherence. Physicians who valued hand hygiene and who considered themselves role models also were more likely to follow recommended guidelines. Unfortunately, most physicians regard hand hygiene as a difficult task, and after decades of education and cajoling, hand hygiene adherence rates remain poor.[1]

B. H. Thiers, MD

Reference

1. Weinstein RA: Hand hygiene—Of reason and ritual. *Ann Intern Med* 141:65-66, 2004.

Eradication of Methicillin Resistant *Staphylococcus aureus* by "Ring Fencing" of Elective Orthopaedic Beds

Biant LC, Teare EL, Williams WW, et al (Broomfield Hosp, Chelmsford, England)
BMJ 329:149-151, 2004
20–5

Background.—Deep infection after joint arthroplasty can be a catastrophic complication, resulting in additional surgery, loss of the prosthesis, disability, and a risk of death. *Staphylococcus aureus* bacteria that possess the *mecA* gene and the penicillin-binding protein PBP2a are resistant to methicillin (MRSA) and oxacillin. MRSA is a particularly challenging organism to treat because of the need for antibiotics that are expensive, potentially toxic, or both. This study investigated the feasibility of a strategy of ring fencing of elective orthopedic beds and introduction of simple infection control measures to reduce the rates of postoperative infection and the number of patients treated.

Methods.—This prospective trial was conducted at 1 district general hospital in Essex in the United Kingdom. All patients undergoing primary hip or knee replacement at this facility between July 1999 and July 2001 were included in the trial. Ring fencing of the elective orthopedic ward and the introduction of simple infection control measures were used in the treatment of the patients. The main outcome measures were the number of patients having joint replacement; the number of all postoperative infections in the participant groups; and the number of cases of MRSA.

Results.—There was a decline in the incidence of all postoperative infections from 43 infections in 417 cases before the introduction of ring fencing to 15 infections in 488 patients after the introduction of ring fencing and simple infection control measures. There were no new cases of MRSA.

Conclusions.—The introduction of a ring fencing to an elective orthopedic ward and the use of simple infection control measures allowed for the treatment of 17% more patients and a significant reduction in the incidence of all postoperative infections.

▶ The authors illustrate the importance of simple infection control measures to significantly decrease the incidence of postoperative infections. Although this study focused on joint replacement surgery, application of the simple principles demonstrated here likely would help prevent infections following dermatologic surgery as well. The treatment of infections associated with surgical implants has recently been reviewed.[1]

B. H. Thiers, MD

Reference

1. Darouiche RO: Treatment of infections associated with surgical implants. *N Engl J Med* 350:1422-1429, 2004.

Postoperative Infection With Meticillin-Resistant *Staphylococcus aureus* and Socioeconomic Background
Bagger JP, Zindrou D, Taylor KM (Imperial College London; Hammersmith Hosp, London)
Lancet 363:706-708, 2004   20–6

Introduction.—Infectious diseases can be associated with social deprivation. The correlation between the incidence of postoperative infection with meticillin-resistant *Staphylococcus aureus* (MRSA) and socioeconomic background was examined in patients undergoing isolated coronary artery bypass grafting.

Methods.—All patients included in the study had an address in the United Kingdom and were admitted during a 5-year period until the start of 1998. Variables relevant to hospital infection were documented and included age, sex, presence or absence of diabetes, obesity, chronic lung disease, corticosteroid treatment, and duration of surgery. The Carstairs score was used to stratify patients by social deprivation, according to postcode.

Results.—In a consecutive series of 1739 patients (313 women), 23 (1.3%) became infected with MRSA (infection of leg wound in 10, sternal wound in 6, respiratory tract in 6, and central line in 1). A graded association between the incidence of MRSA and the social deprivation score was observed: patients from the most deprived areas had a rate of infection 7-fold that of patients from less deprived areas (2.2% vs 0.3%; P = .0040). The incidence of MRSA infection in women was higher than in men (2.6% vs 1.1%; P = .035). Patients who had a postoperative MRSA infection had a mortality rate that was 6-fold that of patients with no MRSA infection (26% vs 4.2%; P = .001).

Conclusion.—Social deprivation greatly affects the risk of a postoperative MRSA infection. Patient from deprived areas may be particularly susceptible to postoperative infections with MRSA.

▶ Patients from socially deprived backgrounds appear to be especially susceptible to postoperative infections with MRSA. These findings do not contradict the assumption that hospital hygiene is important in the control of such infections, but they do help identify an important risk factor for this serious complication of surgery.

B. H. Thiers, MD

Controversies in Perioperative Management of Blood Thinners in Dermatologic Surgery: Continue or Discontinue?
Alcalay J, Alkalay R (Assuta Med Ctr, Tel Aviv, Israel; Hadassah Univ, Jerusalem, Israel)
Dermatol Surg 30:1091-1094, 2004   20–7

Introduction.—Patients treated with blood thinners, especially warfarin and aspirin, may be at risk for excessive intraoperative and postoperative bleeding when undergoing cutaneous surgery. The need to discontinue treatment with blood thinners has been debated but not fully resolved. This issue was examined by a literature search and a review of the authors' own practice.

Methods.—The literature search included articles published in English through October 2003 that related to perioperative use of blood thinners in dermatologic surgery. In addition, 68 consecutive patients receiving warfarin for various conditions and who underwent cutaneous surgery at the study institution between November 1999 and September 2003 were prospectively evaluated. One week before surgery, the anticoagulant effect of warfarin was evaluated by using prothrombin time and international normalized ratio.

Results.—Thirteen of the 14 articles reviewed reported either no documented surgical complications in patients receiving blood thinners or no adverse effects from the discontinuation of blood thinners. Only 1 article found statistically significant higher complications in patients receiving warfarin compared with aspirin and a control population. In data from the authors' practice, 68 of 2790 patients operated on during the study period were taking warfarin for various underlying diseases. Sixty-three underwent Mohs surgery and 5 underwent excisional surgery. No significant bleeding occurred during or after surgery, and bleeding during surgery was easily controlled by electrocoagulation. None of the wounds showed postoperative complications.

Conclusion.—Most dermatologic surgeons have stopped anticoagulant or antiplatelet therapy before the operation, but the findings of this study indicate that intraoperative bleeding can be easily managed. The mean international normalized ratio of patients taking warfarin in this series was 2.49. Values greater than 5 may result in major bleeding, and values less than 4 should be adjusted lower. Aspirin need not be discontinued before dermatologic surgery. All patients undergoing cutaneous surgery with blood thinners should have a well-compressed dressing applied for 48 hours after surgery.

▶ It has been routine practice to discontinue anticoagulant therapy before cutaneous surgery for fear of excessive intraoperative and postoperative bleeding. However, there appears to be mounting evidence that as long as the patient is not over anticoagulated, blood thinners may be continued with minimal risk of bleeding complications. This article reviews the literature on this subject and adds additional data to support this conclusion.

P. G. Lang, Jr, MD

Patients Spend More Time With the Physician for Excision of a Malignant Skin Lesion Than for Excision of a Benign Skin Lesion
Feldman SR, Camacho F, Williford PM, et al (Wake Forest Univ, Winston-Salem, NC; State Univ of New York, Brooklyn)
Dermatol Surg 30:351-354, 2004   20–8

Introduction.—The standard Current Procedural Treatment coding system differentiates between benign and malignant skin lesion excision, with typically greater reimbursement for the latter. However, a Center for Medicare and Medicaid Services proposal would eliminate the difference, assuming that lesions of the same diameter, whether benign or malignant, require the same amount of physician work. Data from the National Ambulatory Medical Care Survey (NAMCS) were analyzed to obtain an estimate of time required to excise benign versus malignant lesions.

Methods.—A search of NAMCS data from 1990 to 2001 centered on unmistakable benign and malignant conditions and excluded visits that had procedures other than excisions or at which multiple diagnoses were addressed. A total of 213 observations of benign lesion excisions and 132 of malignant lesion excisions (from a sample of 5 million visits) were compared for time spent with the physician.

Results.—Physicians spent a mean of 30.4 minutes when a malignant lesion was excised and a mean of 22.9 minutes for a benign lesion. Thus, the time required for a malignant lesion was 7.5 (33%) minutes longer than for a benign lesion. The adjusted (for age, gender, and race) difference was 8.3 minutes.

Conclusion.—Considerably more physician time is involved in office-based excision of malignant versus benign lesions. Factors affecting time required include a deeper margin in malignant lesion excisions, a greater degree of counseling and planning, and more time-consuming wound closure.

▶ In the United States, most cutaneous neoplasms are resected by dermatologists. Efforts have been undertaken to eliminate differential compensation for benign versus malignant skin lesion procedures. This study shows that the time spent with the patient to excise a malignant lesion is approximately 30% greater than when a benign lesion is excised. This undoubtedly is related to the more extensive preoperative counseling and other considerations involved in removing skin cancers. Interestingly, this 30% increase in time corresponds almost precisely to the percentage difference in compensation for excising malignant versus benign lesions of equivalent size.

J. Cook, MD

Factors Influencing the Number Needed to Excise: Excision Rates of Pigmented Lesions by General Practitioners
English DR, Del Mar C, Burton RC (Cancer Council Victoria, Carlton, Australia; Univ of Queensland, Herston, Australia; Natl Cancer Control Initiative, Carlton, Victoria, Australia)
Med J Aust 180:16-19, 2004   20–9

Introduction.—Nevi and seborrheic keratoses are often excised so that a melanoma is not missed. The number of pigmented lesions excised per melanoma can be considered to be the "number needed to treat" (NNT). A low NNT may mean that melanomas are being missed, whereas a high NNT may indicate excessive economic and personal costs of excising lesions. Data on the management of pigmented skin lesions in general practice were analyzed for factors influencing the NNT.

Methods.—General practitioners (GPs) in Perth, Australia were enrolled via mail. Those eligible to participate did not already use cameras to record images of pigmented skin lesions and agreed to permit their practices to be randomized to an intervention or control group and to allow pathology laboratories to provide skin biopsy results. The intervention consisted of the use of a diagnostic algorithm and photographic images. The data reported here were from the baseline period of the study. A total of 468 GPs (39% response rate) from 223 practices provided data on 4741 pigmented lesions excised from November 1998 to February 2002.

Results.—Forty-two lesions were excluded from analysis, which left a total of 4699 (including 62 in situ and 98 invasive melanomas). Two thirds of GPs had excised at least 1 lesion, and the median number excised was 8. The NNT was 29 but fell to 21 when seborrheic keratoses were excluded from the analysis. Recently graduated GPs excised more benign lesions for each melanoma (NNT, 59) than the least recently graduated (NNT, 22). Patient factors associated with a higher NNT included younger age, female sex, and disadvantaged socioeconomic status. The NNT was particularly high among female patients of female GPs.

Discussion.—Observed differences in the NNT according to patient categories suggest that GPs, especially those who are recent graduates, might lower their threshold for excision among older and male patients and raise their threshold for excision among younger and female patients.

▶ As the data were derived from the baseline period of a randomized controlled trial of a diagnostic aid for pigmented skin lesions, presumably none of them was removed for purely cosmetic reasons. Specifying an ideal NNT would be difficult, as a low number might mean that the diagnostic criteria are too narrow and that melanomas are more likely to be missed and a high number may mean that the diagnostic criteria are too liberal and the associated costs of excising so many benign lesions are excessive. It would be interesting to perform a similar study with dermatologists.

B. H. Thiers, MD

Documenting Dermatology Practice: Ratio of Cutaneous Tumors Biopsied That Are Malignant
Green AR, Elgart GW, Ma F, et al (Univ of Miami, Fla; Veterans Administration Med Ctr, Miami, Fla; Yale Univ, West Haven, Conn)
Dermatol Surg 30:1208-1209, 2004   20–10

Background.—The skin biopsy is a cornerstone of cutaneous diagnosis, especially for skin cancer. However, dermatologists differ widely in how often they submit a skin biopsy specimen for histopathologic examination. The percentage of skin biopsy specimens that are malignant (ie, the "malignancy ratio") and the factors that influence the malignancy ratio were examined.

Methods.—The diagnoses of all cutaneous tumor specimens submitted by dermatologists to 1 institution over a 6-month period were reviewed. The malignancy ratio was calculated by dividing the number of malignant lesions by the total number of lesions sampled. The characteristics of the dermatologists submitting these specimens were also analyzed.

Results.—During the study period, 11,072 cutaneous tumor specimens were submitted for histopathologic analysis. Of these, 4613 were malignant, which yielded a malignancy ratio of 41.2%. The malignancy ratio (13.4%-86.6%) widely varied by individual dermatologist, but the overall malignancy ratio was very stable regardless of the practice type, the years in practice, the use of dermatoscopy, or the volume of specimens submitted for examination. Multivariate regression analyses indicated that the only significant and independent predictor of a higher malignancy ratio was the age of the dermatologist. For each increasing year of age, the malignancy ratio increased by 2%. The malignancy ratio for pigmented lesions was 3.8%.

Conclusion.—About 40% of cutaneous tumors undergoing biopsy were malignant. This ratio remained stable regardless of the type of practice, the years in practice, the use of dermatoscopy, and the volume of submissions. Malignancy ratios increased significantly with the dermatologist's age.

▶ The ideal frequency of a malignancy diagnosis in submitted pathology specimens remains uncertain. A malignancy percentage too low obviously suggests a tendency toward performing too many biopsies. Conversely, a malignancy rate too high suggests possible underutilization of the procedure. In this series, malignant diagnoses of tumor biopsy specimens were rendered approximately 40% of the time. It would be interesting to gather data on a larger scale, as insurance companies are certainly interested in effective practice management strategies and the avoidance of excess expenses resulting from overutilization of skin biopsies.

J. Cook, MD

Topically Applied Imiquimod Inhibits Vascular Tumor Growth In Vivo
Sidbury R, Neuschler N, Neuschler E, et al (Children's Mem Hosp, Chicago; Northwestern Univ, Chicago; 3M Pharmaceuticals, St Paul, Minn)
J Invest Dermatol 121:1205-1209, 2003   20–11

Introduction.—The currently available therapies for vascular tumors—which include corticosteroids, vincristine, and interferon-α—require systemic administration and may be toxic. Imiquimod, a potential alternative treatment, is a topically applied inducer of cytokines with local dermatitis as its only significant side effect. The efficacy and mechanism of action of imiquimod was investigated in a mouse hemangioendothelioma model.

Methods.—The model was generated by inoculation of EOMA cells, which result in tumors approximately 5 days later and death at an average of 16 days after inoculation. Imiquimod 5% cream was applied to the flank at the site of EOMA cell inoculation 3 times weekly, beginning on day 1 or day 5 after inoculation. Survival was compared among the following treatment groups: vehicle base control subjects, arachidonic acid control subjects, and imiquimod subjects. Two hours after the last treatment, anesthetized animals had tissue harvested from skin overlying the tumor and from distant untreated skin.

Results.—The application of imiquimod cream, whether at the time of cell inoculation or when tumors became visible, significantly decreased tumor growth and increased survival relative to control groups (Fig 2; see color plate XIX). Findings in the imiquimod-treated tumors included decreased tumor cell proliferation, increased tumor apoptosis, and increased expression of tissue inhibitor of matrix metalloproteinase-1 with decreased activity of matrix metalloproteinase-9.

Conclusion.—The topical application of imiquimod inhibited tumor growth and promoted tumor apoptosis in a mouse hemangioendothelioma model. Effects of imiquimod are similar to the changes seen in the natural involution of the more common hemangioma of infancy. Local irritation at the tumor site was the only noted toxicity of the topical therapy.

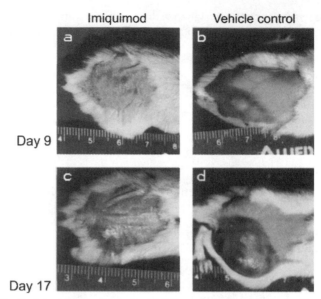

FIGURE 2.—Topical application of imiquimod inhibits tumor growth in 129/J mice. Tumors were photographed serially every 4 days to record the appearance of the tumors and the potential irritant dermatitis. Mice treated with imiquimod beginning day 1 at 9 days (A) and 17 days (C) after EOMA cell introduction. Mice treated with vehicle base beginning on day 1 at 9 days (B) and 17 days (D) after EOMA cell introduction. (Courtesy of Sidbury R, Neuschler N, Neuschler E, et al: Topically applied imiquimod inhibits vascular tumor growth *in vivo. J Invest Dermatol* 121:1205-1209, 2003. Reprinted by permission of Blackwell Publishing.)

▶ The authors describe a possible molecular mechanism underlying the reported utility of topical imiquimod for the treatment of infantile hemangiomas.

B. H. Thiers, MD

Adverse Effects of Systemic Glucocorticosteroid Therapy in Infants With Hemangiomas

George ME, Sharma V, Jacobson J, et al (Children's Mercy Hosp, Kansas City)
Arch Dermatol 140:963-969, 2004   20–12

Background.—Glucocorticosteroids have been used for the treatment of hemangiomas in infants and children for 3 decades. Standard daily doses in these patients have ranged from 2 to 3 mg/kg of body weight; however, some investigators have recently advocated the use of up to 3 to 5 mg/kg with excellent results and mild reversible adverse effects. Previous reports have indicated that systemic glucocorticosteroid therapy is relatively safe for treatment of problematic hemangiomas with minimal short-term adverse effects and no serious long-term adverse effects. However, few data are reported in the literature regarding the issue of adrenal suppression or hypertension in these patients. The short- and long-term adverse effects of systemic glucocorticosteroid therapy in infants with hemangiomas were assessed.

Methods.—A retrospective chart review was conducted of infants treated with glucocorticosteroids for hemangiomas during a 3-year period at a tertiary care children's hospital. All of the patients were treated with a minimum of 1 month of glucocorticosteroid therapy at a minimum starting dose of 0.5 mg/kg per day. The main outcome measures were demographic and anthropometric measurements, starting dose and duration of glucocorticosteroid therapy, subjective parental concerns, complications related to the hemangioma, adjunctive treatment, and morning cortisol levels and/or results of corticotropin stimulation tests.

Results.—Of the 141 patients with hemangiomas, 22 (15.6%) were treated with glucocorticosteroids. The average starting dose was 2.23 mg/kg per day, and the average duration of therapy was 28.1 weeks. Complaints of irritability, fussiness, or insomnia were identified in 16 (73%) patients. Hypertension (3 or more episodes of systolic blood pressure > 105 mm Hg) was observed in 10 (45%) patients. Morning cortisol levels were abnormal in 13 (87%) of 15 patients evaluated. Low-dose corticotropin stimulation test results were abnormal in 2 of the 3 infants tested.

Conclusions.—Glucocorticosteroid therapy for infantile hemangiomas was well tolerated overall, but changes in behavior, insomnia, and gastrointestinal symptoms were common parental concerns. Hypertension and hypothalamic-pituitary-adrenal axis suppression were frequent observations. Infants treated with long-term glucocorticosteroid therapy for hemangiomas should be monitored carefully for these potentially adverse effects.

▶ Systemic glucocorticosteroids remain the most effective treatment for infants with problematic hemangiomas. However, as is well known and further elucidated in this article, such therapy is not without side effects. As with any serious medical problem, risk versus potential benefit should be considered when deciding therapy. The authors emphasize in this article that blood pressure of infants should be monitored during steroid treatment, and parents should be counseled on the potential need for stress doses of glucocorticosteroids for several months after therapy has been discontinued.

S. Raimer, MD

The Key to Long-term Success in Liposuction: A Guide for Plastic Surgeons and Patients
Rohrich RJ, Broughton G II, Horton B, et al (Univ of Texas, Dallas)
Plast Reconstr Surg 114:1945-1952, 2004   20–13

Introduction.—The long-term success of liposuction requires careful patient selection and education. To achieve improvement in body contour after the procedure, patients must exercise, follow a proper diet, and undertake positive lifestyle changes. Results from a survey of 600 patients who had liposuction between 1999 and 2003 were used to create a "road map" for patients and plastic surgeons to achieve successful long-term outcomes.

Methods.—The anonymous self-assessment survey was returned by 209 of the 492 patients who were able to be contacted. Patients were asked about weight gain since the procedure, clothing size, health, physical activity, and overall satisfaction. Postoperative satisfaction was analyzed by time since liposuction (<6 months, 6-12 months, 1-2 years, and >2 years).

Results.—Most responders (54%) had their last liposuction more than 2 years before completing the survey; only 10% were in the less than 6 months category. The 4 time groups did not differ importantly in responses for satisfaction and weight gain. Of the 57% of patients with no weight gain, 46% reported weight loss. Most weight loss (67%) occurred within 6 months of the procedure, and most weight gain (66%) occurred after 6 months. Only 29% of those who gained weight rated their appearance as good or excellent (vs 79% in the no weight gain group). Patients with no weight gain after liposuction were more likely to have exercised more, changed their diet, and had increased productivity compared with patients who gained weight.

Conclusion.—Successful body contouring surgery requires that a patient adopt positive lifestyle habits after the procedure. The relative success rate of liposuction depends on patient education regarding alternatives in diet and exercise. The road map provided shows, for example, that patients who fail to exercise regularly are 4 times more likely to have weight gain and in general to be far more likely to experience dissatisfaction with the results of liposuction.

▶ The more satisfied patients after liposuction surgery are ones who embrace lifestyle habits that augment the success of the surgical procedure—exercise and weight management. I find the title of this article interesting. Much of the pioneering work for tumescent liposuction was done by dermatologists, and data show that a substantial portion of the liposuction surgeries done in this country are performed by dermatologists. Retrospective reviews on malpractice action after liposuction surgery have shown that dermatologists typically fare much better than our plastic surgery colleagues.

J. Cook, MD

Pharmacokinetics and Safety of Epinephrine Use in Liposuction
Brown SA, Lipschitz AH, Kenkel JM, et al (Univ of Texas, Dallas; Mayo Medical Laboratories, Rochester, Minn)
Plast Reconstr Surg 114:756-763, 2004   20–14

Introduction.—The advent of wetting solution and the evolution of wetting solution infiltration techniques have greatly improved the safety of liposuction but have led to increases in volumes of infiltration and lipoaspirate. During large-volume cases, patients are regularly exposed to epinephrine doses greater than 5 to 10 mg. Epinephrine toxicity may have played a role in deaths associated with liposuction, but the link has been difficult to prove. Volunteers were recruited for a study of the pharmacokinetic aspects of epinephrine when administered during large-volume liposuction.

Methods.—The 5 women included in the study underwent 3-stage ultrasound (US) assisted liposuction under general anesthesia with standard fluid resuscitation guidelines. Wetting solution contained 7.3 mg epinephrine, corresponding to 0.09 mg/kg. Blood samples collected at regular intervals from induction through the postoperative period were assessed by high-performance liquid chromatography for total plasma epinephrine and norepinephrine concentrations. Approximate exogenous epinephrine absorption was calculated after correction for estimated endogenous epinephrine production.

Results.—Overall peak total plasma epinephrine concentrations, observed at the final intraoperative reading, were 15-fold greater than baseline. Plasma concentrations of norepinephrine increased significantly from a mean of 46 pg/mL at 0 hours to 114 pg/mL at 3 hours. Peak levels appeared at 4 hours postoperatively (mean, 169 pg/mL), but all levels remained within the expected normal range. Approximately 25% to 32% of infiltrated epinephrine was ultimately absorbed. A reversal of the normal epinephrine/norepinephrine ratio (<0.5:1) was noted intraoperatively (>5:1).

Conclusion.—The time to peak exogenous epinephrine level in these patients was at 2 hours 48 minutes, and peak exogenous epinephrine concentrations ranged from approximately 286 to 335 pg/mL after correction for endogenous epinephrine secretion. Peak levels were comparable to those observed during major physiologic stress. Despite the increase of exogenous epinephrine concentrations during liposuction, none of these patients showed clinical evidence of toxicity. Significant cardiovascular disease, however, is a contraindication to single-stage moderate to large-volume liposuction.

▶ The sensationalistic reporting of liposuction deaths in the lay press has generated much debate about the procedure. Many studies have been published addressing the safety of infused lidocaine and recommended maximum doses. Few, if any, studies have looked solely at the safety of the epinephrine used for hemostasis in the infused solutions. Although this study was very small, it showed peak epinephrine levels comparable to those observed during major stresses, such as larger surgical procedures or exercising to exhaustion. For this reason, the liposuction surgeon may be advised to extend particular caution to patients with concomitant cardiovascular disorder. Smaller volume procedures with less physiologic stress may be indicated in this subgroup of patients.

J. Cook, MD

Absence of an Effect of Liposuction on Insulin Action and Risk Factors for Coronary Heart Disease

Klein S, Fontana L, Young VL, et al (Washington Univ, St Louis; Istituto Superiore di Sanità, Rome)
N Engl J Med 350:2549-2557, 2004   20–15

Background.—Some authorities suggest liposuction as a potential treatment for the metabolic complications of obesity. The effects of large-volume abdominal liposuction on metabolic risk factors for coronary heart disease in women with abdominal obesity were studied.

Methods.—Fifteen obese women were included in the study. The insulin sensitivity of liver, skeletal muscle, and adipose tissue were assessed before and 10 to 12 weeks after abdominal liposuction. Levels of inflammatory mediators and other risk factors for coronary heart disease were also determined. Eight women had normal glucose tolerance and a mean body mass index of 35.1. Seven had type 2 diabetes and had a mean body mass index of 39.9.

Findings.—Liposuction reduced the volume of subcutaneous abdominal adipose tissue by 44% in patients with normal glucose tolerance and by 28% in those with diabetes. Women with normal oral glucose tolerance lost a mean 9.1 kg of fat, for an 18% decrease in total fat. Women with type 2 diabetes lost a mean 19.5 kg of fat, for a 19% reduction in total fat. Liposuction did not significantly affect the insulin sensitivity of muscle, liver, or adipose tissue. This treatment also did not significantly change plasma levels of C-reactive protein, interleukin-6, tumor necrosis factor α, or adiponectin. Liposuction had no significant effect on other risk factors for coronary heart disease—such as blood pressure, plasma glucose, insulin, and lipid levels—in either group.

Conclusion.—The findings demonstrate that abdominal liposuction does not significantly improve metabolic abnormalities associated with obesity. Reducing adipose tissue mass alone does not achieve the metabolic benefits of weight loss.

▶ Although a small study, this interesting article proved that aggressive high-volume liposuction surgery causing a significant reduction of body fat does not impart the metabolic advantages seen when a similar volume of fat is lost through traditional means of weight loss including diet and exercise. For this reason, liposuction surgery cannot be recommended as a method to surmount the health problems associated with obesity, including diabetes mellitus and coronary vascular disease.

J. Cook, MD

Hourglass Deformity After Botulism Toxin Type A Injection

Guyuron B, Rose K, Kriegler JS, et al (Case Western Reserve Univ, Cleveland, Ohio)
Headache 44:262-264, 2004   20–16

Introduction.—In an ongoing study to identify migraine trigger sites, patients had botulinum toxin type A (BTXA) injected into a number of anatomic locations including the temporalis muscle. All 92 patients were found at routine follow-up 4 to 8 weeks after injection to have bilateral depression of the temporal region (Fig 1; see color plate XX) resembling an hourglass. The dose of BTXA was consistent in all patients, but the extent of deformity varied considerably.

Methods.—Patients had received 25 units of BTXA with a 30-gauge needle. The injection was aimed at a point initially approximately 1.7 cm lateral and 0.6 cm cephalad to the lateral canthus. Photographs of the deformity were obtained, and preinjection photographs were compared with postinjection photographs.

Results.—Only 26 of the patients reported depression of the temple area, but the deformity was apparent on examination in all those who received injection of BTXA into the temporalis muscle. The hollowing observed was consistent with disuse atrophy. Patients who seemed to have less atrophy tended to be those with excess soft tissue in the region. Muscle mass was re-

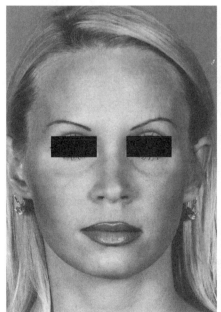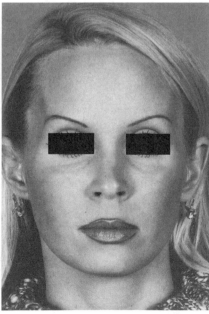

FIGURE 1.—Before and after injection of botulinum toxin type A demonstrating bilateral depression of temples (hourglass deformity). (Courtesy of Guyuron B, Rose K, Kriegler JS, et al: Hourglass deformity after botulinum toxin type A injection. *Headache* 44:262-264, 2004.)

covered in all patients several months after return of muscle function, and no permanent damage to the temporalis muscle was apparent.

Conclusion.—Physicians using BTXA should be aware of this temporary facial side effect. The atrophy at the temporalis muscle location was not noticeable at other migraine trigger sites.

▶ Dermatologic surgeons should inform their patients of this temporary side effect before performing injections of BTXA.

J. Cook, MD

Evaluation of the Radiance FN Soft Tissue Filler for Facial Soft Tissue Augmentation

Tzikas TL (Delray Beach, Fla)
Arch Facial Plast Surg 6:234-239, 2004   20–17

Introduction.—The search for the ideal agent for soft tissue augmentation has led to the development of numerous materials, including biologically derived products and synthetic fillers. All such products, however, have had significant limitations. The 90 patients (85 women and 5 men; ages 25-85 years) reported here underwent subdermal injection for facial soft tissue augmentation with Radiance FN, a new highly biocompatible, calcium hydroxylapatite–based implant.

Methods.—A total of 142 syringes of Radiance FN were used in 103 treatment sessions. Most patients were injected with a special 30-gauge needle with a larger inner diameter. After injection, the material was manually compressed. A long 27-gauge needle was used for lip augmentation. Patients were surveyed after treatment and for up to 6 months for pain, ecchymosis, skin erythema, nodules, softness, appearance, and satisfaction.

Results.—At 6 months, appearance and softness were rated good or excellent by 74% and 80% of patients, respectively. Patient satisfaction was quite high: excellent in 47%, good in 41%, and poor in only 2%. Pain, erythema, and ecchymosis were common immediately after treatment but soon resolved, although some edema continued for months. Four of 7 patients who had visible, persistent nodules required intervention.

Conclusion.—Radiance FN was effective and well tolerated when used for facial soft tissue augmentation. The product is nonantigenic, biocompatible, and does not require sensitivity testing. An additional advantage is ease of use, because Radiance FN is premixed, prefilled, and requires no special handling or storage. Precise technique is required with lip augmentation to reduce the risk of submucosal nodules. After approximately 3 years of use for facial plastic surgery, no adverse reactions have been reported.

▶ This effective new implant further crowds the US market for soft tissue augmentation products. In my experience, it is easy to use and is met with a high degree of patient satisfaction. Like many other alternative products, it appears that perioral injections are more problematic, with a significant number of patients developing nodules that may require intervention.

J. Cook, MD

Nursing Home Quality and Pressure Ulcer Prevention and Management Practices

Wipke-Tevis DD, Williams DA, Rantz MJ, et al (Univ of Missouri, Columbia)
J Am Geriatr Soc 52:583-588, 2004   20–18

Introduction.—Because the prevention of pressure ulcers in long-term care facilities (LTCFs) requires coordinated care, the prevalence of pressure ulcers is a useful indication of the overall quality of the facility. Pressure ulcer quality indicator (QI) scores were measured retrospectively in LTCFs in Missouri to determine the relationship between these scores and risk assessment in the LTCFs.

Methods.—A 16-item survey sent to 577 Missouri-certified LTCFs yielded a response rate of 62.7%. The Minimum Data Set assessment findings and pressure ulcer QI scores were available from 321 facilities. Over a 6-month period (April 1 to September 30, 1999), Minimum Data Set and pressure ulcer QI data were retrieved from 44,502 assessments involving 23,833 residents.

Results.—The mean number of licensed beds at responding LTCFs was 109; 68.0% were for profit and 47.8% were located in a metropolitan county. Most facilities (85.6%) assessed the risk of pressure ulcers within 24 hours of admission, and many (54.3%) performed reassessments weekly. The mean pressure ulcer QI score was 10.9; the risk-adjusted score was 15.7 for residents who were at high risk and 3.1% for those considered to be at low risk. Both the overall mean and the high-risk mean exceeded the upper threshold set by an expert panel. Fewer than 20% of facilities practiced minimizing the head-of-bed elevation to less than 30%, and fewer than 13% used the Agency for Health Care Policy and Research pressure ulcer prevention and treatment guidelines. In addition, more than 40% of LTCFs used a risk assessment tool that was not evidence based. No relationship was noted, however, between pressure ulcer QI scores and the numbers of prevention or treatment strategies.

Discussion.—The best practices for the assessment and prevention of pressure ulcers were not used in these LTCFs. The administration and staff of the facilities need specific training in the use of the Braden Scale for assessment; they need to limit head-of-bed elevation, and they need to provide more frequent repositioning when an ulcer develops.

▶ The authors documented significant problems in pressure ulcer prevention and management practices in LTCFs. Educational and quality improvement programs are clearly needed to maximize the care of affected patients.

B. H. Thiers, MD

Subject Index

Author Index

BUSINESS REPLY MAIL

FIRST-CLASS MAIL   PERMIT NO 7135   ORLANDO FL

POSTAGE WILL BE PAID BY ADDRESSEE

PERIODICALS ORDER FULFILLMENT DEPT
MOSBY
ELSEVIER
6277 SEA HARBOR DR
ORLANDO FL 32887-4800

VISIT OUR HOME PAGE!
www.us.elsevierhealth.com/periodicals

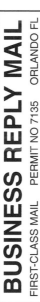

ELSEVIER
MOSBY